f**P**

YOU

Staying Young

The Owner's Manual for Extending Your Warranty

MEHMET C. OZ, M.D.
and **MICHAEL F. ROIZEN, M.D.**

With **TED SPIKER, CRAIG WYNETT,**
LISA OZ, and **MARK A. RUDBERG, M.D.**

Illustrations by
GARY HALLGREN

Free Press
Published by Simon & Schuster

New York   London   Toronto   Sydney

Free Press
A Division of Simon & Schuster, Inc.
1230 Avenue of the Americas
New York, NY 10020

First Free Press hardcover edition October 2007

FREE PRESS and colophon are trademarks of Simon & Schuster, Inc.

For information about special discounts for bulk purchases, please contact Simon & Schuster Special Sales at 1-800-456-6798 or business@simonandschuster.com.

Designed by Ruth Lee Mui

Manufactured in the United States of America

9 10 8

Library of Congress Cataloging-in-Publication Data

You, staying young: the owner's manual for extending your warranty / by Mehmet C. Oz ... (et al.); illustrations, Gary Hallgren.
          p. cm.
1. Longevity—Popular works.   2. Aging—Prevention—Popular works.   I. Oz, Mehmet, 1960–
          RA776.75.Y64 2007
613.2—dc22   2007026480

ISBN-13: 978-0-7432-9256-6
ISBN-10:   0-7432-9256-1

Note to Readers

This publication contains the opinions and ideas of its authors. It is intended to provide helpful and informative material on the subjects addressed in the publication. It is sold with the understanding that the authors and publisher are not engaged in rendering medical, health, or any other kind of personal professional services in the book. The reader should consult his or her medical, health, or other competent professional before adopting any of the suggestions in this book or drawing inferences from it.

The authors and publisher specifically disclaim all responsibility for any liability, loss, or risk, personal or otherwise, which is incurred as a consequence, directly or indirectly, of the use and application of any of the contents in this book.

To all who desire longer life so they can serve more

Contents

Part I

Why You Age and How You Stay Young

YOUNG OLD

INSIDE THE CELL

GENES
TELOMERES
STEM CELLS

MITOCHONDRIA

IMMUNE

GLYCOSYLATION

TOXINS

CALORIE RESTRICTION
(SIRTUIN)

UV RADIATION

ATROPHY

NEUROTRANSMITTERS

WEAR AND TEAR

AROUND THE BODY

NITRIC OXIDE   HORMONES

UNFORCED ERRORS

Introduction

Most of us think aging happens like this: We go on our way, living happily through life, until one day we start to *feel* old, and the symptoms domino right before our cataract-clouded eyes. Our bones creak, our backs hurt, we space on the names of our neighbors, we hate driving at night, we can't play golf anymore, we can't hear what our spouses are saying, and our sex lives pretty much come down to brushing up against the washing machine. Soon we're eating dinner at three-thirty and our primary goal of the day is staying up long enough to catch *Wheel of Fortune.*

To us, that approach means you're drowning in life—not bathing in the beauty of it. We're here to challenge that perception of aging and create a new way of thinking about "antiaging medicine." The traditional focus of the medical community has been on treating chronic diseases and reversing acute illnesses associated with aging—cancer, heart disease, stroke. The assumption was clear: Since heart disease and cancer alone account for over 50 percent of all deaths, you could live maybe 50 percent longer if you could avoid the big killers. As it turns out, this isn't what would happen. As devastating as these diseases are, wiping them out as your killer increases your average life expectancy by only about nine and a half years—not the thirty to forty years that you would expect. Why? Because something else takes their place.

To add serious years to your life—and life to your years—you have to lower your risk for *all* diseases. And the only way to do that is to slow your rate of aging *on the cellular level.* Curing cancer or any other disease does not necessarily do anything to change the nature or speed of your bodily aging process. That's because

3

What Is Your RealAge?

aging and disease—although they interact with each other—aren't the same thing. As we grow older, all of our systems slowly deteriorate, which makes us more vulnerable to disease. By slowing the aging of our cells while simultaneously preventing disease, we can enjoy not only a higher quality of life but a much longer one as well. This is where we're taking YOU.

Of course, the reason why aging is so intimidating isn't because it appears to sneak up on you like a first-rate mugger. In reality, aging is more like a savvy bank robber who's spent months casing the joint. Why the discrepancy? Because there are huge delays between the cause of the problem and the effects you actually see in your life. And that means you have to start building defenses in your thirties, forties, and fifties against attacks that may not occur until your sixties, seventies, and eighties.

Fortunately, science has finally figured out most of the spectacular biological processes that control aging. And by learning about such things as mitochondria, telomeres, sirtuin, nitric oxide, and the vagus nerve—which you will do in this book—you'll appreciate how to apply these remarkable discoveries to your own life. As we take you inside your own body, you'll learn about the shoelacelike chromosome that affects memory loss. You'll discover the body's cellular energy factories that play a role in damaging and preserving your arteries (and you thought it was all due to the buttered biscuits). You'll even figure out whether you're a good candidate for hormone therapy as you age and understand how your third eye controls your sleeping pattern (yes, we said *third*). Ultimately, by understanding the science behind your body, you'll slow your rate of aging—to live long and strong. While science holds the keys, only you have the power to unlock your potential longevity.

After all, aging may be inevitable, but the rate of aging is certainly not.

Your Body, Your City

Perhaps the best way to explain the dynamics of aging is to take a look at another complex system that's subjected to the same forces as your body: a city. Some cities remain beautiful and elegant in their old age (think of old but elegant European cities like London), while others that may not even be so old look worn down, beat up, and in need of an urban ICU. Every city experiences the ups and downs of aging; how well the city managers and residents adapt largely determines whether the city will age gracefully or end up on the wrong side of spray paint, riots, and urban decay (see Figure Intro 1).

Now, every city has its own genetic code, just as you have yours. For a city, genes are geography—whether it's built on a river, or whether it's located in a hot or cold climate, or whether it lies directly in a prevalent hurricane path. The city's geography can't inherently change. But the city can adapt to that environment, with earthquake-proof construction, underground tunnels for walking in wintertime, or a ferry system for commuting. The adaptation the city makes to survive and to thrive is what's crucial to its vitality. The same goes for YOU.

Just because you've been dealt a genetic hand that predisposes you to heart disease or diabetes or needing pants as large as a parachute doesn't mean that you can't mitigate the effects of those genes. One of the major things we'll teach you is that while you can't change your genes, you can change whether they are turned on or off, or how you *express* them. Not every aggressive detrimental gene needs to be turned on, and not all of your sleepy protective genes have to remain dormant. Just like a city, you can compensate elegantly if you understand your options. After all, Rome is called the *eternal* city.

While some cities can deteriorate if they're not managed well, others can be maintained and revitalized if the right resources and investments are made available. That's the way you, too, can live gracefully and passionately with a fundamentally older infrastructure. Throughout the book, you'll learn many ways to manage your personal metropolis. You'll see that your immune system is your

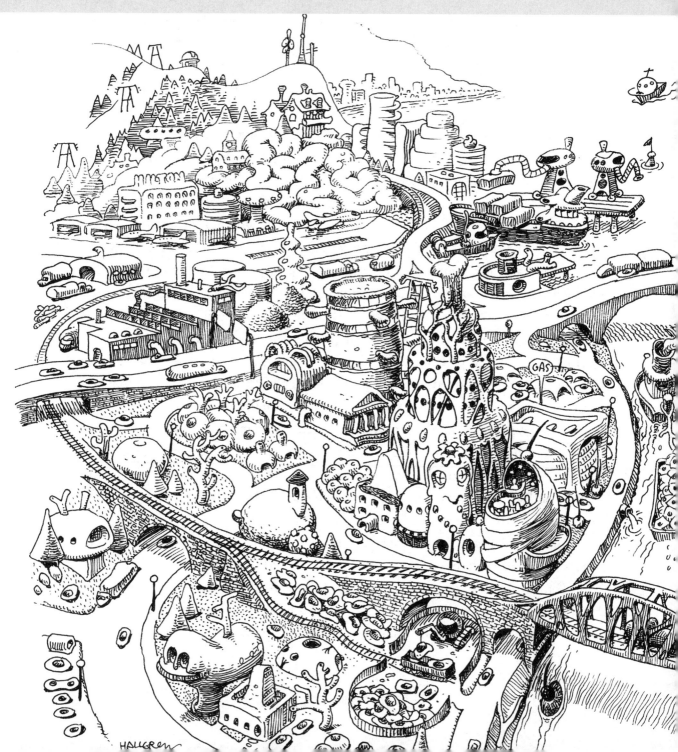

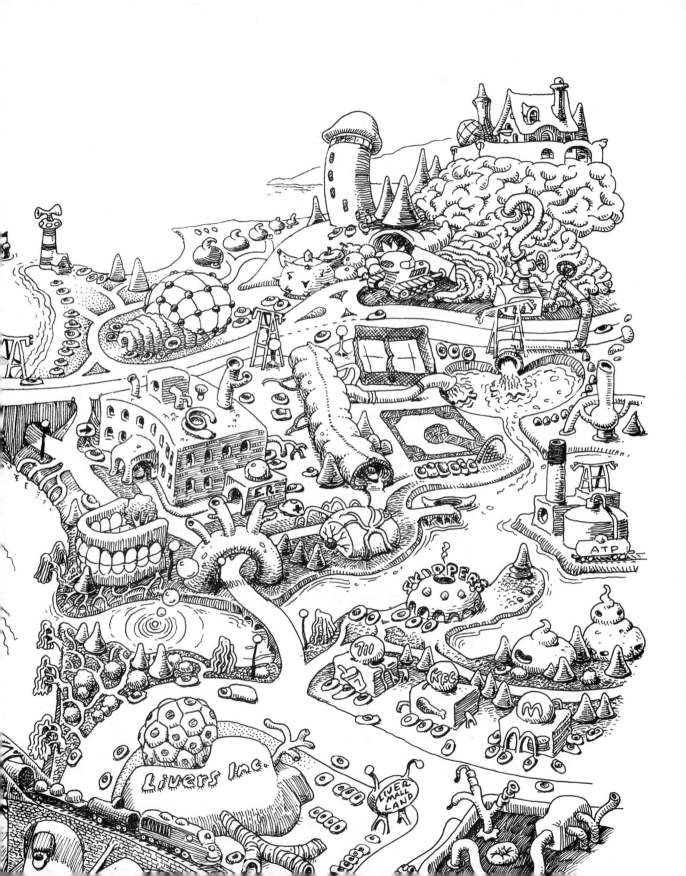

body's police force. Your arteries are like roadways that can be clogged, blocked, or worn down by years of abuse. Your brain is like the energy grid that supplies power to the entire city; it can be knocked out here and there if you let neurological branches fall on your power lines. Your skin, in many ways, is like a city's parks and green space, contributing to the overall sense of beauty and vibrancy. Your fat? Yep, landfill.

You? Consider yourself the mayor, with the power to make all the decisions about what's best for your biological city.

Our ultimate goal isn't just to keep your biological city from naming tumbleweed as the town flower—in other words, to keep you from dying (though that sure is a biggie). Our goal is to put your body at the top of the "ten best cities to live in" list. It's to make it vibrant and hip, with lots of resources and good management of those resources. Perhaps most of all, it's to give it the ability to adjust rapidly to changing times—to reinvent itself.

How will you get to know your city and all of the things that influence it? Here's how we're going to introduce it to you: Science has pointed to fourteen major processes that drive almost all of the aging we experience. Those causes of aging—everything from wear and tear to neurotransmitter imbalances—indicate the tools you'll need to get at what you really want: to help your body live younger and stronger, and to have more energy than a Labrador puppy.

Throughout the book, you'll encounter these causes of aging in special sections titled "Major Ager"; in the chapters between, you'll discover exactly how the Major Agers affect various parts of your body and find specific, practical suggestions about how you can counteract their effects. Understanding the reasons for aging will give you insights into the action steps for extending your own warranty, which we unveil in the last chapter.

Along the way, look for these features to help you learn about your body:

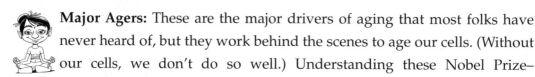 **Major Agers:** These are the major drivers of aging that most folks have never heard of, but they work behind the scenes to age our cells. (Without our cells, we don't do so well.) Understanding these Nobel Prize–

winning processes will make you a lot wiser as you wade through the littered terrain of antiaging therapies. At the very least, they'll make you sound smart around the water cooler. Take a look at our crib sheet on page 17, which summarizes these Major Agers so you can see which ones can tip the youthful scale in your favor.

YOU Tests: The beginning of each chapter will start with a quick test that you can take to assess where you stand on the aging scale. These interactive moments will give you new insights into your own body—and how young it's working.

YOU Tips: At the end of each chapter, we'll list a bunch of actions and strategies to keep your body working as vibrantly at sixty as it was at thirty-five. These tips—some admittedly controversial—will provide information about simple changes you can make to alter the complexities of your body. Whenever the science gets thin because we can't accurately extrapolate fifty years into the future, we offer the advice that we would give our families.

YOU Tools: On page 334 and throughout the book, we've created programs that you should implement in your life. They'll help you decrease stress, stop smoking, get the right lab tests, deal with anger, and so many other things. In addition, you'll get a special chapter on ways you can improve your body (and mind) with workouts that work for everyone.

YOU Tools
Detailed programs that will help you live longer

Anger-Management Plan	page 84
Quit-Smoking Plan	page 134
Deep-Sleep Program	page 186
Medical Tests You Need	page 336
Ultimate Workup	page 339
Deep Breathing and Meditation	page 350
Stress Management	page 353
Vital Vitamins and Supplements	page 356
De-Tox Plan	page 359
The YOU2 Workout	page 366
Chi-gong Workout	page 377

The YOU Extended Warranty Plan: At the end of the book, we'll provide a fourteen-day plan for doing the little things every day that make a big difference so that you can live longer and live younger. This plan will serve as the blueprint for your future decades.

YOU: The Principles of Longevity

It turns out that one of the best predictors of aging isn't how slowly you drive in the left-hand lane or whether or not you wear plaid pants. It's your own perception of how healthy you are. So indulge us for a moment and answer this question:

How healthy are you compared to other people your age?

- ❖ Excellent
- ❖ Very good
- ❖ Good
- ❖ Fair
- ❖ Bad

If you selected fair or bad, you're thirty times more as likely to die in the next two years. If that's not enough to scare the Pop-Tart right out of your mouth, then we're not sure what is. But we're not in the business of trying to frighten you to make changes; we simply want you to see that you're responsible for making your own "most livable city" list. Are you happy in your body? Do you want to live there? Where do you rank your own health? Would it top anyone's list?

The answers to these questions provide the ultimate answer to how long and well you will live. Why? Because the truth is that you likely have a gut feeling about how well you're living; about how healthy you are and about your personal weak links. Your innate feelings about your body may lead to the ultimate insight—that you may not be headed in the right direction. Luckily, science is here to help. And given what science has uncovered recently (recently, as in, some of this stuff could never have been talked about ten or even five years ago), you're going to be able to make the changes.

Before we jump into the book with explanations about these wondrous biological processes—and the specific conditions and aging-related problems you can control—let's explore what, in fact, science has found. Once you understand these new principles of longevity, you'll be better equipped to shift your actions. These five principles will change the way you think about the way your body ages.

1. Aging Is Really About Trade-offs

Despite what you think, aging—in the traditional way that we think of it, with everything slowly and painfully shutting down—isn't "meant to be." It's not an effect of life. It's actually more of a side effect of a grander plan for humans.

A lot of people think that creaky joints, craggy nails, and cranky bowels are simply part of the deal. You get to live to eighty-something; then, in exchange, you're going to have your fair share of misery along the rest of the way. Horrible being old, eh? Hold on. Yes, there is a trade-off, but it's not that one. If you take a look at every biological process that happens in your body, there's an evolutionary reason why it works that way, and that reason, without fail, is to ensure the survival of the species. That is, evolution has deemed the perpetuation of your genes to be much more important than the perpetuation of your individual life. Your biological processes are designed to protect you only long enough to reproduce and to raise your young. In fact, it wasn't until the mid–twentieth century—at least in developed countries—that human beings could expect to live much beyond their reproductive years.

Those processes that make perfect sense for reproduction may not work in your favor as you get older. That's aging. The systems designed to protect you until you finish reproducing (whether you're actually reproducing is unimportant) can be maladaptive as you age. When you look at aging through the lens of the gene, rather than the lens of the individual, it all makes much more sense.

These trade-offs are what we'll occasionally refer to as the YOU-nified theory of aging—the fact that aging isn't some master plan for life but, rather, an offshoot.

2. Aging Isn't About Breaking Down as Much as It Is About Repair

Stuff breaks. Cars, computers, and relationships all have their own breaking points. And to suggest that stuff will not break either through acute injury (a five-alarm fire or a torn knee ligament) or from wear and tear over time (a fifty-year-old roadway or an overused back) would be misleading. While it's obviously important to keep your biological systems from breaking down, the real secret to longevity isn't whether or not you break; it's how well you *recover* and *repair* when you do. Our bodies, in fact, weren't designed not to break down (legs as thick as redwoods may not break, but they wouldn't be very nimble). They were designed with a great efficiency and ability to repair themselves.

As with a car, you'll get a lot more mileage out of your body if you perform routine maintenance. Aging is essentially a process in which your cells lose their resilience; they lose their ability to repair damage because the things you might never have heard of (until now), like mitochondria and telomeres, aren't working the way they should. But it's within your power to boost that resilience and keep your vehicle going an extra couple hundred thousand miles.

3. Aging Happens from Both the Inside Out and the Outside In

Many of us like to think that aging is a magical process that happens deep within our bodies; that some so-called gremlins of gerontology ratchet down our cells and our systems so we grow old. You'll learn in this book that aging is not only about those cellular processes, but, more important, it's how you respond, adapt to, and deal with the stressors that affect you from the outside—things like sun and stress and slippery sidewalks. What does that mean? It means that aging is really about the *rate* of aging—specifically, how the outside and inside factors accelerate or decelerate your aging. Here's the big secret about aging: Your rate of aging doubles every eight years. So, if we were able to maintain a forty-year-old's rate of aging for the rest of our lives, we would live past age one hundred twenty and "die of old age." While inside out and outside in both play a role—and both influence each other—your job is to try to manage both forms, so that you slow the real culprit in growing old: the rate of aging.

4. Aging Is Not About Individual Problems but Compounded Ones

Spend any time at a deli counter, and you know that Swiss cheese has two different looks. Big holes or small holes, all in random order and patterns. A good way to think about aging is to imagine yourself looking through a dozen slices of stacked-up Swiss cheese (see Figure Intro 2, page 14). If the holes are small and the slices are thick, you can't see through the stack. Now pretend that each of these Swiss cheese slices represents a layer of protection that your body provides to prevent aging. People who are vibrant and strong may have small holes in their system—stuff that lets through a few problems, but nothing too major. Maybe they've got a little hole in their slice of heart health, and a few little holes in their slice of brain health, and a medium-sized hole in their slice of chromosome health. Nothing major lets you see through the stack.

> **FACTOID**
>
> Currently, there are approximately forty thousand centenarians in the United States—although this is difficult to estimate precisely, since there was no national birth registration system in the United States until 1940. Approximately 85 percent of them are women.

As aging takes effect, however, those holes can get a little bigger, or the cheese can get a little thinner. When big holes from one slice perfectly align with big holes from another slice, then, in effect, you've got big problems. That's a little bit what aging is like: The small problems may not have a big effect here and there, but when they grow, and when they interact with other problems, then you've created what we like to call a (*cue scary orchestra music*) web of causality. That's when seemingly small health problems spiral into bigger ones—all possibly triggered by several different causes.

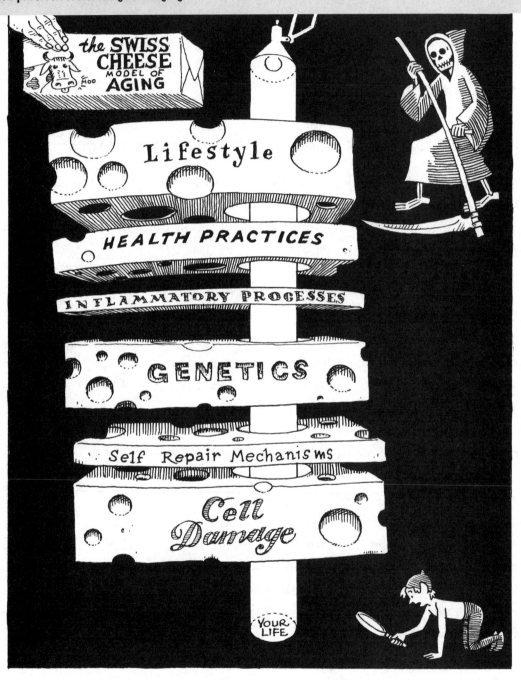

5. Aging Is Reversible—All You Need Is a Nudge

Most people think aging is a landslide of a process, that we're destined to use walkers and hearing aids and thick glasses no matter what. And while we're not saying that you will absolutely avoid all the bumps (big and small) along the way, we are saying that aging isn't as inevitable as a morning trip to the bathroom.

What you will learn in this book is how to nudge your systems so that they work in your favor, to create leverage points in life. And the great thing is that it's never too early or too late to start making these changes. You don't need a complete overhaul, because, frankly, your body is a pretty fine piece of machinery. What you'll ultimately do is find and fix your own personal weak links—the things that make you most vulnerable to the effects of aging. The cumulative effect of those nudges, though not major from a behavioral or even a biological perspective, can be huge when it comes to increasing the length and quality of your life.

The truth about aging is that you—right now—have the ability to live 35 percent longer than expected (today's life expectancy is seventy-five for men and eighty for women) with a greater quality of life and without frailty. That means it's reasonable to say that you can get to one hundred or beyond and enjoy a good quality of life along the way. While relying on the talents, skills, and knowledge of others may get you out of a medical jam, what you really want is to avoid it in the first place. Restricting calories, increasing your strength, and getting quality sleep are three of nature's best antiaging medicines. Together, these activities—as well as the other actions we recommend—control 70 percent of how well you age. Wouldn't you want to hold the power of your future in your hands, rather than put it in someone else's?

Just because you've made mistakes in the past doesn't mean you can't reverse them. Even if you've had burgers for breakfast or fried your brain cells with stress, you're not necessarily destined to wear husky pants and forget birthdays. No matter what kind of life you've already led, aging is reversible: You can have a do-over if you want it. If you perform a good habit for three years, the effect on your body is as if you've done it your entire life. Even better, within three months of changing a behavior, you can start to measure a difference in your life expectancy.

As we said, aging is inevitable, but the rate of aging is not. Consider this fact: Only 10 percent of people are classified as frail when they're in their seventies. By the time people reach one hundred, almost 100 percent are considered frail. What we're trying to do is make sure that percentage stays lower for longer. We want you to feel as good at the end of the race as you do at the start.

Our goal here is to ensure that you have a high quality of life until whatever time—forgive our bluntness—you drop dead. That's the ideal scenario, right? Nobody wants to spend their golden years on diets of Jell-O, suffering from bedsores, or not remembering the previous nine decades. You want to feel like you're thirty even when you're eighty. You want to have the wisdom of a grandparent without feeling like one. So our goal isn't to get you to 120—unless those 120 years come with quality.

After all, living longer shouldn't be about "taking longer to die," which is what so many people think it means. It should be about enjoying every moment of a longer life—and taking longer to live.

You want to live long and live well. You want to feel alive while you're living.
You don't want to grow old. You want to stay young.
This is the way.
Now hup to it.

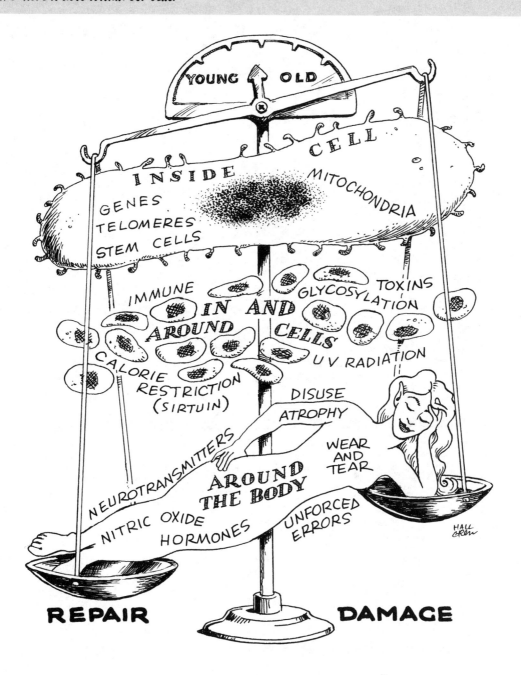

Bad Genes & Short Telomeres

How Genetics Influences Aging—and You Control Your Genes

As we get older, it's easier and easier to pass the blame for our own health problems on to other people. Recently diagnosed with high cholesterol? Aha, three grandparents and two great-uncles all died of heart disease. Accidentally put the ketchup in the freezer the other day? Oh yes, Aunt Matilda had a touch of dementia. Battling a weight problem for most of your life? Yup, Pops and his brothers believed in the three food groups of cheese ravioli, meat sauce, and multiple helpings.

In fact, many of us buy into a very similar theory of aging: We're born with our health destiny. That is, our genes—the chromosomal alphabet soup that includes ingredients from our parents, their parents, and so on—are primarily responsible for determining whether we'll get heart disease, cancer, Alzheimer's, or any of the other diseases or conditions that can turn a grade-A quality of life to spoiled ground chuck.

But that's simply not the way aging works. Your genes are important, especially when it comes to one of the most powerful age-related problems: memory loss. Your genetic destiny, however, is not inevitable.

What do we mean by that? Think back to the city that we outlined for you in the introduction, and consider your genes as the physical location of that city. Some characteristics you simply can't change. Chicago is windy, Minneapolis is snowy, San Francisco is built on fault lines, Cape Hatteras is in the path of tropical storms. A city's location serves the same function as your body's genes. Your genetic traits make you more or less predisposed to health-related windstorms, snowstorms, earthquakes, and hurricanes. But just as you can modify cities to adjust to natural geography and natural occurrences, you can also protect yourself from abnormalities in your genes if you're unhappy with how you've been genetically programmed.

When it comes to your body, here's what we know, primarily through studies of identical twins: Your longevity is based one-quarter on your genetics and three-quarters on your behaviors and lifestyle choices. It's not about what genes you have but how you express them. Genes work by manufacturing proteins, but whether or not a specific gene is turned on or off is largely under your control.

Think of the ability to manipulate your genes as developing a set of city building codes to adapt to the circumstances you're in. It would be like a coastal town requiring houses to be built on stilts to protect against surging tides or office buildings in San Francisco using earthquake-resistant materials to better protect against an architectural crumble. You adapt and adjust to deal with whatever nature throws your way. That's the way your body works. As the mayor of your physiological city, you can create different codes to mitigate the effects of the genes you've been dealt. For example, exercise isn't good for you just because it helps burn fat and assists with bikini satisfaction, but it can also alter the expres-

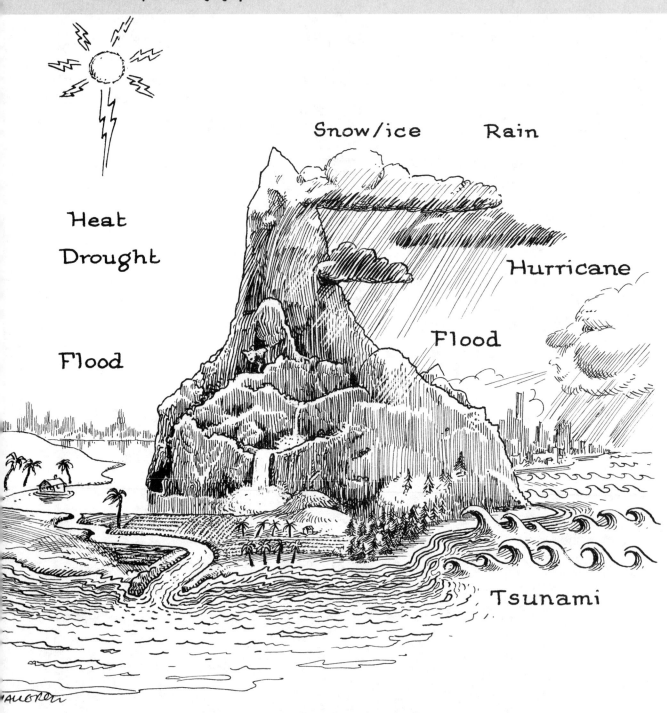

sion of your genetic codes to decrease your risk of getting cancer. That means you do have some control over how your genes manifest themselves in your body and how they control the rate—and way—that you age.

Maybe you've been dealt a bad hand of genetics, but that doesn't mean you can't exchange a few cards, or at least change how you play them. Another way to think about your genetic inheritance: It's stored information, the factory-installed info that comes with your biological system. You have the power—with your behavioral software—to alter that information along the way. But if you don't take any action, then the stored information is what dictates how those genes play out.

Which of Your Genes Is Turned On?

Controlling your genetics can help you avoid the major age-related diseases and improve the chances that you'll spend more time with your grandkids than you will in doctors' waiting rooms reading large-print magazines that are three years old.

If you remember our Swiss cheese model, it makes sense: By fixing one thing about your body—like adding a daily thirty-minute walk—you'll end up (perhaps unintentionally) fixing many others along the way, so that the holes of aging don't line up and cause total system failure. And by making small changes, you'll reach that goal of adding years and quality to your life.

So how do you change the function of your genes? One way is through the rebuilding of chromosomes. Your chromosomes, the little rascals, have small substances on the ends called telomeres (see Figure A.2). Think of them as being like those little plastic tips of shoelaces (which are called aglets, in case you want to show off in your next Scrabble competition). Every time a cell reproduces, that telomere gets a little shorter, just as the shoelace tip wears off with time. Once the protective covering on the tip is gone, your DNA and shoelace begin to fray

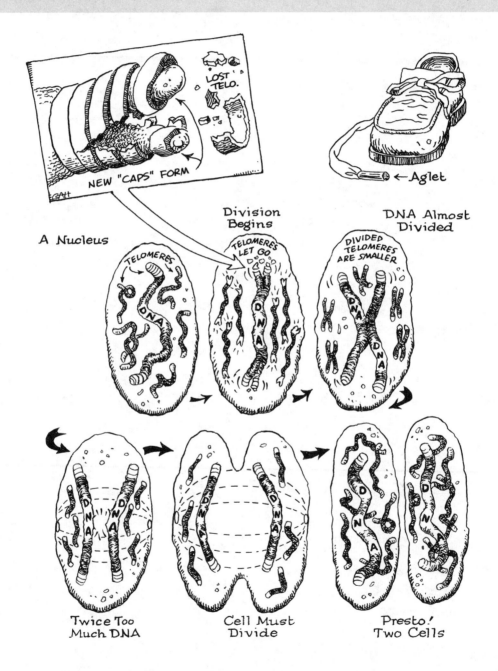

LOST TELO.

NEW "CAPS" FORM

←Aglet

A Nucleus

Division Begins

DNA Almost Divided

TELOMERES

TELOMERES LET GO

DIVIDED TELOMERES ARE SMALLER

DNA

DNA

DNA

Twice Too Much DNA

Cell Must Divide

Presto! Two Cells

and are much harder to use. That's what causes cells to stop dividing and grow-ing and replenishing your body. The cell realizes that it is no longer helping the body and commits suicide (that's called apoptosis), which can contribute to age-related conditions. But your body also has a protein—called telomerase—that au-tomatically replenishes and rebuilds the ends of the chromosomes to keep cells (and you) healthy. However, lots of cells in your body don't have telomerase, meaning that many of them have a reproduction limit—thus putting a cap on how well your systems can be replenished. (Telomerase, by the way, is overactive in 85 percent of cancers. That makes sense, right? Rebuilding the aglet that allows cells to divide helps those cancer cells reproduce and spread.)

The amount of telomerase depends on your genetics, but we're now starting to see that we can influence the size of those little tips, the telomeres. For exam-ple, researchers have found that mothers with chronically ill children have short-ened telomeres, indicating that chronic stress can have a huge influence on how cells divide—or fail to. The implication is that if you can reduce the effects that stress has on you, through such techniques as meditation (see page 350), you can increase your chance of rebuilding the telomeres and decrease the odds of having your cells die and contribute to age-related problems.

Yes, you're stuck with the genes you were given, just as you're stuck with the decisions your parents made about where you grew up, and you can't return your genes for a complete refund. You can, however, change the way they function. We're starting to uncover more and more ways that you can change how your genes function, which we'll detail in the following chapter about your memory. For example, just ten minutes of walking turns on a gene that decreases the rate of cancer growth, and resveratrol (the ingredient found in red wine) turns on a gene that slows or stops a dangerous inflammatory process that happens inside your body. And in the very near future, we're going to be able to develop medi-cines tailored to individuals whose genes work differently from others'.

Because each of us has a unique genetic fingerprint, the detection, prevention, and treatment of diseases can be difficult. But as we start to unlock the ways that we and modern medicine can dramatically manipulate our genes, we're going to start seeing how we can make our genes work for us, not against us. Perhaps the best example of how genes affect us is our memory, which is goal one—in part so you can remember the rest.

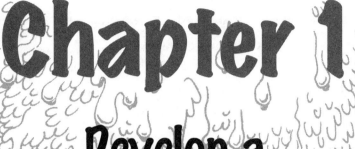

Chapter 1
Develop a Memorable Memory

YOU Test: Mind Game

GCHC F ANA BHD FDHEGHEHNEDBNA F BHGCHDE BGAHECHN FGNB
A BDCACEGH FH FHDN HBCE BDNEHGNH FGAC FNCHDE AHAGFDBHA
BCE FHDANHC FGDHA EHBNCHGDGFNEHB E BDHCACHD FGF AHNE
B EHNHNGBGDA FHCEHD FHE AGHGCBNBNCAHD F BNE AH FDGHC

Photocopy this page so that you can do the test twice. Have somebody time you. As quickly and accurately as you can, take a pencil and cross out all the *H*s in the above pattern, moving left to right and starting from the top line. Average the time it took on both of your tries. This test helps measure mental acuity.

(*continued on next page*)

Results:

Count the number of *H*s you knocked out. The total number is thirty-six. See where you fell with the averages below.

Age	Average Seconds	Number Missed
Under 30	40	1
30–45	41	1
45–50	42	2
50–55	43	2
55–60	44	2
60–65	46	2
66–70	46	2
71–75	47	3
76–80	50	3
81–85	51	3
86–90	52	2
91–95	53	2

Credit: Letter cancellation used with permission from Bob Uttl.

Our brains sure do have a way of messing with our minds.

One moment, you can be spitting out the names of your entire third-grade class, the batting statistics from the 1974 St. Louis Cardinals, the color dress you wore to the eighth-grade Sadie Hawkins Day dance, or the entire script from your favorite *Seinfeld* episode. The next minute, you space on the name of your cat.

Call them what you want—senior moments, doomsday to dementia—but the truth is that we all experience these neurological hiccups as we age. And we all wonder exactly what they mean. Some of us write them off to stress, fatigue, or some kind of neurological overload that's caused by the ogre who signs our paychecks, while others worry about whether a moment of forgetfulness means that we have a first-class ticket on the express train to Alzheimer's.

No matter what we may think causes our decline in mental acuity, most people share a pretty big assumption about our gray matter: Either our brains are genetically determined to be Ginsu sharp for the duration, or we're eventually going to live life putting on our underwear last. That is, we believe that our genes, the very first Major Ager, *completely* control our neurological destiny.

That simply isn't true.

While many diseases and conditions have genetic elements to them, memory conditions have some of the strongest genetic indicators. For example, a PET (positron-emission tomography) scan, which records images of the brain as it functions, reveals evidence of early Alzheimer's when it identifies that the brain is misusing energy. This abnormality is caused by illness of the mitochondria (more details on this Major Ager on page 48), which is genetically determined. But the truth is that even if your genes have decided to give you a life of serious forgetfulness, you do have the ability to control those genes so your mind is strong, your brain functions at full power, and you remember everything from the crucial details of your life to whether or not you turned off the oven—even when your birthday candles reach triple digits. Plus, we have lots of data from twin studies saying that less than 50 percent of memory is inherited, meaning that if you get a head start on the action steps we're going to cover, you can alter how your genes are expressed. In the end, genetics loads the gun, but your lifestyle pulls the trigger.

Clearly, the brain is the most complex organ in your body. In fact, if the brain were simpler, we wouldn't be smart enough to understand it. But we are. Think of

Vice Is Nice

Though there's some evidence that nicotine (in the form of a patch, not the kind you smoke) plays some role in improving awareness, research also supports the memory-boosting effects of a less dangerous vice: caffeine. About five cups of coffee a day protects against cognitive impairment from both Alzheimer's and Parkinson's diseases. (Remember, if you experience side effects like migraines, abnormal heartbeats, anxiety, or acid reflux, the benefits may not be worth the side effects.) By keeping you alert, caffeine will also help you assimilate knowledge and deposit it in your memory bank efficiently, improving the chance that you'll recall it correctly.

your brain as the city's electrical grid. Your brain's nerve cells, or neurons, are constantly firing and receiving messages in much the same way that power plants send signals and homes and businesses receive them. Power may originate from a main source, but the connections then branch out every which way throughout the city. Your brain functions the same way: Messages are sent from one neuron to another across your neurological grid. When those neurons successfully communicate with one another through the sending and receiving of neurological impulses, your brain can file away your memories.

But what happens when a storm, an accident, or a chainsaw-wielding hoodlum knocks out the power lines? You lose connections, so you lose power—maybe to a particular neighborhood or maybe to a large segment of the city, depending on which ones got fried. Same goes for your brain. If something knocks out those neural connections, then small or large parts of your brain can experience a blackout, and you freak because you can't remember that you left the car keys on the back of the toilet.

Certainly, many things can cause malfunctions in your neurological grid. Some are acute and immediate, like a concussion arising from a brain bruise. Others are more chronic, as in the case of a genetic malfunction that can cause your power lines to be rickety so they easily fritz out. These are the ones that we're mainly going to address here.

Your Memory: Don't Fuggedaboudit

Part of our job as doctors is to tell you things straight up, because when we don't tell the truth, people get hurt. No sugarcoating. No BS (that really stands for *no bad science*). No "Win One for the Gipper" speeches. When it comes to your brain, here's a fact that's harsher than a Buffalo winter: The research shows that, eventually, everyone in America will either get Alzheimer's or care for someone who has it.

In some way or another, we're all going to be affected by serious change-your-life memory problems. But the Gipper side of that statistic is this: Memory disorders aren't as uncontrollable as they seem, and the way to attack potential brain problems is by using your brain to understand them. For starters, here are some things you should know about your noggin:

Play Doc

When trying to determine if a family member is having serious memory trouble, ask him what he had for dinner or to describe current events, or give him three objects to remember and five minutes later ask him what they are. If he has trouble with any of those questions, it's an indication that something's going wrong with his short-term memory—one of the signs of a serious cognitive dysfunction.

- ❖ We actually experience a mental decline a lot earlier than we realize. Memory loss starts at age sixteen and is relatively common by forty. One way you can see this is through research done on video game players. People start losing their hand-eye coordination and the ability to perform exceptionally well on video games after the age of twenty-five. The fascinating part of this research isn't that you'll rarely beat your kid in Mario Kart: Double Dash; it's that even if your brain knows what to do when presented with an animated hairpin turn at 135 mph, your brain can't fire those messages fast enough to your trigger-happy thumbs. There's a natural slowing of the connection—the power line—between your brain and your body.

- ❖ Men and women not only differ when it comes to movie tastes and erogenous zones, but also differ when it comes to mental decline. Men usually lose their ability to solve complex problems as they age, while women often lose their ability to process information quickly. That split shows us a couple of things. One, that there's certainly a strong genetic component to memory loss. And, two, that there are specific actions you should be taking to combat that genetic disposition. While there are some places where you're naturally going to decline because

Develop a Memorable Memory 29

of your sex, there are other areas where you're going to have an advantage. That means your job isn't only to try to rebuild the area that's breaking down but to preserve the areas that excel. But across the board, both genders lose competency in the areas in which they are weak to begin with. So women lose spatial cognition, and men suffer verbal losses. Though it's certainly not true for everyone, it may give you clues as to what areas of your brain to concentrate on as you age—or it may help you play to your strengths. (Those with poor memory recall can use organizational skills to compensate, for example.)

❖ You don't have to have an elite brain to know that your three-pound organ has more power than a rocket booster. It controls everything from your emotions to your decision making, and it gives you the ability to understand why the baseball in Figure 11.1 on page 220 is pretty darn funny. But when we discuss memory loss, we're essentially focusing on three specific brain functions: sensory information (your ability to determine what information is important), short-term memory loss (quick, what's the title of this chapter?), and long-term memory loss (that's your bank of recipes, trivia, names, and every piece of information you've known, read, and stored during your life).

Whether you've seen it on the news, on TV shows, or within your own family, you know how dementia looks from the outside: People forget faces, names, where they live, and information that seems—to the rest of the world—so easy to remember. The most frequently seen problem: getting lost on a walk home. To really control your own genetic destiny, you need to take a look at what memory loss looks like on the inside. For the record, age-related memory loss is classified in several ways. Conditions such as Alzheimer's, dementia, and mild cognitive impairment are all technically different. For our purposes, we're tackling them all together as age-related memory problems because of the similarities in how they change people's lives.

Your Brain: Mind and Matter

Before we crack some skulls and dive inside the brain, let's quickly look at what memory really is: Essentially, it's the process of learning information, storing it, and then having the ability to recall it when you need it—whether to solve problems, tell stories, or save yourself on the witness stand.

Learning begins with those power connections in your brain: neurons firing messages to one another. Your ability to process information is determined by the junctions between those neurons, called the synapses. The ability of brain cells to speak to one another is strengthened or weakened as you use them. We'll spare you all the biological miracles that take place between your ears, but essentially, the more you use those synapses, the stronger they get and the more they proliferate. That's why you may have strong neural pathways for your family history or weak ones for eighties music trivia. That also gives you a little insight into how you remember things. If something's exciting to you, then you learn it faster—and train those synapses to make strong connections. But if the information seems more boring than the sexual habits of an earthworm, you can still learn and build those connections with repeated use.

Problems arise when synapses lie dormant: The less you use certain connections, the greater chance they have of falling into disrepair (like losing fluency in a foreign language if you don't use it for a long time). Technically, we actually learn by weakening underutilized synapses and repairing and strengthening the synapses we commonly use. So if you cook a lot and enjoy it, you'll eventually know the recipes by heart—and learn them faster because it's enjoyable. You build a large connecting wire, which allows for the faster flow of information. By contrast, lesser-used pathways fall into disrepair, so you lose or disable those connections. If you haven't exercised your 1970s TV trivia synapse in a long time, then you're

> ## FACTOID
>
> Type 2 diabetes (the kind associated with being overweight) increases the risk of Alzheimer's, probably by increasing inflammation or arterial aging, but also because too much of the hormone insulin in the brain can stimulate beta-amyloid buildup. In fact, Alzheimer's is now being called type 3 diabetes.

not going to remember the name of the kid who played Bobby Brady on *The Brady Bunch* (ten points if you said Mike Lookinland before we did).

To keep your memory functioning at optimal power, you'll need to focus on three aspects of your biology.

Your Brain. Let's peel back your scalp and look through a peephole in your head. From the toupee's-eye view, you can see that your brain has 100 billion nerve cells, and each cell receives one hundred messages per second. Yup. In the time it takes you to read this sentence, your brain cells have been doing more processing than the IRS's computer server.

Your neurons—the cells that transmit information—look like mops with shaggy strings that reach out to one another, while the handles of the mops act like cables that carry the information. These neurons talk with one another with the frequency of eighth-grade girls at a slumber party; a lot of information is exchanged very quickly.

The hippocampus, which is shaped a little like a seahorse and is buried deep inside your brain (see Figure 1.1), is the main driver of memory. (The other two memory-related areas of the brain are the prefrontal cortex, which controls the executive function of your brain, and the cerebellum, which controls balance.) Your hippocampus processes information before it is stored. It works best when you're either emotionally interested in the material or alert when you're learning about it. That's one reason why coffee may aid memory; it seems to increase your alertness the first time you learn something, which increases the chance you'll deposit it in your long-term memory bank.

But for the purposes of aging, we're mostly concerned about what happens to the power lines within your brain. So flip on your hippocampus (or grab a cup of coffee) and remember this: There are protein fragments in your brain that sound like the name of a *Star Wars* droid—beta-amyloid—and they're responsible for gunking up your power lines like overgrown vegetation or fallen branches. They're likely responsible for causing Alzheimer's. The primary defect in Alzheimer's affects the input and output power lines of the hippocampus. Memory

Figure 1.1 **Storage Units** Memories are stored in the hippocampus. The other two major memory-related areas of the brain are the prefrontal cortex (controlling the executive function of your brain) and the cerebellum (used for balance). Craving memories are found in the insula.

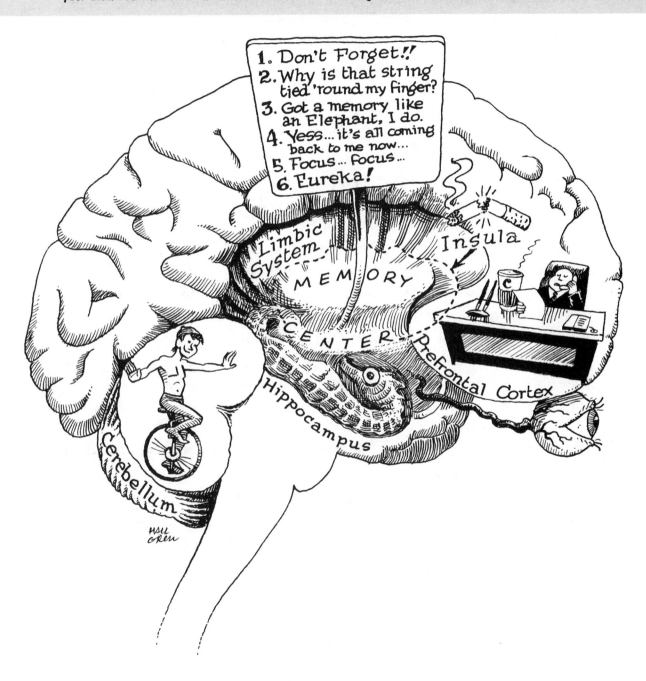

starts to fade. (The other physiological sign of Alzheimer's is the buildup of what are called neurofibrillary tangles. They're insoluble twisted fibers that build up inside neurons, like power lines getting crossed up and sending energy to the wrong location. These tangles influence intelligence.) Now, a downed branch here and there won't do much to disrupt the flow of energy through your entire city, but what happens when a lot of branches or shrubs or trees fall on the same part of the grid? You're out of commission.

In general, genes control how much beta-amyloid you have. Some branches may be knocking out those notes from your course in eighteenth-century Roman history, while others may be causing you to forget to pick up the very thing that you went to the supermarket for in the first place. But your genes don't have complete control. You can alter the amount of gunk you have gooping up and weighing down your power lines by altering the expression of one of your genes: the Apo E gene, to be exact. Apo E protein acts like the power company crew that removes the branches and sap from the power lines after the storm. It sweeps through and removes the beta-amyloid so that your synapses can keep functioning and you don't lose the ability to remember how many career touchdown passes Dan Marino threw (420), or what year Diane Keaton won an Oscar for best actress (1977). Whenever we create new synapses to help our brain improve itself, some of this beta-amyloid remains behind, and the Apo E workers clear the gunk to ensure a clean connection.

One group in the union, however, local Apo E4, sabotages the effort to restore power and even gunks up the power lines further (see Figure 1.2). Research shows that an elevated level of the E4 protein is correlated with a higher incidence of Alzheimer's. Fortunately, there are things you can do to turn down the activity of the E4 gene and allow the rest of the Apo E team to clear your power lines. Eating turmeric, which is found in Indian foods, seems to reduce expression of the E4 gene (India, by the way, has a relatively low incidence of Alzheimer's). Exercise has a similar effect.

Your Blood Supply: While there's a strong genetic component to memory problems, we'd be remiss if we didn't address the arterial component of an aging

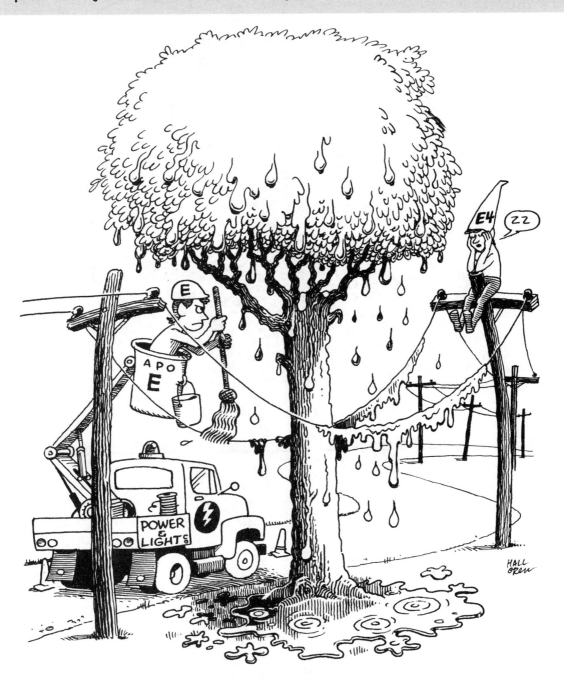

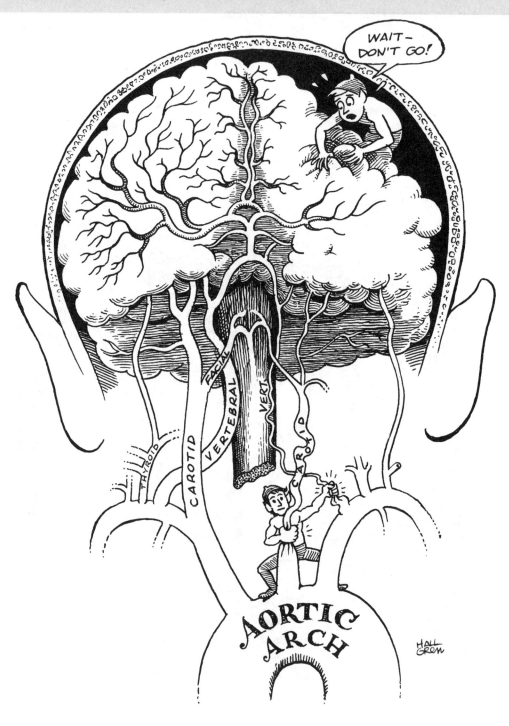

Brain Pills?

It'd be nice if there were such a thing as mental Viagra—just swallow a pill and get a little lift where you need it. But the verdict's still out on many pills, supplements, and vitamins that purport to make your memory stronger. Here's our take on the ones that get most of the attention:

Pill	Do We Recommend It?	The Fine Print
Aspirin	Yes	Research shows a 40 percent decrease in arterial aging, a major cause of memory loss, for those who take 162 milligrams of aspirin a day. Though science isn't sure of the mechanism protecting against memory loss, it may happen because aspirin helps decrease that gunky beta-amyloid from your wiring, and because it improves circulation.
Vitamin E	In your diet, ideally	People who consume the highest amount of vitamin E are 43 percent less likely to get Alzheimer's. You can get the vitamin E you need by eating just 3 ounces of nuts or seeds a day (about 15.5 milligrams), which is our preferred method. Alternatively, you can take a 400 IU (international unit) supplement daily if you take it with vitamin C and are not taking statin drugs like Lipitor.
Vitamins B_6, B_{12}, folic acid	Yes	Without B vitamins, your neurotransmitters don't work efficiently. To compound matters, without B vitamins, your homocysteine levels rise, and that doubles the risk of developing Alzheimer's. Homocysteine is an amino acid associated with stroke, heart disease, and Alzheimer's. Although no study has demonstrated a benefit of supplementation to your thinking process, the products are generally safe, and anecdotal evidence is enticing. We recommend a supplement with 400 micrograms of folic acid, 800 micrograms of B_{12}, and 40 milligrams of B_6 a day.
Aceytl-L-carnitine/ alpha-lipoic acid	Not yet	There are lots of strong theoretical reasons why this should enhance brain health—specifically, by improving mitochondrial activity and reducing mitochondrial DNA decay, resulting in higher neutrotransmitter function—but there's not enough evidence in humans.
Rosemary, roses, and mint	Yes	Not to ingest, but to smell. Research suggests that inhaling these three aromas at the time of learning a new task can enhance recall when you're exposed to the scent at a later time.

Ginkgo biloba	If you want to	Though there are no large studies to support its use, there's some promise that this very commonly used supplement is effective in helping improve cognition. It can also thin the blood, which can be helpful in folks with blood vessel disease but dangerous for those with clotting disorders or anticipating surgery. Because it's considered a safe antioxidant supplement, we're comfortable with you trying 120 milligrams daily to see if it has any positive effects.
Huperzine A	Maybe	This ancient Chinese herb was used for memory loss even before we knew that it increases acetylcholine levels by blocking a chemical that devours this precious neurotransmitter. If you have mild cognitive impairment, we recommend 200 micrograms twice daily and suggest that your doctor help titrate the treatment if other pharmaceuticals with similar effects are being used.
Vinpocetine	No	There's not enough evidence that this supplement from a periwinkle plant helps, and it can reduce your blood pressure too much, so we would rather wait for more clinical trials.
Phosphatidylserine	If you want to	About 70 percent of our cell membranes are made from this, and as we age, the level of phosphatidylserine drops, and the membranes become brittle. This supplement seems to strengthen cell membranes and the phospholipid sheathing around nerves, protecting the cables that transfer information from shorting out. Since risks are few, taking 200 milligrams daily is reasonable.
Coenzyme Q10	Yes, but for other reasons	This supplement has a beneficial effect in protecting against Parkinson's disease (a neural disease that can be caused by trauma, as in the case of boxers, or through viruses and genetics). As a potent antioxidant, it may help prevent inflammatory damage to the brain, but this remains unproven. The ideal dose is 100 milligrams twice a day (some research says that 300 milligrams four times a day is even better for Parkinson's). This is one supplement where more than 90 percent of what's sold doesn't contain the real thing, so look for products that have actually been shown repeatedly to have in the bottle what's on the label. The website to check to see if it contains what's on the label: www.consumerlab.com.

brain. A lack of healthy blood flow to the brain is one of the other main causes of forgetfulness. Each side of the brain has a separate blood supply that looks like several large trees during winter. Between the twigs at the tips of the major branches are areas of brain that are dependent on blood from each of the surrounding trees. The area farthest from two blood-supply lines is the watershed area where we tend to have ministrokes when the branches of surrounding trees are pruned by atherosclerosis or the tree trunks themselves wither from poor maintenance (see Figure 1.3). Cholesterol-lowering statin drugs may help maintain memory by preserving tree architecture, while also reducing inflammation that ages the brain cells directly (more on arterial health in the next chapter).

Your Neurochemicals: Nerve cells communicate with one another via neurotransmitters, chemicals that ferry information from neuron to neuron across the synapses between them. The most common neurotransmitter is called acetylcholine. When levels of this chemical fall, especially in the hippocampus (the part of the brain that controls our memory), we develop cognitive impairment. Many of the treatments for Alzheimer's are aimed at increasing the amount of acetylcholine in the brain.

> **FACTOID**
>
> Those neurofibrillary tangles associated with Alzheimer's disease contain aluminum (an element that makes up 14 percent of the earth's crust). While there's no evidence suggesting that aluminum causes memory problems, it's better to try to avoid it. One way to reduce the aluminum you absorb: Use sea salt instead of table salt, which is processed with aluminum to avoid caking. Other things that contain aluminum include nondairy creamers, antacids, cans, certain cookware, and antiperspirants.

The other chemical that plays a significant role in memory is called brain-derived neurotrophic factor (BDNF, or just neurotrophins if you prefer), which works like Miracle-Gro for your brain. During infancy, BDNF helps develop nerves that help us learn, but as we get older, things like inflammation and stress can decrease its levels. Research shows that you can do things to improve your levels of BDNF, such as consuming the spice curcumin (a component of turmeric), restricting calories, doing exercise, being in love, and taking some of a class of antidepressants known as selective serotonin reuptake inhibitors, or SSRIs. Not surprisingly, you can decrease BDNF by eating high levels of saturated fats and refined sugars, as well as by not getting enough of the natural antidepressant tryptophan (sure, it's found in turkey, but there's twice as much in spinach) in your diet.

So what's the biological effect of all this? Well, if you have serious memory-related problems, the gray matter in your brain actually shrivels faster than a centenarian sunbather. And the connections that are so important to maintaining memory get blocked and broken and detoured so that your memory function is slowed—or sometimes lost. In the end, that can cause you to lose the power lines that go to the neighborhood of fashion trivia or to the office complex of phone numbers or to the cul-de-sac of your anniversary date.

Luckily, as you'll see, there are several simple ways to restore those power lines, regrow those neural connections, and preserve one of the most powerful things you can pass along to the generations that follow: your memory. And your wisdom.

YOU TIPS!

Like babies and brats, all your brain wants is this: attention. Feed it, challenge it, care for it, and you'll smack a bad genetic destiny square in the face with five knuckles of good information and smart action. One of the key things to do is constantly stretch your mind—be it through crosswords, Scrabble, chess, or learning how to speak Chinese (if you don't already). Thankfully, there are many ways to keep your brain operating at maximum efficiency, maximum power, and maximum quality.

YOU Tip: Teach a Lesson. In life, we have all kinds of teachers—first-grade teachers, basketball coaches, ballet instructors. While they may have been responsible for teaching us how to read, how to shoot a ball, or how to do the perfect plié, they also taught us perhaps one of the most important lessons about aging: Teaching can save your brain. You're far more likely to retain information if you have to explain it to somebody else. The degree to which you can effectively explain information indicates how well you've actually learned it. The lesson: Take advantage of mentoring opportunities, whether it's instructing a class in your favorite hobby at a community college or inviting the neighborhood teens over to teach them how to change a tire or make a soufflé. Teach the next generation, and you'll power up your own generator.

YOU Tip: And Be a Lifelong Learner. Yeah, sure, we know what your ideal picture of retirement looks like: one hammock, one baby-blue ocean, four naps a day. That's great and all, but one of the best ways to insure that your mind doesn't liquidate into the consistency of a piña colada is to continue to give it a reason to function. Work it. Challenge it. Teach it new things. Just take a look at a massive study done on a population of more than three thousand nuns. Researchers measured the daily mental and physical activities of living nuns and autopsied those who died during the study. They found that 37 percent of the nuns who died had confirmed Alzheimer's disease—at least according to what was happening pathologically in their brains. The nuns who fared the best were the ones who were better educated. The nuns with Alzheimer's were, as young adults, less mentally and physically active outside their jobs than those without the disease. That's important because Alzheimer's disease takes decades to develop. The amazing part was that even if the nuns showed pathological signs of Alzheimer's, they had no clinical symptoms. The point: Although these neurological tangles may be genetic, your ability to resist the effects of them is not.

When you increase your learning during life, you decrease the risk of developing memory-related problems. That means your brain has a fighting chance if you keep it active and engaged, if you keep challenging it with new lessons, if you learn a new game or new hobby or new vocation. You have to challenge your mind—even making it a little uncomfortable by pushing yourself to learn tasks that may not come naturally. Doing tough tasks reinforces the neural connections that are important to preserving memory. Like a clutch athlete, your mind has a way of rising to the occasion. Challenge it, and it will reward you.

YOU Tip: Stop and Think About Thinking. Like breathing, thinking is designed to be an automatic process. Don't believe us? Then do this: Don't think of a bruised banana. Don't picture it. Don't let the image cross your mind. Ha! The only thing you can think of right now is that darn potassium-loaded phallic symbol. The other vantage point here is that you can't do anything but think when you're thinking. Thinking is an involuntary reflex; while you can often control what you think about, thinking is as natural as an ocean's ecosystem—stuff just kinda floats around and goes where it wants to go.

Now, try this when you're doing a simple activity, like waking up: Instead of just rolling out of bed, splashing water on your face, and dreading your eight o'clock meeting, think about your surroundings. Listen for birds, notice the drips of water beading down your leg in the shower, savor the sips from your OJ, think about every tooth you're brushing. It doesn't take any more time; it just helps train your brain. We're not trying to go all philosophical on you; thinking about the thought process is really about awareness and is one of the tools you can use to strengthen your neural connections.

YOU Tip: See If Your Genes Fit. If you have a family history of memory-related problems and are comfortable with genetic testing, you can have your level of Apo E4 protein checked. That will help you determine whether you're more or less predisposed to clearing that gunky beta-amyloid from your neural wiring. You can find out more about the test on www.aruplab.com, www.athenadiagnostics.com, or www.realage.com. No matter what your result, know that obesity and alcohol intake increase expression of the gene, while exercise decreases the amount of Apo E4 in the blood.

YOU Tip: Live in the Moment. We all know what life is like when the dog's barking, the phone's ringing, the baby's crying, Nickelodeon is on high volume, and your spouse is trying to explain by goodness why the toilet seat wound up in the up position again—and you're worried about what you need to do tomorrow and haven't done today. When it comes to your brain, stress acts as a massive amount of noise in your system—only it comes in the form of nagging tasks, job dissatisfaction, bills, and fights about who's going to which family's house for the holidays. Oy. One of the keys to having a healthy mind is to live as much as you can in the moment; that is, thinking about what you're doing right now, not worrying about the mistakes you made yesterday or the headaches that await you tomorrow. That actually helps reduce the noise in the system.

Evolutionarily, you can see how it works: When you're aroused by stress (saber-tooth bearing down fast), you have a very narrow functioning cognitive ability: run, fight, or die. Good for survival, sure, but that acute function actually shortens the telomeres on your chromosomes (remember the first Major Ager?) and contributes to memory problems. In the modern age, more stress means the inability to concentrate, and that's been shown to contribute to a shrinking of the prefrontal cortex. Is living in the moment hard to do? Of course it can be, but it's a behavior you can learn with practice, similar to our previous strategy of thinking about thinking. Example: When you're playing with your kids and letting tomorrow's workday weigh on you, force yourself to concentrate on Candyland, making it a great experience for your kids rather than a distant one for you. It takes some time and effort, but in the end, the act of living in the moment rewards not only you but the people around you.

YOU Tip: Feed on Brain Food. While physics would dictate that your food travels down after you eat it, a certain amount travels up to your brain (via arteries after it's been through the digestive process, of course). Among the best nutrients to help keep your cerebral power lines strong are omega-3 fatty acids—the kinds of fat found in fish like salmon and mahi-mahi. These healthy fats, which have been shown to slow cognitive decline in people who are at risk, not only help keep your arteries clear but improve the function of your message-sending neurotransmitters. Aim for 13 ounces of fish a week, or, if you prefer supplements, take 2 grams of fish oil a day (metabolically distilled), or DHA from algae (where fish get their omega-3s), or an ounce of walnuts a day. DHA is the omega-3 that seems best for the brain.

YOU Tip: Try Chi. Chi-gong, an activity that looks like slow-mo martial arts, can not only help improve your physical well-being but can serve as a mind-clearing exercise. This slow, gentle series of movements can help reduce the noise and is especially great if you have aches and pains that hold you back from your normal routine. We offer a sample plan on page 377.

YOU Tip: Load Up on Salad. The veggies, not the fat-laden dressing. It's been shown that vegetables—any kind, any place—slow cognitive decline even more than fruits. Eating two or more servings a day (*just two!*) decreases the decline in thinking by 35 percent over six years. Pass the sprouts, please.

YOU Tip: Add a Dash of This and That. Several substances have been shown to help cognitive function. These are the ones we recommend:

❖ Carotenoids and flavonoids, which are vitamin-like substances that can act as antioxidants. Not essential for life, they tend to give color to fruits and vegetables.
❖ Lycopene and quercetin. Good sources include tomatoes, pink grapefruit, watermelon, leafy green vegetables, red apples, onions, cranberries, and blueberries.
❖ Resveratrol, found in red wine, although the high doses that have been researched might require too much alcohol (like 180 bottles a day), so also consider a high-dose purified product as a supplement.

- A variety of flavonoids found in dark chocolate made with at least 70 percent pure cocoa (just don't overdo it, because chocolate is high in calories).
- Turmeric and curcumin, spices found in Indian and curried foods. Mustard also contains turmeric and can reduce Apo E4 levels.

YOU Tip: Go with the Flow. Your blood feeds your brain nutrients. No nutrients, no brain. No brain, no Super Bowl party this year. So one of your big goals should be to keep your arteries clear and flowing (details in the next chapter). Reducing high blood pressure to normal improves cognitive function and slows Alzheimer's progression substantially. If you have a diastolic blood pressure of over 90 (that's the bottom number), then you have a five times greater risk of getting dementia two decades down the line than if it's below 90. If you have elevated blood pressure, it may be because your arteries are constricted, often as a result of cholesterol plaques, and limit the amount of blood and nutrients that reach a particular area. In the case of the brain, not having sufficient blood supplied to that watershed area between the two main arteries is what elevates the risk of stroke. We'll offer tips for reducing blood pressure and cholesterol plaques in the next chapter.

YOU Tip: Consider Your Hormonal Options. Early research on menopausal women showed that boosting estrogen levels delays Alzheimer's. Newer research is less clear, so we don't believe that's reason enough to start taking estrogen. But if you're considering taking it for other reasons, it could be one additional positive factor. See our complete thoughts on estrogen on page 203.

YOU Tip: Get into the Game. It's no surprise that exercise is good for your heart as well as for your modeling career, but it's also an elixir for your mind. It seems that more intense exercise preserves neurocognitive function by decreasing the expression of the Apo-E4 gene to help clear the beta-amyloid plaque that gunks up your power lines. Exercise has also been correlated with increased telomere length. Our suggestion for a brain-boosting workout: Once or twice a week, choose an exercise that requires not only your body to work but also your mind, such as Bikram yoga or a game of singles tennis. The sports or exercises that engage you in the moment can really help clear your mind at the same time. You don't need to overdo it. Just thirty minutes of walking a day plus our YOU2 Workout a couple times a week will help you burn the 2,000 to 3,500 calories a week—the amount shown to increase telomere length.

YOU Tip: Detox Your Life. If you know the original story of the mad hatters, you're familiar with how they got their name. Workers in hat factories were exposed to a lot of mercury when molding felt for the hats, and they eventually turned crazier than an unneutered pit bull. This historical nugget illuminates how toxins in our environment can have a profound influence on our mind and memory. If you're experiencing memory problems that are causing you alarm, eliminate some key chemicals from your lifestyle first, before adding anything new. That includes such things as artificial foods (like sweeteners), MSG, and even shampoo (better to make sure the inside of your head is clean, isn't it?). Finally, despite their lifesaving benefits, statin drugs can uncommonly cause reversible memory loss, a discussion that you should pursue with your doctor if you are more concerned about your memory than your heart. Surprising tidbit: Even over-the-counter cold and allergy medications can contribute to memory problems; in fact, injecting lab animals with the active ingredient in Benadryl (diphenhydramine) is a research model for memory loss that immediately simulates Alzheimer's.

YOU Tip: Learn to Tell a Joke. There's lots of evidence that a good laugh can help improve your immune system, and humor can also have a valuable effect on your memory. Humor requires what the laugh doctors call conceptual blending—that is, the ability to relate the expected to the unexpected; we laugh when something surprising happens. Having a sense of humor is a sign of intelligence. Telling a joke, like being a teacher, is another way to challenge your brain. You have to be able to play mental hopscotch from one word to another to make sure that the story, joke, riddle, or pun combines a set of expected circumstances and unexpected ones (in other words, what happens once the guy walks into the bar?). And ultimately, if you tell it right, you have to have a fair amount of social intelligence as well—the ability to maximize the tension and mystery of the joke until the very last second.

YOU Tip: Map Your Mind. One way to strengthen your mind is by flexing parts that you don't use often—like perhaps those associated with imagination. So try this trick from our friend psychologist Tony Buzan the next time you're feeling overwhelmed by a task (see Figure 1.4). Map out your to-do list rather than actually listing it. That is, draw a picture of your issue in the middle of a piece of paper, then branch out from that centerpiece with smaller subsections and keywords related to that issue. For example, if you want to lose 25 pounds, draw a picture of yourself on a scale in the middle. Instead of making a list of ways to do it, draw lines from the center to things like food, exercise, pitfalls, supports, and other broad categories that will help you. Then branch out from there with subcategories (food may include such branches as "Eat breakfast," "Eat five small meals a day," and "No more doughnuts"). Why is this helpful? For one thing, starting in the center gives your brain freedom to spread out in different directions; for another, a picture flexes your imagination muscles and also keeps you focused and able to concentrate better. And the branches work because your brain works by association. Connect the branches, and you will understand, remember, and act on the problem much more easily.

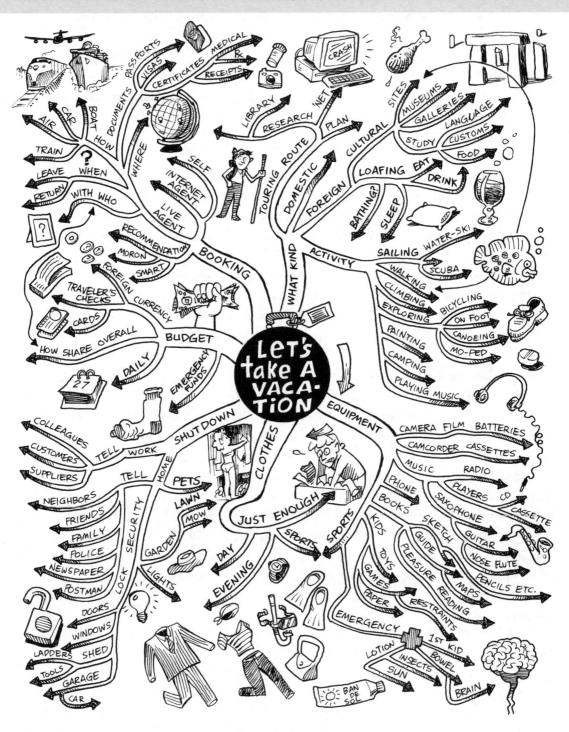

YOU Test: Quick Thinker

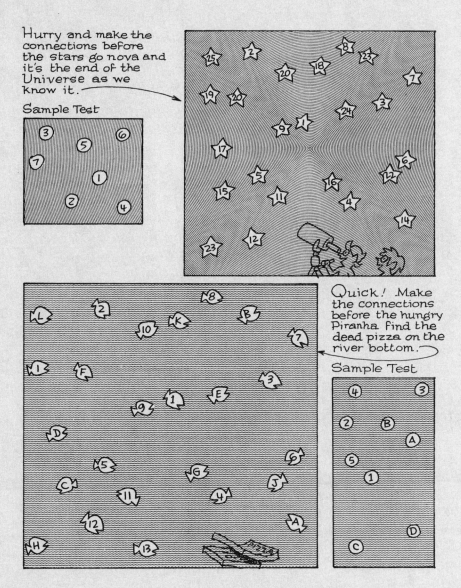

Figure 1.5 **Score!** Connect the dots in the sample test without lifting your pencil and using straight lines (just go through numbers that are in the way). In the first test, connect all the numbers in order. In the second, move from 1 to A, A to 2, 2 to B, and so on. Race the clock to determine your physiological brain age. Have someone else time you, and add up your times on both tests to determine how your mental acuity ranks against others your age.

Age Range	Time in Seconds
20–29	122
30–39	113
40–49	145
50–59	148
60–72	228

Oxidation & Inefficient Mitochondria

Keep the Energy Factories of Your Body Running Smoothly

When you live the kind of life so many of us do—having a job and a family, and running around like a preschooler with a Kool-Aid high—someone's bound to ask you where you get all that energy. Instead of answering with a laugh, a thank-you, a shrug, or "More Snickers than I should," do your part to increase the biological IQ of our society.

Tell them that your body gets its energy from the same place theirs does: from mitochondria.

We know you remember (perhaps vaguely) mitochondria from tenth-grade biology, but we don't expect that you remember all that much about what mitochrondria do and why they're important.

Think back before iTunes, even before eight-tracks, and well before our ancestors made music by banging rocks. That's the time when mitochondria used to be independent single-celled organisms—essentially parasites that lived symbiotically with their host. But at some point in our evolution, they were swallowed by our regular cells, thus becoming a part of every cell rather than existing on their own.

Mitochondria (you have hundreds of those per cell) convert nutrients from the food you eat into energy that your body uses in order to perform all of the functions it needs to. They are the fundamental drivers of metabolism. They make sure that what you eat fits into how you perform. Plus, their function (and dysfunction) serves as the backbone for one of the major theories of aging.

The problem is, when mitochondria turn your food into energy, they produce oxygen free radicals—molecules that cause dangerous inflammation in the mitochondria themselves as well as in the rest of the cell when they spill over. Think of them as the power plants of our bodily city. Just like an old factory (see Figure B.1), aging mitochondria spill more industrial waste into the environment. The damage this inflammation causes to your cells and to the mitochondria within your cells is responsible for many aging-related problems. This oxidation, for example, is what causes a "rusting" of your arteries, which is some of what ages your cardiovascular system. So let's take a closer look at how mitochondria work.

Mighty Mito: The Body's Power Plant

If you look at mitochondria from an aerial view (don't try this at home), you'd see something a bit like a labyrinth or maze. Those jagged little edges you see in Figure B.2 are called cristae. You have hundreds of mitochondrion per cell and dozens of strands of mitochondrial DNA per mitochondrion. That means that every cell contains thousands of strands of mitochondrial DNA.

Now think about your bodily city and picture these mitochondria as your body's nuclear power plants. They give off a lot of energy but also have the potential to cause a lot of damage. As you'll see many times throughout the book, most things that are powerful enough to help you are also powerful enough to hurt you.

If something bombs your power plant, it's not just the physical plant that suffers damage; a whole lot of collateral damage takes place as well. In the case of

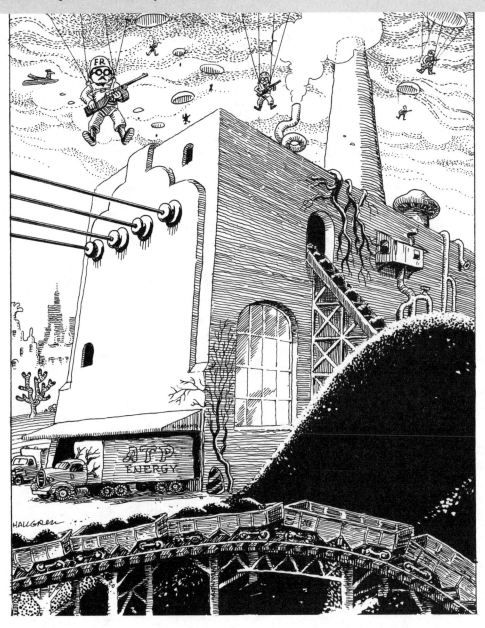

Factory Jobs Mitochondria are our energy factories and continually pump barrels of ATP into the cells as it travels through the circulatory system. They look like a maze with jagged edges called cristae. Mitochondria are especially hardy to withstand the dangers of being near free radicals that can be generated with high-powered energy production.

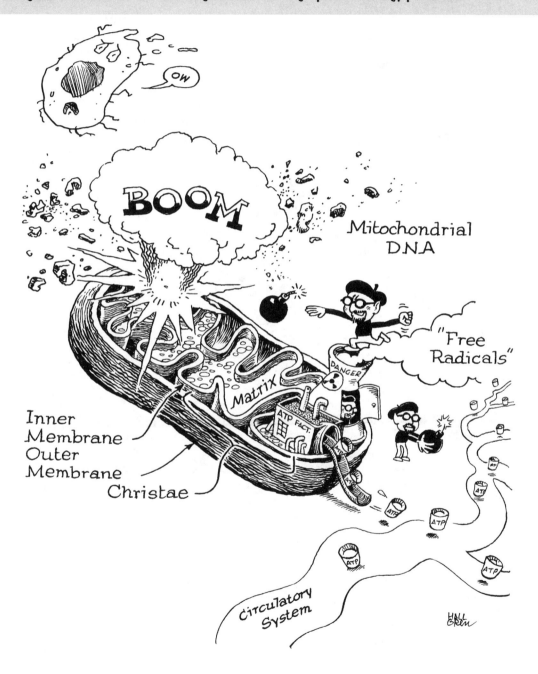

Figure B.3 Radical Demonstration Oxygen free radicals are created when a pair of electrons is separated while spinning around the nucleus of a cell. The odd man out becomes disruptive as it seeks another partner.

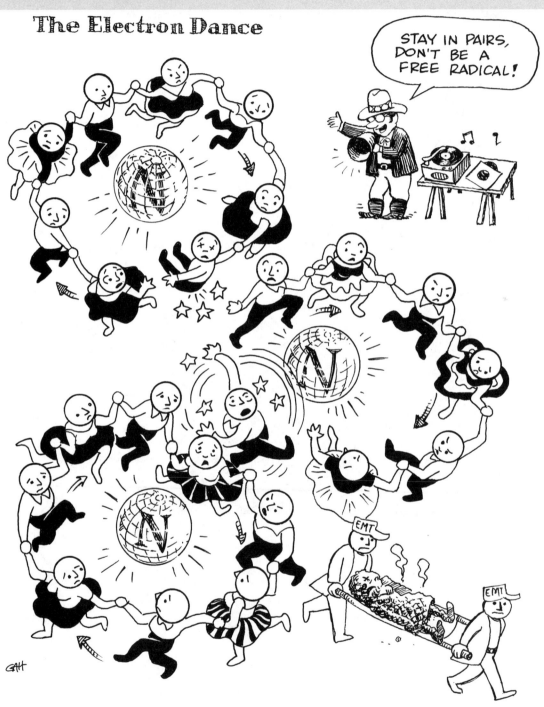

The Electron Dance

the power plant, it's radiation that seeps into surrounding neighborhoods and towns. In the case of mitochondria, it's those inflammation-causing oxygen free radicals, which also decrease the ability of your mitochondrial DNA to convert energy. Both forms of damage spin into a cycle of destruction to your body's cells: Inefficiencies in mitochondrial function cause increased production of free radicals. Well, guess what? More free radicals cause more damage to the mitochondrial DNA, which makes them more inefficient, and so on.

Maybe you're thinking, So what? So what if my mitochondrial DNA is a little slow on the ol' energy conversion process? What's that mean for me?

Well, for a business, inefficiency may mean losing money. For a student, inefficiency may mean pulling all-nighters. For a quarterback, inefficiency may mean life as a third-string clipboard holder. But for mitochondria, inefficiency means you're that much closer to booking a bed at the extended-care facility.

Think about it. If your body can't produce energy efficiently, it means that mitochondria are not getting the most energy out of the oxygen and sugar that their furnaces are fed. So even if you have good nutrition in what you eat, lower levels of your body's energy currency, called ATP (adenosine triphosphate), are made.

We know that mitochondrial damage in the heart happens when your body no longer consumes oxygen and glucose efficiently. We also see mitochondrial damage in brain-related disease and in diabetes, where it influences the pancreas's ability to make insulin. In fact, mitochondrial damage may serve as a contributing factor to certain types of cancer, because the more oxidative damage that takes place, the more DNA is damaged, and that damaged DNA, when it's replicated over and over again, can evolve into a cancer.

Damage Control

Like a politician who gets bad press, your body can also perform damage control. Over time, those furnaces (the cristae) in your mitochondria swell and become lazy fat cats—they don't do a whole lot of work. At the same time, young, small, but efficient mitochondria that are continually born become the energy work-horses of your body.

In a city model, the big-cristae mitochondria would be the high-salaried bu-reaucrats who spend all day preventing city government from being reinvigorated by young whippersnappers who could replace them, cut through red tape, and do a lot of work for a lower price. In your body, the turf battle happens because the large ones (the bad ones) have the power to survive at the expense of the little ones (the good ones).

It turns out that you can tolerate a lot of damage to your mitochondria because mitochondrial DNA is resilient. This special Marine Corps brand of DNA is used to dealing with the damage that happens when you bombard them with oxidative substances. In a way, they are a little like parents. The mitochondria can tolerate quite a bit, but eventually they blow a gasket. And that's when the real damage begins.

This all happens as a natural part of the aging process. In fact, people older than sixty have a 40 percent lower mitochondrial efficiency than people younger than forty. But remember, what's natural is not necessarily inevitable. As you'll see in our next chapter on the muscle that uses the most energy, that means this: While these seemingly uncontrollable cellular battles may be taking place deep in-side your body, you still have the power of an anatomical puppeteer—to control the ways that your cells function. But when the system starts to spew toxic waste and you can't keep up with the oxidation in your cells, your arteries begin to rust, which puts heat on quite a few organs, including the heart.

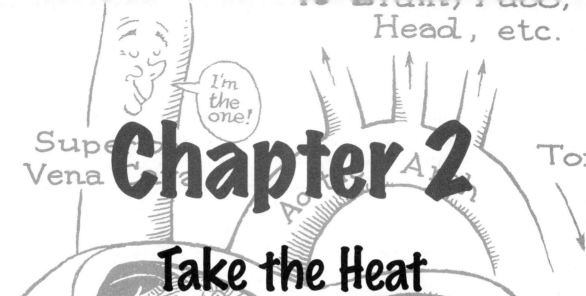

Chapter 2

Take the Heat off Your Heart

YOU Test: Beat Up

During your next intense cardiovascular workout (and with your doctor's consent), bring your heart rate to 80 percent or more of your maximum heart rate (that's 220 minus your age). After you stop, how long does it take for your heart rate to drop to 66 beats less than your 80 percent max?

A. Less than 2 minutes
B. Less than 4 minutes
C. Oxygen, STAT!

Results: If you recover quickly enough to have your heart rate drop 66 beats in less than 2 minutes, you're in primo cardiovascular shape, and your RealAge is at least 8 years younger than your calendar age. Anything longer means you have some work to do.

We all know the things that make our hearts skip a beat (first loves and bases loaded in the bottom of the ninth). We all know the things that make our hearts pound faster than a collegiate drum line (horror flicks and being six minutes away from a train that pulls out in five). And we all like to think that we know the kinds of things that will make our hearts stop forever: cigarettes, sausage links, and cyanide.

But when we think about aging-related heart disease, we have to go beyond the basic assumptions that either we're born with bad genes that destine us for cardiac troubles, or we create our own by gunking up our arteries with forty-five years of holiday cheese balls.

The damage that we do to our hearts—whether through genetics, life-style choices, or both—is caused not solely by genes or cheese balls, but also by a double-whammy Major Ager of mitochondria-induced oxidation and inflammation that happens within your arteries.

Inflame Shame: Your Heart and Arteries

You may have about as much tolerance for blood as you do for drivers who don't use turn signals, but to understand how to protect your heart, you have to get a wee bit sanguine. If you were to sneak a peek inside a chest (c'mon, a little closer now), here's what you'd see: a twisting muscle that looks like the coiled back of a boa constrictor. That's your heart. Not only does its twisting motion keep you alive, but it's also the mechanism through which your body gets the nutrients it needs.

Here's how the process works: The heart muscle is stimulated by pacemaker cells to eject blood through the aortic valve. It doesn't push out blood like a balloon emptying air, but like a towel being wrung out of water. That blood pulsates into the aorta—the body's largest artery—which delivers oxygen-rich blood to the rest of the body, as well as to the coronary arteries surrounding the heart.

Much of heart disease happens in your arteries—the tunnels that feed both nutrients and toxins to all your organs—rather than in your heart itself. Made of three layers (a cellophane-like exterior shell, a muscular middle, and a thin, smooth inside layer that allows blood to slide through), your arteries serve as the site of the inflammatory process that's responsible for many kinds of heart disease (see Figure 2.1).

How? Well, it all starts with cholesterol, which as you know comes in healthy (HDL, or high-density lipoproteins) and lousy (LDL, or low-density lipoproteins) forms. The smooth inside layer of your arteries is pummeled by a variety of things: high blood pressure, cigarettes, excess sugar. When that happens, your body sends lousy LDL cholesterol (remember it by its first initial) to those damaged areas in an attempt to heal the wounds. Your immune cells in the damaged area swallow up the LDL cholesterol and burrow into the inner layer of your arteries.

Your body then reacts to the wounds and the cholesterol with a low-grade inflammation. Makes sense: Inflammation is how your immune system deals with many problems, like splinters, unwanted bacteria, insect venom, or other foreign invaders. Meanwhile, as part of your homeland security team, your healthy HDL cholesterol works to clear that LDL cholesterol out of the area. Think of your LDL as a bus carrying loads of hooligans and dropping them off in your arteries to do damage to them, while your HDL serves as a high-speed paddy wagon that zips through your arteries to get the rogue elements off the streets. HDL is mostly made in intestines and looks like a plastic baggie that wraps cholesterol so that it can be more easily excreted.

Like TVs, toy trucks, and lingerie, cholesterol comes in different sizes. But the

Your Own Meth Lab

A process in your body called methylation may sound like it's illegal in forty-nine states, but it's one that your body depends on. The process—changing a molecule by adding a methyl group—helps detox your body, repair DNA, and form new cells. As you age, the reduced ability to methylate is associated with heart disease as well as Alzheimer's and diabetes. What can you do? Make sure you're getting cofactors for methyl transfer like those found in fish and whole grains. Also, taking B_{12} and folic acid (see chart on page 357 for doses) seems to help methylation by reducing levels of homocysteine.

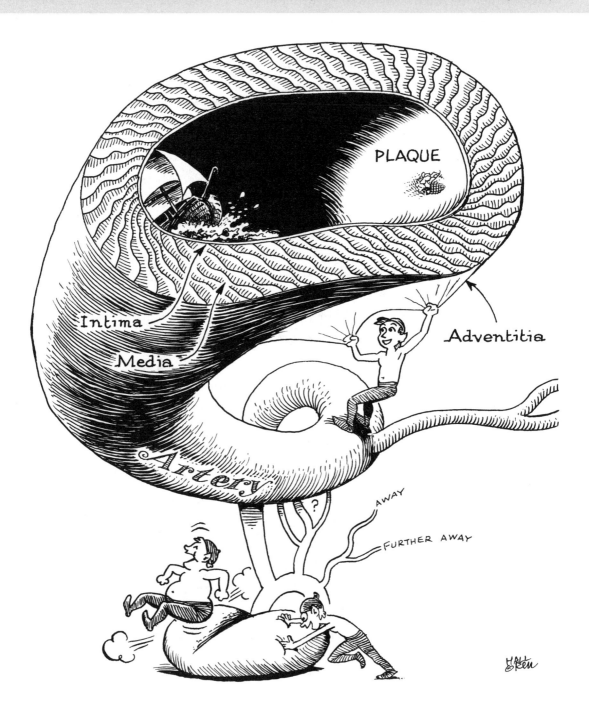

most dangerous kind is the smaller kind. The smaller the particle, the more likely it is to nestle itself into the arterial wall, cause damage, and trigger the inflammatory process (see Figure 2.2). To clear the arteries, we need to increase the function as well as the size of the healthy HDL cholesterol. Help can come in the form of niacin, omega-3 fatty acids, and vitamin B_5, as well as some new-generation fibrate and statin drugs.

Meanwhile, the low-grade inflammation occurring in response to LDL cholesterol (which, combined with inefficient mitochondria, causes the Major Ager of oxidation) sounds the alarm that summons your body's reinforcement immune cells called macrophages. These macrophages eat the LDL cholesterol, becoming engorged with fat and blowing up like marshmallows, then attach to the arterial walls. Pathologists call them foam cells, as they clog the artery walls. An arterial plaque is born.

As the plaque grows, it reduces the nutrient-rich blood supply through the arteries. And when the marshmallow cracks—that is, when the plaque runs out of blood supply—there's a big-time supersonic explosion as a clot fills up the plaque like a bloated tick. The sudden clot formation, like a scab on any cut, closes off the artery. Think of a six-lane bridge going into a city: If one of the lanes is shut down, traffic can still get through, albeit a little slower. But if an explosion on the bridge takes out all the lanes, no traffic can get through. That's why arterial plaques are so dangerous. No test can tell whether you have just one lane closed or a potential tanker that's waiting to explode.

When talking about heart disease, you often hear the word *calcification*. That has little to do with dietary cal-

> ## FACTOID
>
> Supplements that seem to reduce inflammation include: nettle leaf extract (900 milligrams), bromelain (2,000 milligrams), ginger (900 milligrams), and curcumin (1,200 milligrams). There's not a lot of human data on this point, but there is enough science to suggest that they can be helpful.

> ## FACTOID
>
> Men with short telomeres may have a higher risk of developing coronary heart disease. While we know that stress can shorten telomeres, we don't know if the shorter strips of DNA are a marker for a problem or play a role in disease development. In any case, it does seem that men with shorter telomeres respond very well to statin drugs. So if you get your telomeres measured and they are shorter than you'd like, consider a statin.

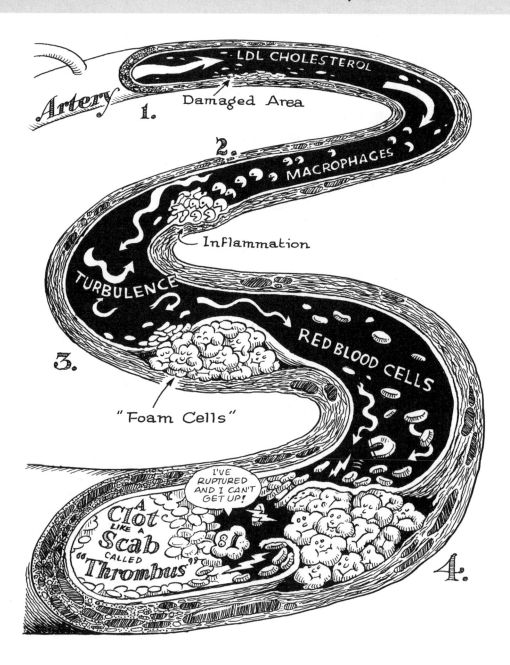

Figure 2.2 Shutoff Arteries respond to cholesterol with an inflammatory reaction, so your body calls in immune cells called macrophages. They eat the cholesterol that forms the plaque and bloat up like marshmallows. The resulting foam cells hinder the blood supply to the plaque and increase inflammation, so it cracks—and results in an arterial explosion.

A Valve Check

While most cardio talk is about clots and clogs that tie up traffic in your heart and arteries, there are also toll booths involved—the valves that accept blood coming into and leaving your heart. About 30 percent of people have significant valve disease by the age of eighty-five, just from the wear and tear of shuttling blood into and out of their hearts for all those years. When valves experience a little bit of turbulence over time, they get scarred with calcium and can get stuck like a door with a rusted hinge, disrupting blood flow. You can hear the difference between a good valve and a malfunctioning one through a stethoscope: Instead of a *rub-dub* beat, it's more of a *rub-woooosh* sound as blood passes through the diseased valve. (Diagnosis, though, comes after an echocardiogram.) Statins delay the process, and surgery can repair or replace valves. Even better, researchers are developing ways to make those repairs without opening your chest, which cuts back on suture costs, not to mention the ICU stay.

cium and the amount of double-dip chocolate cones you've snorted down in your life. Calcification in arteries is the body's attempt to heal those inflammatory plaques in your body. The calcium stabilizes the plaque like cement reinforcement of a plaster wall. About 90 percent of men with atherosclerosis have calcified arteries, as opposed to women, who calcify their plaques only 30 percent of the time. This means that women respond to heart disease reversal programs even better than men, since their arteries are not lined in a cast of calcium, but it also might mean that their plaques are more precarious and prone to rupture and sudden clot formation. The big point in all of this: You can't become healthy by testing yourself; you have to live healthfully to prevent the sudden explosions that cause heart attacks and strokes.

Inflammation plays a role in lots of kinds of heart disease. For example, in atrial fibrillation (an abnormal heart rhythm), the heart's small upper chambers, which are supposed to receive blood and gently propel it downstream, start looking like bags of worms (see Figure 2.3). Because blood isn't pushed completely out of the atria, it may pool and clot. Atrial fibrillation is frequently caused by inflammation of the heart wall, and the damage is done by those oxygen free radicals produced by inefficient mitochondria. Arrhythmias can also be caused by a number of other things, including pressure on the walls of the atria or hormonal

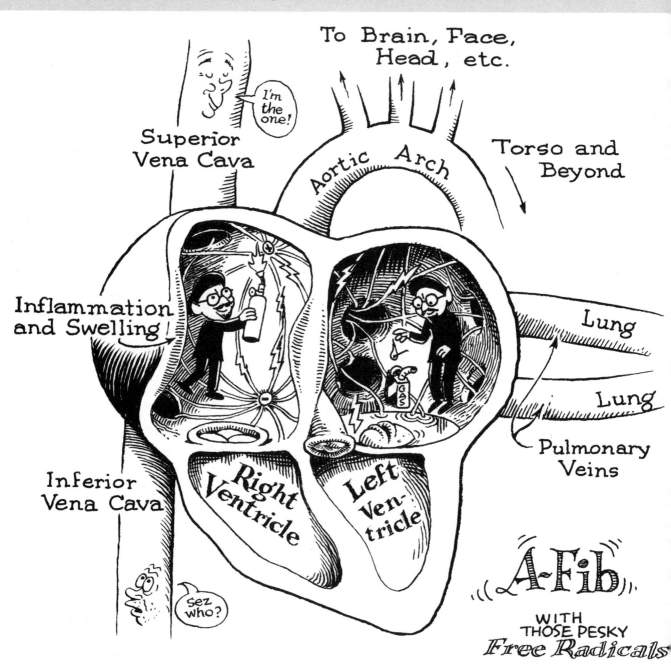

Figure 2.3 Bad Beat Irritation caused by inflammatory cells in the right and left atrial chambers of the heart makes the wall swell and electrical circuits short-circuit. The abnormal heart rhythms then cause blood to pool, so clots form, which can lead to strokes.

The Chelation Sensation?

You may have read about a development called chelation therapy—basically an arterial Drano. In the process, a solution is injected into your veins, and it is supposed to bind with the calcium that hardens arterial plaque and subsequently clear it through your urine. The theory that chelation therapy works to diminish the calcium in your plaque has never been proven, but there's anecdotal evidence that it can help clear arteries in some people. It's very enticing but still experimental. An even better Drano promises to be a new drug that is a super HDL called alpha-1-Milano. Look for it in the next few years if it passes the scientifically rigorous clinical trials.

abnormalities, and can be linked to general inflammation of the heart. No matter the cause, the delicate cables that conduct electricity throughout your heart become swollen and start short-circuiting. You can actually feel arrhythmias as a fluttering of the heart (unassociated with love pangs, of course). Steer clear of bad trans-fat- and saturated-fat-laden fries, burgers, and textbook-thick pieces of pie.

Your goal to protect your heart is not only to cut down on the things that chip away at and clog up your arteries, but to take action to strengthen your heart muscle and decrease your risk of cardiovascular disease. You have firefighters standing by, in the form of antioxidants, which your body produces to keep the Major Ager of oxidation from wounded mitochondria in check. And medicine can help too. Statins work by decreasing the inflammation in the plaque, which slows the progression of the clogging process and reduces sudden ruptures that can lead to clot formation and sudden closure of arteries.

Ultimately, though, many of our recommendations are aimed at adding to your firefighting unit so it stays fresh and is able to quench the small fires and occasional meltdowns that occur within your arteries.

FACTOID

When you're over sixty-five, HDL is more important than LDL. Although statin drugs can be life saving, the net effect is that some choices may reduce healthy HDL cholesterol too. So you may want to try an alternative, like taking niacin, vitamin B_5, and omega-3 fatty acids, and exercise for lowering your LDL while keeping your HDL high.

YOU TIPS!

It'd be easy for us to sit here and scold you: no more fried chicken, no more smoking, no more popping scoops of M&M's every time you walk by the cupboard. We believe that you're fully aware that candy, fried anything, and cancer sticks aren't exactly cardiac elixirs. So without taking away all your joys, here are the steps that you should do to let your heart perform its main job: moving blood through your body—with no obstructions.

YOU Tip: Feed Your Heart. These days, you don't have to be a dietitian to know that certain foods will create some serious roadblocks on your arterial highways. Saturated fats and trans fats are two of the things that accelerate and magnify the inflammatory process. That chili-drenched hot dog doesn't just add to your lousy LDL cholesterol; it also stimulates your genes to produce more inflammatory proteins to make the tissue irritation a whole lot worse. Thankfully, the following foods are good not only because of the heart-healthy nutrients they deliver but because they have strong anti-inflammatory effects.

❖ *Fruits and vegetables.* Many fruits and vegetables—specifically red grapes, cranberries, tomatoes, onions, and tomato juice—contain powerful antioxidants called flavonoids and carotenoids. Found in colorful foods, flavonoids and carotenoids are vitamin-like nonessential substances that seem to decrease inflammation by handcuffing those damaging oxygen free radicals and stimulating your body to take them out of your system through urine.

❖ *Garlic.* While it is still being debated, we believe a clove a day can help thin your blood and lower your blood pressure. (Plus, it helps keep people away, to lower your stress level.) If you don't like the taste or the fact that coworkers shrink away when they pass you in the hall, you can also take garlic in pill form (called allicin) at 400 milligrams a day (though the odor may still emerge through your sweat glands).

❖ *Olive oil.* The "extra virgin" kind contains lots of healthy phytonutrients as well as monounsaturated fats, which help raise your good HDL cholesterol. Aim for 25 percent of your diet to come from healthy fats like those found in olive oil. That will reduce your RealAge by more than six years.

❖ *Omega-3 fatty acids.* These fatty acids (found in fish or the plants fish eat, like certain algae) are the handymen of your arterial system, because they can do a whole lot of fixing up. They reduce triglyceride levels in your blood (high triglycerides are a big cause of plaque buildup), and they help reduce the risk of arrhythmia after a heart attack. In addition, they decrease blood pressure and also make platelets less sticky, to reduce clotting. Aim for three portions of fish per week. Best choices: wild, line-caught salmon; mahi-mahi; catfish; flounder; tilapia; and whitefish.

❖ *Alcohol.* If you don't have a problem with alcohol, having one alcoholic drink a night (4 ounces of wine, 12 ounces of beer, or 1.5 ounces of spirits) for women—up to two for men—seems to have a beneficial effect on your heart by raising levels of that healthy HDL cholesterol. It also helps you to wind down, so your blood pressure can do the same. Our preference: red wine, because it also contains antioxidants.

❖ *Foods with magnesium.* Foods like 100 percent whole-grain breads and cereals, soybeans, lima beans, avocado, beets, and raisins help lower blood pressure and reduce arrhythmias by dilating (expanding) the arteries. Get 400 milligrams a day. A serving of lima beans contains about 100 milligrams, ½ cup of spinach contains 80 milligrams, twelve cashews contain 50 milligrams, thirty peanuts contain 50 milligrams.

❖ *Foods with soy protein.* Getting 25 grams a day of soy protein in foods like tofu and other soybean products decreases your bad LDL cholesterol and triglyceride levels.

❖ *Stanols and sterols.* Good plant cholesterol in foods like the spread Benecol or Take Control helps your arterial health by displacing the lousy cholesterol in your arteries.

❖ *Dark chocolate.* Recent studies show that eating dark chocolate may lower blood pressure as effectively as the most common antihypertensive medications and may increase HDL cholesterol and lower LDL cholesterol. Interesting fact: The Kuna Indians, who live on islands near Panama, have little age-related hypertension. They drink more than five cups of flavonoid-rich cocoa a day.

YOU Tip: Get Your Clothes Wet. We may not like to see sweat on treadmills or public speakers, but we want to see it on you. While we recommend different kinds of physical activity in different circumstances (including resistance exercise, walking, and stretching), the way to improve heart function is to sweat more than a kid in the principal's office. Why? Cardiovascular activity lowers both the top systolic (the pressure being exerted when your heart contracts) and the bottom diastolic (the pressure in the arteries when the heart is at rest) numbers of your blood pressure. Cardiovascular exercise may also be helpful because it makes your blood vessels more elastic by forcing them to dilate. In addition to thirty minutes of daily walking, aim for a minimum of sixty minutes a week of cardiovascular or sweating activity—ideally in three twenty-minute sessions—in which you raise your heart rate to 80 percent or more of its age-adjusted maximum (220 minus your age) for an extended period of time.

We recommend low-impact activities like swimming, cycling, or using an elliptical trainer to get your heart rate up without compromising the quality of your joints in the process (and to change activities, so you don't get repetitive use injuries from doing the same activity over and over). We also recommend interval training—that is, alternating periods of maximum effort with periods of recovery—for the maximum benefit of your heart. (Check with your doc beforehand; she may want to try it in the controlled setting of a stress test first.) Even doing one minute at the end of every ten with maximum effort can be beneficial.

One way to do it: After warming up, go for maximum effort for a minute, and then slow down to 60 percent of maximum (recover) for two minutes. Then go to 80 percent of maximum for seven minutes.

Then cool down. As you progress, you can do intervals, alternating between intense effort and effort that allows you to recover—one minute fast, two minutes slow, and so on.

YOU Tip: Kick Yourself in the Aspirin. Of all the things that you shovel down your throat, we think aspirin should be one. As a huge anti-inflammatory agent, aspirin works as the chief of the fire company called in to put out the inflammation response. Speak with your doc about making it part of your regular routine, just like brushing your teeth or walking the dog. We recommend half a regular aspirin or two baby aspirins (162 milligrams total) every day if you're a man over thirty-five or a woman over forty. Why? Many studies of primary prevention have shown that two baby aspirins decrease the risk of heart attack by 36 percent. It's thought to work by making platelets less sticky to avoid clotting, and by decreasing arterial inflammation. You can reduce potential gastric discomfort by drinking a half glass of warm water before and after taking aspirin; the pills dissolve faster in warm water and are less likely to cause stomach irritation and ulcerations and bleeding. One note of caution: If you begin bleeding more during flossing or from a shaving cut, or if you notice that you're more susceptible to bruising, the aspirin is the likely culprit, and you may have to cut back.

YOU Tip: Supplement Your Diet. These vitamins and supplements have the most potent effects on strengthening your heart:

Pill	Do We Recommend It?	The Fine Print
Folic acid, vitamin B_6, vitamin B_{12}	Yes	Folic acid, vitamin B_6, and vitamin B_{12} work by reducing levels of homocysteine, a body chemical that's related to increased risk of heart disease. You should get 800 micrograms of folate a day. Most folks get half of that in their diet, so add an additional 400-microgram supplement. Get 50 milligrams of vitamin B_6 and 800 micrograms of B_{12}.
Coenzyme Q10	Yes	Mitochondria convert glucose into electric energy, and one of the molecules carrying electrons in this process is coenzyme Q10. Taking it as a supplement seems to protect against heart failure and other inflammatory processes by improving the efficiency of the mitochondria. The usual dose is 200 milligrams a day (100 in the morning and 100 in the

Coenzyme Q10 (*cont.*)	Yes	afternoon). It's especially helpful for people who take statin drugs, because statins decrease levels of CQ10, which may be why statins can be associated with muscle cramps and pain—your arteries are literally being starved of energy and are crying for help.
Niacin (vitamin B₃)	Sometimes	A dose of 500 milligrams can lower LDL cholesterol and lower triglycerides, and help raise HDL. Take it with aspirin when going to bed to help decrease the risk of hot flashes, a common side effect. You can take a higher dose but need to talk to your doc because higher doses often need to be prescribed (Niaspan). Niacin is rarely associated with liver problems.
Vitamin D	Yes	Recent research suggests that D isn't just good for your bones and immune system, but is good for your heart. Try 800 IU daily if under the age of sixty, 1,000 IU if age sixty or over.
Pantothenic acid (vitamin B₅)	Yes	It's a water-soluble vitamin that's essential for metabolism and for forming HDL cholesterol. We recommend 150 milligrams twice a day.
Red yeast rice	Not necessary	It's been touted as a supplement that can help lower cholesterol and triglyceride levels, as well as increase healthy HDL cholesterol. The rumors are true because the active ingredient is identical to a commonly used pharmaceutical statin drug. But because herbs are harvested without tight controls, you don't know exactly what you're getting inside the pill. For the same cost, you're better off using another supplement such as niacin or pantothenic acid.
D-ribose	Yes	It's been shown to improve blood pressure and exercise tolerance in patients with congestive heart failure. It seems to work by getting ATP energy to heart and skeletal muscles. The dose is 5 grams once to three times daily.

YOU Tip: Know the Ratio. We could spend an entire book talking about the fat around our waists (oh, wait, we already did that). But we also need to spend some time talking about the fat in our diet. Most of us know that dietary fats come in two general forms: Either they're good for us, or they're more destructive than tank treads on armadillos. And most of us know that we should avoid the bad kinds the way we avoid telemarketers.

But if we dive a bit deeper into the story of good fats, we can also realize that it's more than just a get-good/avoid-bad argument. Research suggests that omega-6 fatty acids (found in cereals, some nuts, whole grains, and vegetable oils) can be harmful to us if we don't have the proper ratio of omega-3 (found in oily fish, walnuts, certain algae, and flax) to counterbalance those fats and provide a protective effect against heart disease. The ideal ratio: Omega-3s, especially DHA, should be one-quarter of omega-6s.

YOU Tip: Get Between the Cracks. Despite the pleading from dentists, doctors, and people who notice that ill-placed broccoli floret, 85 percent of men and 65 percent of women in the United States still don't floss regularly. Dentists consider it even more crucial for preventing tooth decay and periodontal disease than brushing. But it's also crucial because flossing—which gets rid of inflammation-causing bacteria—helps prevent heart disease. But you've got to know how to do it.

The right way: The floss should barely pass between each tooth and should gently touch the gums.

The wrong way: You can't get into certain openings, so you hack away, which causes so much gum bleeding that your bathroom looks like a scene from *Psycho*.

Now, if you don't floss, remember to save up enough money to buy the dentures you're going to eventually need, and to pay the deductible on the cardiac bypass operation you'll eventually face.

Stem Cell Slowdown

What You Can Learn—and Use—
from Stem Cells to Keep Your Body Strong

Say the words *stem cell* and you've triggered almost as much controversy as any other two words in the English language (besides maybe *Barry* and *Bonds*). While some may argue that you can't strip away the moral issues from the science of stem cell research for the study of aging, the fact is, that's exactly what we're going to do. Your body naturally already uses its own stem cells to make you stronger, healthier, and more resistant to the conditions that have the potential to slug away at you day after day and year after year (see Figure C.1). Your stem cells are an incredibly powerful tool—independent of what you believe we should be doing in the laboratories. And part of the reason why is that stem cells play a key role in how we recover from stress. The problem is, we lose stem cells as we age, whether by using them to repair damaged organs or because they're destroyed by such toxins as chemotherapy or radiation or oxygen free radicals—leaving us vulnerable to stress-related conditions.

Stem cells come in two varieties:

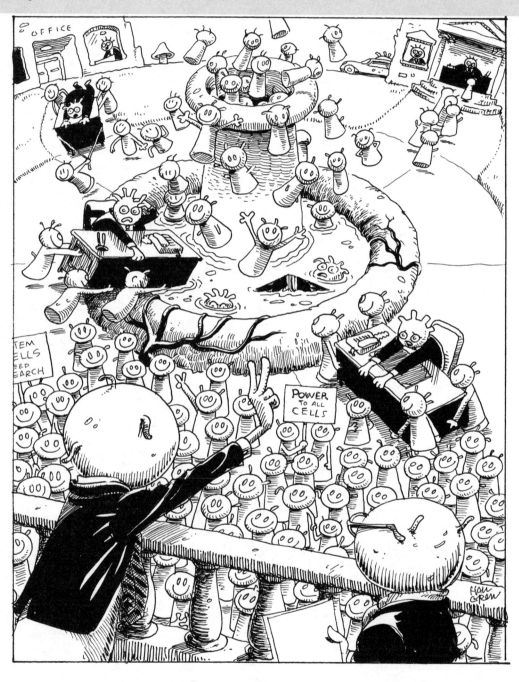

Blastocysts (often mistakenly called embryonic, a charged word that has created a political and moral brouhaha): When a fertilized egg turns four days old, a cluster of specialized stem cells walls itself off to create an inner cell mass. These cells have the amazing ability to reproduce indefinitely, and, *if they become embryos,* they have the ability to mature, grow, and differentiate themselves into every tissue that forms every piece of your bodily puzzle. But they aren't embryos yet; they cannot go on unless they implant. At this stage, they are blastocysts, or *pre*-embryonic. These immortal blastocystic stem cells retain their natural and quite spectacular ability to differentiate into any and every organ. In other words, they have the luxury of deciding what to become when they grow up. Do they mature into heart cells, liver cells, or brain cells? Because of their plasticity, these cells have the greatest potential to cure diseases, especially those associated with aging, such as Parkinson's.

Progenitor cells (also called adult stem cells): Now, some of those blastocystic cells, like kids living at home when they're thirty, stay right where they are and don't mature into other tissues and organs. Instead, they hang back and set up shop in the bone marrow. These adult stem cells retain the ability to grow into other kinds of cells. Why is this so exciting from a medical and scientific perspective? If your own stem cells—the cells you currently have—can be used to regenerate new tissue to replace broken-down or diseased tissue and fix your own organs, then you have the opportunity to punch frailty right in the face.

One of the goals of stem cell research is to harvest some of these universal cells, grow them in laboratories, and then use them to undo the damage done by such things as heart attacks, strokes, diabetes, Alzheimer's, and many other diseases associated with aging. How do we know that this process has potential? Well, just look at the work that's been done on the heart. Cardiology was one of the specialties most resistant to the potential power of stem cells, and the damaged heart was considered representative of the key organs that could not regenerate themselves. In research involving heart transplant, scientists studied groups of men who were transplanted with a female heart (in heart transplantation, the

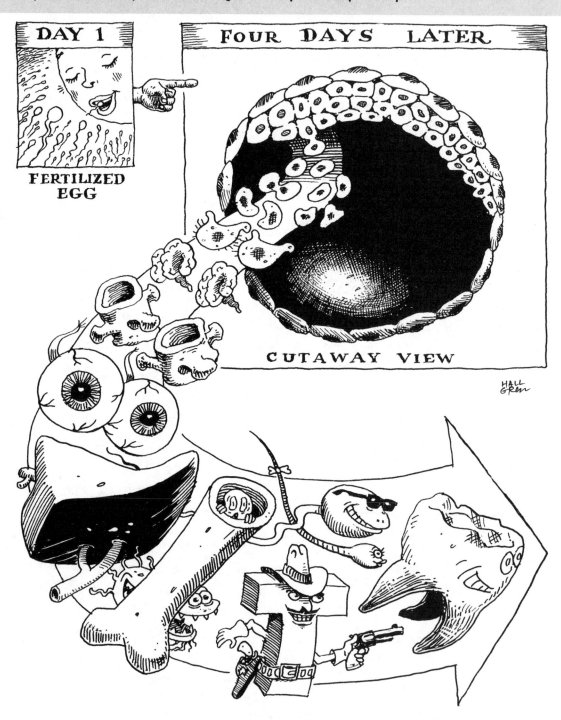

sex of the heart doesn't matter, but, rather, the size). In theory, the cells of a female heart, when transplanted into a man, should have only their original double-X chromosomes, with no male Y chromosomes in them at all. But when researchers examined the hearts only a few months after transplantation, they actually found Y chromosomes in the heart—meaning that the male stem cells were migrating from the bone marrow to the heart to make periodic repairs. Similar reinvigoration of almost all of your organs continually occurs with your own full-time stem cell repairmen.

At all stages of your life, your body responds to damage by recruiting stem cells. When you smoke, stem cells are sent to the lungs to respond to damage. Or when your skin burns from the sun, stem cells go there to make repairs. But—and this is a big *but*—there are two unfortunate consequences of all that repair, and it's another example of how a valuable process has the power to flip you upside your head. First, the more stem cells you send in for repair (say, the more times you burn your skin from lying out by the pool unprotected), the more stem cell reproduction occurs. The more reproduction, the higher the chance that something will go wrong during cell division—meaning that your stem cells have a higher chance of differentiating into a tumor cell. Stem cells know how to replicate quickly, so, *boom,* you've got cancer. (That's why repeated damage to an organ—via smoking, sunburn, alcohol abuse, or inflammation from saturated fat or just being fat—predisposes you to cancer.) Second, if your stem cells are constantly repairing sunburn, then there won't be enough of them available to aid in maintaining other organs.

Add to the equation the reality that as we age, our bone marrow releases fewer stem cells, meaning that we have less ability to repair damage. And that's really why we worry about your stress level. Not because we don't want you angry, panicky, or more tense than a first-time public speaker. It's because stress can disable your telomeres (remember the first Major Ager) and handcuff your stem cells, further weakening your ability to repair damage that happens as you age.

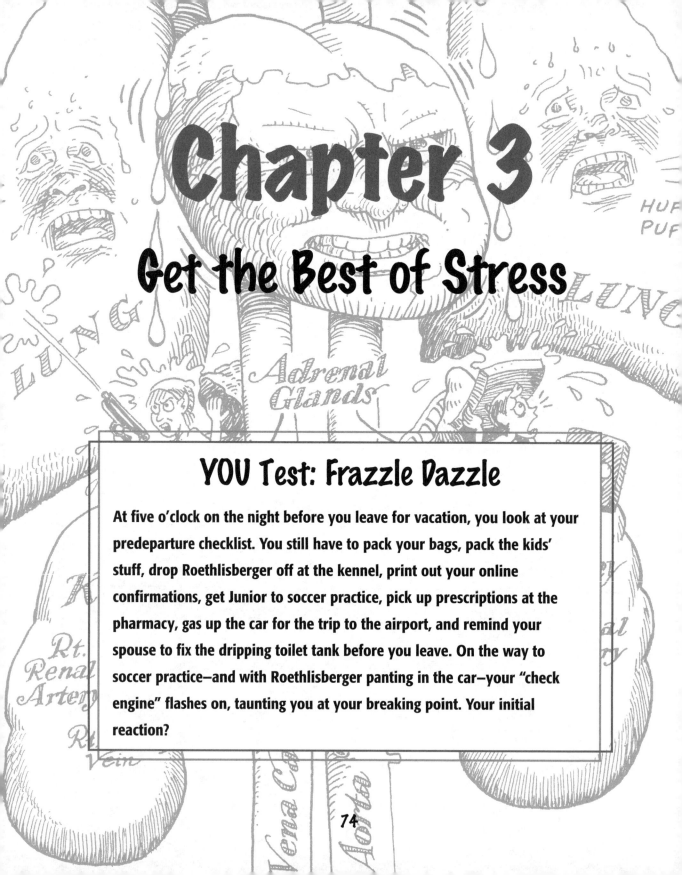

Chapter 3
Get the Best of Stress

YOU Test: Frazzle Dazzle

At five o'clock on the night before you leave for vacation, you look at your predeparture checklist. You still have to pack your bags, pack the kids' stuff, drop Roethlisberger off at the kennel, print out your online confirmations, get Junior to soccer practice, pick up prescriptions at the pharmacy, gas up the car for the trip to the airport, and remind your spouse to fix the dripping toilet tank before you leave. On the way to soccer practice—and with Roethlisberger panting in the car—your "check engine" flashes on, taunting you at your breaking point. Your initial reaction?

74

A. You bawl like an underfed infant.

B. You pummel your intestines with fried cheese.

C. You drive to the nearest shop for an automotive diagnosis, then systematically knock off everything else on your list.

D. You repeat, "Tomorrow, the Bahamas, tomorrow, the Bahamas . . ."

E. You curse car manufacturers, throw your cell phone against the windshield, and lash out at poor Roethlisberger for the time he peed on the carpet four months ago. The filthy bleeping mutt.

Results: If you answered C, it shows that you have a healthy stress response. D is not so bad either. Other responses make you more prone to stress-related aging.

In the old days, we typically knew one kind of stress: life-or-death stress. It may have come in the form of a stalking tiger or a thirty-day famine, but that's the way life was. You hunted, you cooked, you danced by the fire, you told stories, you whittled wood, you procreated. With all due respect to Ms. Hilton and Ms. Richie, *that* was the simple life.

These days, your energy and your attention are pulled in more directions than a piece of gum on the bottom of a shoe. Your boss wants you, your kids want you, you've got telecommunications gadgets that beep and buzz in symphony, you've got deadlines, you've got bills, you've got meetings, you've got twenty-minute traffic backups, you've got six appointments in four hours, and you've got about *wee* much patience to juggle it all. And, oh yeah, how about a little lovin' for your neglected honey-poo?

While Calgon may have achieved advertising immortality with a slogan that capitalized on our overstressed society, most of us are so beaten and bruised and burdened by stress that we've actually gotten used to it. But here's the thing: We like to write off stress as an element of life that we just live with. It is what it is, and we deal. Because it's intangible, it can't be bad for us, right? Nope. Stress is as concrete a condition as any of the others we cover in this book. While we all know that stress is unpleasant, many of us don't realize how unhealthy it is for our bodies—and how it makes us age.

In this chapter, we want you to understand the biology of stress: how it works, why it's important to combat it, and how your stem cells are weakened by it. But we also want you to learn how to manage stress not just in the temporary take-a-bath kind of way but for the long term. We'll teach you how to handle and redirect your stress, not necessarily eliminate it. As you'll learn in a moment, stress isn't all bad. After all, the only time you're free of stress is when you're dead.

Worry Words: What Is Stress?

We tend to think that stress is like a pair of slippers—one size fits all. Either we're stressed or we're not. But the fact is that stress comes in different shapes, sizes, and levels of intensity. Some of us certainly worry more than others, and some of us are much better equipped to cope with exploding dishwashers than others. But the danger is that stress—which often increases as we age—is a major driver of health problems. Stress wears on our immune system. Stress alters the variability of our heart rates, which leads to arrhythmias and even fatal heart problems.

In general, life's stressors can be grouped into three categories, which all have different implications for your life and for your health.

Ongoing Low-level Stress. You work, you have a family, you interact with people who sometimes sneeze without covering their mouths. Life generates a constant hum of stress, no matter who you are or what you do. To expect that you can eliminate all stress is not only unreasonable but unhealthy because, as you'll see in a moment, your ability to respond to stress can make you stronger.

Nagging Unfinished Tasks. One of the most influential forms of stress comes in the form of a chisel that chips and chips and chips and chips and chips and chips away at your brain cells a little bit at a time. Until. You. Can't. Take. It. *Any-freaking-more!* Whether it's a cluttered closet, or cracked bathroom tiles that have been staring at you for years, or weekly paperwork that gnaws at you every Friday, these nagging unfinished tasks (we call them NUTs) are much more destructive than the low levels of stress we expect from life.

Major Life Events. You don't need us to tell you the kinds of things that fit this category; things like a divorce, a move, a job change, a death in the family, a sudden illness, and bankruptcy aren't exactly on the same level as a cell-phone battery dying. The stats show that three major life events in a one-year period will make your body feel and act as though it were thirty-two years older in the following year—meaning that it's especially important to develop coping strategies and support systems to sustain you in times of crisis.

How do these types of stress affect us? Typically, the first kind of stress does its part to wear us down and fatigue us but really won't be all that harmful healthwise. The last two kinds of stress are the ones that do the most damage. Understanding how they do—which we'll now explain—is the first step in understanding how to stop it.

Frazzle Dazzle: The Biology of Stress

Stress is good. There, we said it. Instead of calling us crazier than a four-headed firefly, hear us out. Stress heightens all of our biological systems so that we can deal with an impending threat, be it an enemy, a natural disaster, or the fact that

Yo-ga! Yo-ga! Yo-ga!

These days, yoga gets more love than whoever's starring in *The Bachelor*. And for good reason: Yoga could very well be the ultimate de-stress technique. It lowers blood pressure and heart rate, decreases stress hormones, and increases relaxation hormones like serotonin, dopamine, and endorphins. You can get the benefits of yoga in a single pose or in a full-fledged class.

some idiot built the fire too close to the cave. Changes occur inside our body that give us the strength or the sense to fight a predator or high-tail it out of there. What happens to your body during high-intensity stress? Your concentration becomes more focused than a microscope, your reaction time becomes faster, and your strength increases exponentially. Historically, stress was good—as long as you could survive it.

The big difference between stress today and stress yesterday isn't the fact that cavemen didn't have e-mail; it's that their stress was fleeting. They had periods of high-intensity stress followed by low (or no) levels of it. Today we're drowning in a sea of stress, with wave after wave after wave knocking us over. Those heightened biological reactions work in our favor for short periods, but when stress continues unabated, those biological reactions turn wacky.

Too much stress can lead to a host of ultimate stress-enders, like heart attacks, cancer, and disabling accidents. Plus, stress destroys your sleep patterns, which can lead to unhealthy addictions to food, alcohol, or 3:00 A.M. infomercials. How? Through a series of chemicals that are produced in your brain, travel through your blood, and affect just about every system in your body.

That's your stress circuit.

Specifically, your stress circuit is the interaction between your nervous system and your stress hormones—the hormonal system that sounds like a *Star Wars* galaxy: the hypothalamic-pituitary-adrenal (HPA) axis. The stress hormones cycle among these three glands in a feedback loop. When you're faced with a major stressor like a mugger, a looming deadline, or a chocolate shortage, the cone-shaped hypothalamus at the base of your brain releases CRH (corticotrophin-releasing hormone), which then does a hula dance on your pituitary gland, stimulating it to release *another* hormone called ACTH (adrenocorticotropic hormone) into your bloodstream.

ACTH signals your adrenal glands to release cortisol and facilitates production and then release of norepinephrine (also known as adrenaline, the fight-or-

The True Life Force?

When it comes to the human body, we can talk about energy in terms of calories, and we can talk about energy in terms of the cellular energy that's generated by mitochondria, called ATP. But there's a different level of energy that we should all think about: energy fields. It's a part of medicine that we don't fully understand, this relationship between the energy inside the cell and the energy outside the cell. It's the energy that allows us to see force fields in electromagnetic photographs of an amputee's "phantom limbs" in the place where the limbs once were. It's the energy that allows one part of the body to have an effect on another, even though there seems to be no clear chemical connection—for instance, through acupuncture or reflexology. And if you hang around long enough, we might even identify an underlying energy to prayer. It's these energy fields—your life force, your chi, your intangible aura—that we believe will be the next great frontier of medicine. Your nerve cells, in fact, touch stem cells in the liver, which might explain a more direct connection between the mind and self-healing. Many people believe that it's through these energy fields that prayer may work for them—and, thus, how the mind-body connection works. And it may go on to explain why other things work, like the aging process.

flight chemical). As you see in Figure 3.1, these four chemicals serve as your body's SWAT team—they respond to emergencies. Adrenaline increases your blood pressure and heart rate, while cortisol releases sugar in the form of glucose to fuel your muscles and your mind. Then, to close the loop, cortisol travels back to the hypothalamus to stop the production of CRH. Stress over, hormones released, body returns to normal. But only if the stress stops as well.

In addition to giving you the chemical tools to beat the dickens out of your stressors, stress hormones also work throughout various regions of the brain to influence everything from mood and fear to memory and appetite. And they also interact with hormonal systems that control reproduction, metabolism, and immunity. See where this is going? The HPA axis is like a curious two-year-old, touching everything in its path. That's OK in short spurts, but not when you overfill your hormonal systems. That's why stress is so highly correlated with bad health. Specifically, this is what happens when you let the hormones in the HPA axis run crazy:

❖ An overactive HPA axis can mean that your body is unable to turn off your stress response. So? That can lead to anxiety and depression,

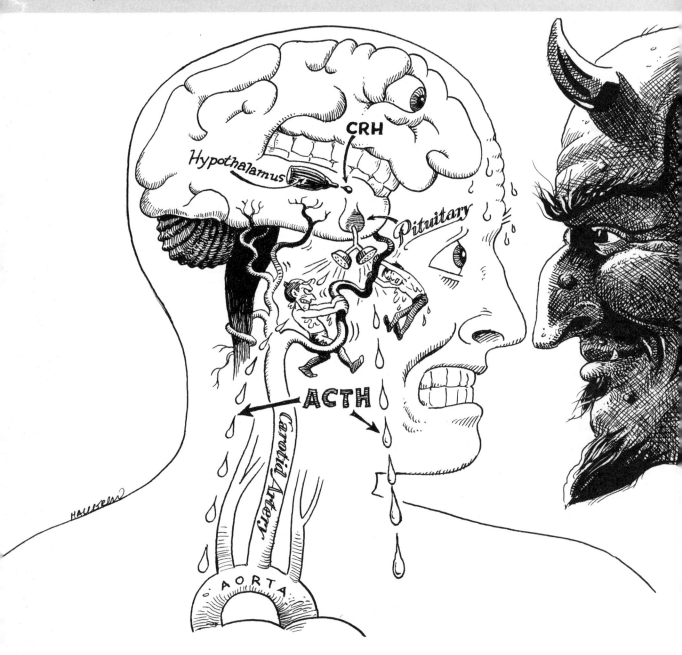

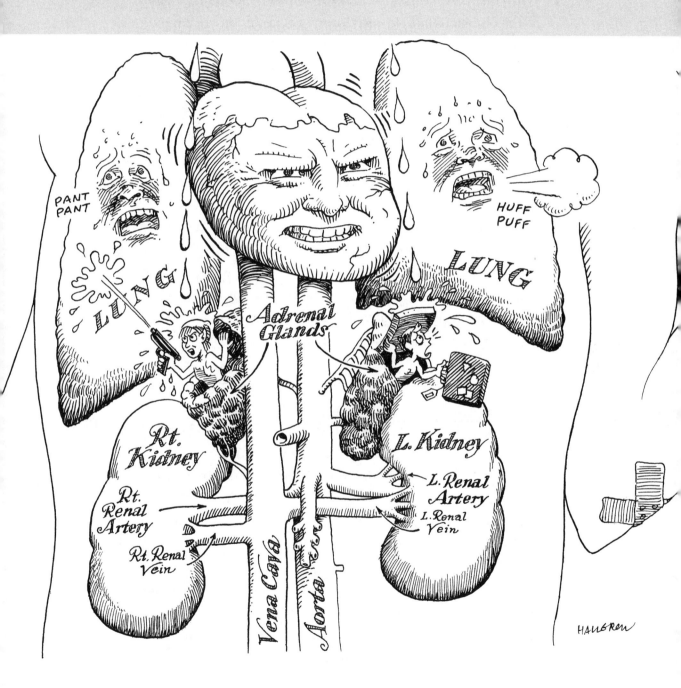

which are further manifested through such things as low sex drive and high blood pressure—both associated with aging.

❖ When the HPA axis is flooded, we also experience other potentially fatal health problems, like elevated lousy LDL cholesterol or triglycerides combined with reduced healthy HDL cholesterol. Part of this risk comes from a stress-related surge in chemicals called cannabinoids (discussed on page 161), which cause us to eat and can eventually lead to such conditions as diabetes and the biggie, literally, obesity.

❖ Cortisol prevents the release of chemicals that strengthen your immune system (see Figure 3.2). That's why you tend to get sick when you're stressed out. Too much cortisol essentially suppresses your immune system and decreases your ability to fight infection. Stress also makes you more susceptible to diseases that you rely on your immune system to hold at bay or eradicate, like cancer. Men have a pretty quick rebound from the cortisol release during stress, but women often sense a lingering impact of the hormone, which is why men are so chipper the day after a lover's spat that they have already forgotten it, while women retain perfect recall of the event, together with the emotional undertones.

❖ CRH prevents the release of a hormone that controls all the hormones responsible for reproduction and sexual behavior, including those that control ovulation and sperm release. Indeed, reducing stress is one of the tactics used by couples with fertility issues. They're relaxing not just for some mumbo-jumbo reason but to try to make their bodies better equipped hormonally for conception. Makes evolutionary sense, right? Why would you want to produce babies in the middle of a drought or when fighting off hairy four-legged neighbors?

❖ If the HPA axis is activated for too long, it hinders the release of growth hormone. As you'll learn in future chapters, you need your growth hormone to help combat some aging-related diseases and conditions and to build lean muscle mass.

❖ If you keep the axis activated for too long, it can develop an exhausted response—and that produces a wiped-out feeling when stress does come.

So what role does our Major Ager of stem cell slowdown play in all of this? Well, the stem cells' regenerative properties are crucial here because of the damage that our environment and the resultant stress can do. Stress is all about adapting to the challenges of life. It is not the strongest or the fastest who wins the game of life, but the most adaptable. When stress hormones damage tissues, cells, and organs in the ways we talked about above, stem cells replace damaged cells and make the repairs. It's one of the reasons why we can't constantly be mentally revved; we need to idle our brains to allow the stem cells to do their job and replenish those cells and tissues that have been battered by bosses, bullies, or brats. So when a toxic food has shriveled our liver, or having a baby has reduced our heart function, or we have damaged an artery by overreacting to a sloppy coiffeur, stem cells come to the rescue to rebuild us *as good as we were before.* To boot, stress shortens those telomeres and turns down telomerase, so that the fastest-producing cells—stem cells—have the most difficulty keeping up.

Even five years ago, we didn't know this stem cell replenishment was true for most organs, but now we know that every organ seems to recruit backup stem cells from the bone marrow to resuscitate itself. These emergency relief worker cells lay the groundwork for re-creating our organs.

Stress has a cascading effect on many aspects of our health. It increases the risk of arterial aging, it damages our immune system, and it also makes us prime candidates for life-altering (or life-ending) accidents—many accident victims admit to having been stressed and angry before the mishap—not to mention affecting our mental health. Stress also releases steroids, which, when given in higher prescription doses, are a legally defensible reason for a rage response. Stress isn't just something you write off as a need for spa treatments; it's a major biological driver of aging.

Now, your response to stress is somewhat hereditary. We all have differences in our genes that control the HPA axis, meaning that some of us never have a

Your Belly: Stress Barometer

When our ancestors faced periods of famine, they stored fat in their bellies with an organ called the omentum. We do the same thing: When we face chronic stress, we eat more food than we need, and we store it in our omentum for quick access to energy. The steroids released by the HPA axis are also sucked up by the omentum and help grow it as big as the muscles on a weight lifter who is dabbling in similar chemicals. That process proves to be damaging because the toxins from our omentum fat are pumped directly into surrounding organs. But it also offers a tangible way to gauge our stress levels: The bigger our bellies, the bigger our burden.

strong response to a threat, while others have a full-fledged response to even a minor threat. (Sound like anyone you know?) But that hereditary predisposition can be altered at any time by extreme stresses. With major stresses early in life, your response becomes stronger, making you better able to handle future stresses. We see an example of this with our response to something called heat shock. When exposed to extreme heat, all animals, including humans, learn to adapt to the temperature so they can respond to it the next time they encounter it. It's the biological basis of the mantra that what doesn't kill us does indeed make us stronger. There are plenty of other techniques that can help minimize the internal damage caused by the pressures from the external world.

YOU Tool: Anger Management

It's no secret that anger doesn't help anyone. Not the fellow motorist you're swearing at. Not the intern you're making cry. Not your kids, who are seeing you lose it. And most of all, not you. Anger has been shown to lead to a higher incidence of heart disease and other health problems. Part of the problem is that we're misinformed about the best way to handle our anger. (By the way, there's a difference between anger, which is frustration at a poor driver, and hostility, which is hoping he runs into the concrete divider.) While you may think that lashing out or hitting a pillow or punching bag helps you release tension, the opposite is true. It teaches you to develop a behavior pattern: Get mad, punch. Get mad, get even. Get mad, harbor stress until it eats away at you like ants on crumbs. Instead, use behavior and mental techniques that have been shown to reduce anger and anxiety, as well as the chronic heart problems associated with them. If you're one of the sixteen million Americans who have anger issues, try these techniques to make a change that we'll all be thankful for:

Do the Opposite. Research has found that "letting it rip" with anger actually escalates anger and aggression and does nothing to help you (or the person you're angry with) resolve the situation. In general, to cope with an emotion, you have to do the opposite. The opposite of anger isn't to withdraw or lash out, but to develop empathy. So instead of swearing at the guy who cut you off, think that maybe there's a reason he did so—like, he just got a call that his wife is in labor or his mom tripped over his child's toy and can't get up. It helps to remind yourself that few people are jerks on purpose. Getting angry just forces you to justify your actions, so you act out to make sense of how crazily you just acted.

Find Your Pattern. Keep thought records with no censorship of all the emotions you feel (and why) during the day. This helps you identify and find a pattern in the core beliefs that are associated with your anger. Do you get angry at a lack of respect, or wasted time, or insults?

Do Push-ups. Somehow, you do have to acknowledge that you are experiencing a physiological response to your anger. Telling yourself to "stay calm" is one of the worst things you can do (second only to being told to "calm down"), because we're *supposed* to act out when we feel threatened and are angry. So act out in a way that doesn't burn bridges, by doing push-ups or stretching or deep breathing. This dissipates the physiological burden of anger.

Choose Smart Words. Be careful of words like *never* or *always* when talking about yourself or someone else. "This machine never works!" or "You're always forgetting things!" are not only inaccurate, they serve to make you feel that your anger is justified and that there's no way to solve the problem. They also alienate and humiliate people who might otherwise be willing to work with you on a solution. Another important distinction is making sure that you have realistic expectations—and are not blaming yourself for things that aren't under your control, with a string of woulds, coulds, and shoulds.

YOU TIPS!

Breathe in. Hold it. Hold it. Hold it. Now release *slooooooooowly.* Feel better? Good. (The nitric oxide is working. You'll learn about that soon; see page 228.) But that's not the only antistress solution you should have. First and foremost, put stress in context. Allow us a few moments of philosophical waxing. Say that you're afraid of public speaking. You tense up and sweat, and your stomach turns into a butterfly museum. But the truth is that when you're that tense, the task becomes more painful and difficult to accomplish. Anticipating the horror of the talk is much worse than the actual reality. So if you retrain your mind to relax, as difficult as it is, by using some of our techniques, and tell yourself that the universe will run its course in the right way, you'll have mastered the first step of decreasing stress.

YOU Tip: Create Your Backup Plan. As we said, stress isn't all bad. It's what gives you the concentration and ability to finish a project or meet a deadline. But stress can linger around like week-old leftovers and create its own kind of stink. So in periods of high stress, you need to have a plan that works for you. Such things as exercise and meditation work for some people, and both of them will help you manage chronic stress through the release of such feel-good substances as nitric oxide and brain chemicals called endorphins. But in the heat of the moment, at peak periods of high intensity, you should be able to pull a quick stress-busting behavior out of your biological bag of tricks. Our suggestions:

❖ Scrunch your face tightly for fifteen seconds, then release. Repeat several times. This repetitive contraction and relaxation helps release tension you're holding above the neck.
❖ Breathe in, lick your lips, then blow out slowly. The cool air helps you refocus and slow down.
❖ Cork it. Hold a wine cork vertically between your teeth. Putting a gentle bite on the cork forces your jaws—a major holder of tension—to relax. (Don't fight stress by emptying the bottle of wine into your body first.)

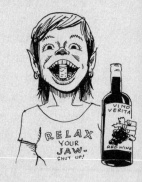

YOU Tip: Lean on Him, Her, or Whomever. Friends aren't just good for borrowing sugar from or for telling you that you have wing sauce on your cheek. Friends are the ultimate de-stressor. Friends can remove over 90 percent of the aging penalty you face after a major life event accelerates your aging. Research shows that one of the most vital elements in reducing the negative health effects of stress is to have strong social networks. So gossiping, playing poker, having girlfriend spa days, playing golf, and going to happy hour aren't all just fun and games. They're mental medicine. So are religious and church groups. We recommend that you talk to friends or extended family daily as a way to strengthen those networks. Of course, your posse isn't just good for managing chronic stress. In periods of major stress, they can be the anchor you need when you're rocking in stormy seas.

YOU Tip: Chop Big Pieces into Small Ones. You know how mountain climbers get up Everest or marathoners get through Boston? One step at a time. They don't think about the big picture, they think about making it through the next stride or step. When you're facing a seemingly insurmountable task, do the same thing. Instead of thinking about your stressor as one insurmountable hurdle, break that unmanageable task into smaller, more manageable ones. Those are the ones you can accomplish. Before you know it, you'll have reached 29,035 feet.

YOU Tip: Work, Work, Work. The theory goes like this. At the end of a long career awaits the ultimate stress reduction plan: retirement. Sure, there's some appeal to sleeping in, taking aquatic therapy classes, and becoming the over-sixty-five county shuffleboard champion. But retirement may not be the mental hammock that everyone expects it to be. Take three parts of the world where people have a greater chance of living to one hundred: Sardinia, Okinawa, and Costa Rica. In each of those areas, people have found ways to cope with stress. The communities have strong traditions of walking, building family strength, playing with kids, and being active. Plus, there's no such thing as retirement. Now, we're not recommending that you subject yourself to the same corporate punishment that's graying your hair and beating you down. But we are recommending that even in retirement, you find a way to continue working—either as a volunteer or for pay—at something you enjoy. It'll help you stay active physically and mentally, give you a life-enhancing sense of purpose, and help you maintain the strong social ties that are so necessary for stress management.

YOU Tip: Be Money Smart. One of the biggest drivers of stress is financial woes. Not coincidentally, health problems are the major driver of bankruptcy, and then bankruptcy cycles back to be a major driver of more stress-related health problems. That's why it's important to create some kind of emotional comfort zone with money—that is, just the feeling that you have some sort of nest egg can ease your stress. And that's why socking away 10 percent of your income every month (or at least $100 every month) can start the process of giving you a backup plan. And, of course, with credit card debt exceeding the national debt, having a good frame of mind about your plastic is important. Use your cards for the convenience of paying your bills, not to avoid paying them.

YOU Tip: Make Additions. Two de-stressors to add to your home: pets and plants. Plants have been shown to decrease infection rates in nursing homes and lower blood pressure, while people who get a pet after having a heart attack are less likely to have another heart attack, especially if they walk that pet. In fact, just *imagining* that you have a pet and walking it can reduce your stress.

YOU Tip: Act Out. People who experience high levels of chronic stress typically fall into a very common cycle of destruction. We're stressed, so we eat onion rings. We're stressed, so we don't have to time to exercise. We eat terribly and don't get up from our desk, so we're stressed. It's a cycle that makes us fat, lazy, and depressed—and depressed that we're fat and lazy. While we know we need to change, many of us just can't seem to get motivated. But here's how you can. Instead of waiting for motivation to change your actions, do something to stimulate motivation (like taking a ten-minute walk or doing stretches at your desk). You may find that when you act out something healthy, the willingness then follows.

YOU Tip: Get a Day Planner or Use That PDA. Part of what makes life so stressful is uncertainty. It's why heavy traffic, computer crashes, and customer-service reps who could care less about customers are so #@&!-ing frustrating. Because so much of life is unpredictable, it helps to maintain a regular schedule and track all your responsibilities that lie ahead. Better to clutter a piece of paper with a to-do list than to clutter your brain with how-will-I-do-it-all worries. While you're at it, the other thing you can do with your pen is a nightly gratitude journal. Write down one or more things every day that you appreciate. The action helps puts your stressors in perspective.

YOU Tip: Enlist the Pros. Some things are easy to do alone (we'll let your imagination figure that one out). But dealing with life's major stressors isn't one of them. In the face of trauma, depression, or grief, many of us retreat into our own thoughts and lives and become more inaccessible than a bank vault. But that's the time when you most need therapists and support groups. Treat depression like it's a broken leg, because it's every bit as much of a physical problem as any other health issue.

Major Ager

Declining Defenses

Why Bacteria and Viruses May Be Your Most Powerful Enemies

The word *infection* means different things to different people. For a city, infection can be bad publicity. For your body, it can mean green mucus oozing from nostrils or ingrown toenails that are more inflamed than an irate boss. Parents may think of ear infections, women may think of yeast infections, and teens usually think of the zitty infections that can ruin a day, a date, or some very fragile self-esteem.

All of those examples certainly fit our classical definition of infection: when some foreign invader is attacking our bodies, and our bodies are working hard to show it the anatomical exit door.

When it comes to aging, however, we're concerned not only with the acute infections—the bacteria and viruses that make you sick. We're also concerned with the chronic infections: when bacteria and other germs trigger a behind-the-scenes inflammatory response in your body that ages your entire system. This kind of inflammatory response predisposes you to more cell replications, which increases the risk of mutations that can lead to cancer. As you see in Figure D.1,

Tainted Image An infection is like bad press for a city: News spreads and spreads, and infects the image of the city for a long time. The reverse is also true; "best cities to live in" lists give towns years and years of good publicity.

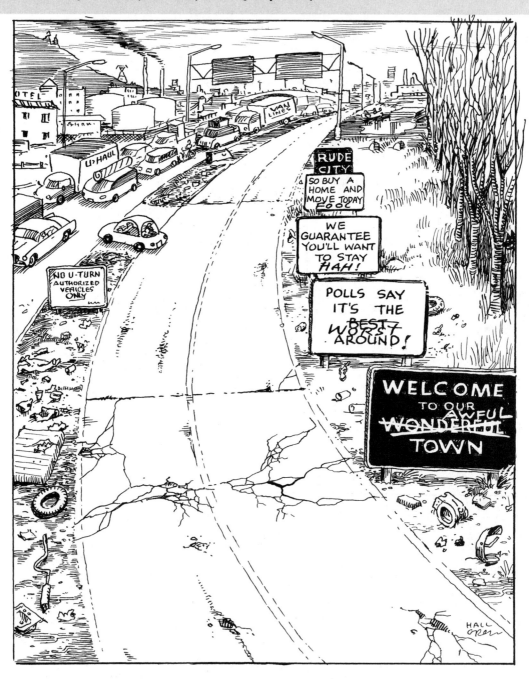

just as a plague scares away visitors from our metaphorical city, you may not want to live in your own body after a while.

Much of the aging process is a side effect of defense mechanisms that our body has designed—and infection might be the best example of all. Historically, infections are what killed us, and even fifty years ago, pneumonia was called an old man's best friend. Viral infections still cause cancers, like some lymphomas, cervical cancer, and perhaps prostate cancer, while bacterial infection of your gums can increase your risk of pancreatic cancer, heart disease, and stroke.

Believe it or not, more than 90 percent of the cells in your body are not actually yours but belong to foreign organisms. Even though our bodies have ten trillion cells, our intestines alone have ten times that many foreign cells. You're actually just a minority stakeholder in your own body. Not only do these cells outnumber us, but we cannot live without them; after all, it's the bacteria in your gut that help digest your food. One of the real secrets of controlling aging is learning how we can make peace with foreign cells and have more influence over them.

Adaptation—the process of making evolutionary changes based on our changing environment—does allow us to respond to whatever bacteria may be attempting to invade us, affect us, or eat our innards in a bacterial seven-course meal. But you know what? We can't keep up; it's almost as if we're running in place. As soon as we zig, the bacteria zag. That's because infectious agents replicate themselves and evolve much faster than we do, so they're always two or three steps in front of our immune system. Biologists call this the Red Queen Principle (see Figure D.2), based on the Red Queen's observation to Alice in Lewis Carroll's *Through the Looking Glass* that "it takes all the running you can do to keep in the same place." Go ahead and trot that tidbit out at the Thanksgiving dinner table when conversation turns to Aunt Fran's chronic bladder infections. Biologically speaking, we've changed very little in the hundred thousand

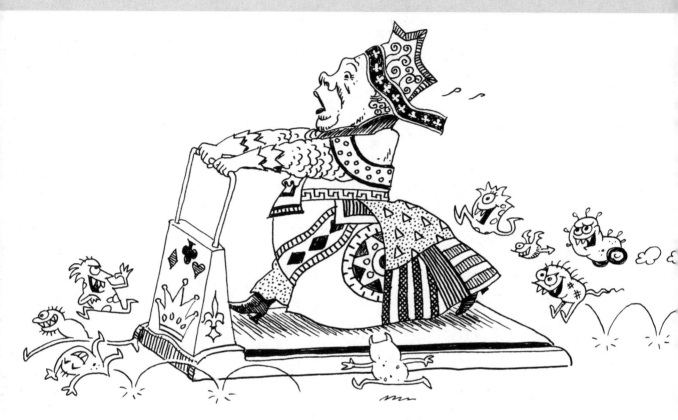

years since modern humans emerged on the African savanna. That's a long time, but not so much in evolutionary terms—it's equivalent to only three thousand generations, which isn't enough time for many serious adjustments. Most bacteria, on the other hand, can crank out three thousand generations well inside of a week. That faster generation of generations has another effect: Bacteria tend to mutate frequently, which is why they become resistant to antibiotics.

While acute infection today ranks as the fifth leading cause of death in the Western world, it's number one for the rest of the world and for most of mankind's history, thanks to the microbes that caused plague, scarlet fever, smallpox, tuberculosis, and the ever-popular infectious diarrhea. Even in relatively recent history, infection was a leading generation killer. The influenza pandemic of 1918, for example, killed forty million people worldwide. And today epidemiologists are worried that with the rapid spread of SARS and bird flu, another pandemic might be in the making. In response, we have to develop a way to combat those foreign invaders. Certainly, many infections today are fought with antibiotics or prevented with vaccines, but from an evolutionary perspective, we also had to figure out a way to get ourselves off that internal treadmill where bacteria was keeping us running in place. The answer? Sex.

Sexual reproduction is crucial to keeping up with the constant cycle of one-upmanship between pathogens and you, their human hosts. If we reproduced asexually, all of us would be identical to one another, with the same set of disease fighters; if smart bacteria figured out that we lacked the antibody mechanisms necessary to kill them, then they could kill all of us.

Sexual reproduction allows for the mixing of genes among different groups, ensuring that we have a diversity of disease-fighting cells to keep pace with the faster-evolving pathogens.

The Good Side of Bad Effects

Now, imagine you had a bad strep infection. Your symptoms might be a headache, sore throat, fever, loss of appetite, even anemia. Of course, our natural reaction is to treat the symptoms with food, aspirin, supplements, Mom's soup. And while this all may be perfectly appropriate, it also makes sense to understand whether these literal and metaphorical headaches are actually doing us some good. Fever, for example, is a calculated response to stop bacterial invaders in their tracks, so when we take fever-reducing drugs, we actually thwart our body's defense mechanism. The bacteria hate the heat, but our immune cells are resilient and continue to replicate even during high fevers. In one study, people with colds took either acetaminophen (Tylenol) or a sugar pill. Those who took the sugar pill had a significantly higher antibody response and much less nasal stuffiness. And what about taking an iron supplement to treat the anemia that comes with chronic illnesses? Not so fast. This may be exactly what the bacteria want you to do. Iron is a key resource for bacteria, and our bodies have evolved several different ways to keep it away from them. When we become infected, our bodies produce a chemical called leukocyte endogenous mediator (LEM), which decreases the amount of iron in our bloodstream. So, ironically, while the blood test tells us we're anemic, this intentionally low iron level is helping keep the bacteria in check.

That's especially important in the body's response to infection. For example, the bubonic plague was very deadly in the Middle Ages because the bacteria would enter our macrophages (white blood cell scavenger system) and thrive due to their high iron content. But in people with hemochromatosis (iron-loading disease), which is now the most common genetic abnormality in northern Europeans, bubonic bacteria had trouble surviving, since the macrophage iron level was so low. Although abnormal iron loading leads to premature death in people with hemochromatosis, the sufferers of this genetic condition do not die of bubonic plague. So when a quarter of the European population was killed during the first plague, our ancestors with hemochromatosis survived. Subsequent bouts of the plague were much less devastating because of this change.

So infections have shaped our genes through natural selection and have forced humans to jump through hoops in developing complex systems to protect ourselves. Aging can weaken our well-honed immune function, which becomes one of the first places we see an obvious change in our health. Sometimes we catch things we used to duck, and sometimes these meticulous defenses go awry. Next we'll explain how to keep your immune system a loyal fighting machine.

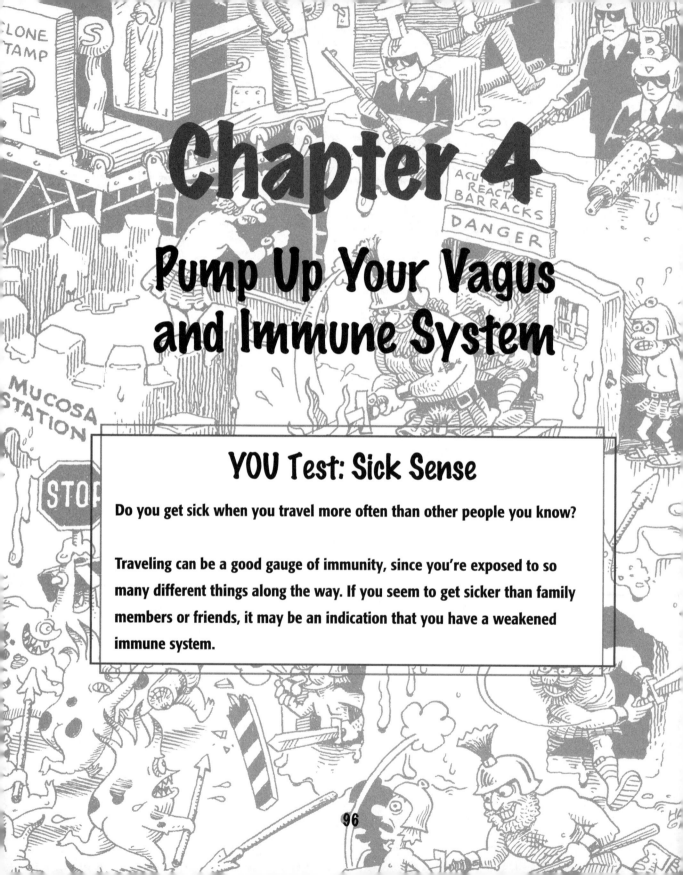

Chapter 4
Pump Up Your Vagus and Immune System

YOU Test: Sick Sense

Do you get sick when you travel more often than other people you know?

Traveling can be a good gauge of immunity, since you're exposed to so many different things along the way. If you seem to get sicker than family members or friends, it may be an indication that you have a weakened immune system.

We all know the kind of destruction a computer virus can cause. It can lock down your computer, fry your hard drive, and send you swirling in a sea of profanity that can be heard three counties over. Anyone whose computer has ever been slowed or shut down by a foreign invader knows what she needs to do: protect any future ones from entering.

In our bodies, we can't firewall ourselves with complete virus protection—that's the price we pay for not living in a bubble. We interact with all kinds of germs, bacteria, viruses, fungi, parasites, and other invaders that want to feed off our insides. Their main points of entry are the skin, the lungs, and the gut, which is why those organs have developed mechanisms to protect us from personal invaders.

Most of us know the stakes: When invaders get the best of us, we're more vulnerable to colds, infections, and more serious disease. As we age, our immune system weakens, making us even more vulnerable. Then it becomes a Major Ager. That's why diseases like cancer become more common as we age—they grow because we have decreased surveillance (and decreased protection) in our bodies. The issue of immunity really comes down to how we manage all the foreign invaders coming at us. We already know that bacteria are responsible for ulcers and a lot of reflux, and viruses are linked to cervical cancer (and, most likely, prostate and bladder cancers). Interestingly, it's not in an invader's best interest to actually kill us, since that would leave it homeless and vulnerable and unable to reproduce. But it is in an invader's interest to gulp up or take over our good cells for themselves.

The whole issue really comes down to protection—protecting our good cells from the thugs, protecting our organs from the hungry enemies, protecting our

FACTOID

Some people may say there's no harm in taking antibiotics if you feel bad, but if you're fighting off a viral infection like the flu, antibiotics can hurt you more than they can help. That's because overtreating with antibiotics can cause collateral damage. You'll kill off all the bacterial allies in your gut and leave the evil virus untouched. If you do have to take antibiotics for a bacterial infection, protect your gut by eating probiotics, simple foods low down on the food chain that bacteria love and that can help reduce inflammation.

health by strengthening our immunity. But it also comes down to making peace with the right allies: the friendly bacteria that are willing to live in harmony with us. If we have the right bacteria in our gut, for instance, they inhibit the bad guys from setting up shop. And we also have to strike the perfect balance: making sure we have enough immune response, but not so much that our immune responders fight back against us.

One of the secrets of controlling our immunity comes in the form of something that few of us have ever heard of, though it could provide the most useful insights into how we can control the aging process: the vagus nerve.

The vagus nerve provides a T1 line of information to the brain from the gut, where battles with bugs are continually raging. Knowledge of the vagus's role was a mystery until very recently, but we now know that you can learn about your body from your vagus.

Vagus, Baby!

Mind over matter. We see it in magicians. We see it in Tibetan monks who pass a test into monkhood by generating enough heat from their bodies in freezing temperatures to make a cold, moist blanket placed over their shoulder dry out. And we see it in a feat of the feet—firewalkers who can slowly walk over burning coals barefoot. Many of us tend to write off these seemingly supernatural behaviors as some freaky sixth sense or some tricky camera manipulation.

But we believe there's a much more concrete explanation for jaw-dropping mind-over-matter missions. It comes in the form of the vagus nerve, the longest nerve directly from the brain, which sends messages to and receives messages from your gut and every other organ in your body (see Figure 4.1). Because 85 percent of this huge nerve carries information back to the brain, it's the main mecha-

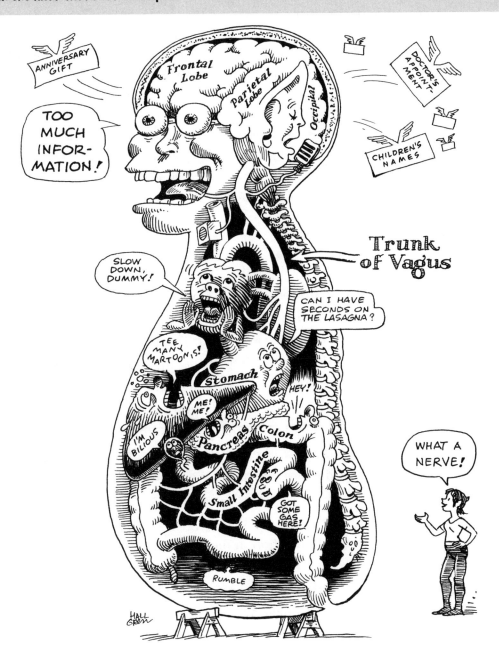

Give Me a V

Vaccines are a kind of immuno insurance policy. Although the body comes stocked with millions of different antibodies, there is always the chance that the one you need won't be available when you need it. Vaccines—typically, weakened strains of viruses or parts of bacteria—cause the body to produce antibodies for that specific infection. So rather than the usual delayed immune response that allows a cold virus to take hold, the antibodies produced by a measles vaccine are ready to knock out that disease before it ever gets started. Of course, sometimes vaccinations create side effects (though the benefits far outweigh the risks for the immunizations we recommend). In a very small percentage of cases, vaccines decrease the chance of other illnesses caused by a revved-up immune response, including heart attacks. Why? Because part of the immune response to real infections is to assume that the invader penetrated the skin. So whereas you really get the flu, your body assumes that you have a cut and quickly moves to create a blood clot by activating your sticky thrombosis cells. These cells also travel to the heart and brain, where they wreak havoc and cause inappropriate clots in minor cuts and plaques in these critical arteries. Yearly flu vaccination prevents this and is an easy part of the YOU Extended Warranty Plan.

nism by which your brain audits your body. The remaining 15 percent takes information from your brain to your body. One of the key processes in this message system involves toll-like receptors, which stimulate an immune response once invaders have breached an area like the skin or gut. The bacteria colonizing our gut work to block new bacteria from moving into the neighborhood. The toll receptors are able to distinguish effectively between pathogen cells and host cells, and they work as a sort of smoke alarm for your body by putting your immune system on alert when foreign cells have invaded, so that the immune team can take care of them before any damage takes place (see Figure 4.2). However, this early warning system is a very primitive defense and lacks the sophistication of some of the other immune cells (T and B), which we'll discuss in a moment.

From experiments with rats we know that the vagus plays a role in overall immunity. When they're given an infection in the gut, the rats go into septic shock. Their blood pressure drops, their organs fail, and then they die. Now give the rats the same exact infection and cut the vagus nerve. What happens? Bingo. They live. By cutting (or controlling) that message system, you haven't eliminated the infection, but you've altered the rat's brain's response so that it doesn't get the message

Figure 4.2 Taking Toll The immune system has very primitive early response "toll receptors" that provide the front line of a continuous battleground foreigners are always passing through: the intestinal tract. These medieval guards can quickly triage invaders, but when the threat is real, the more corporate B and T cells are created in a regimented fashion—and bring the big guns to smack down invaders.

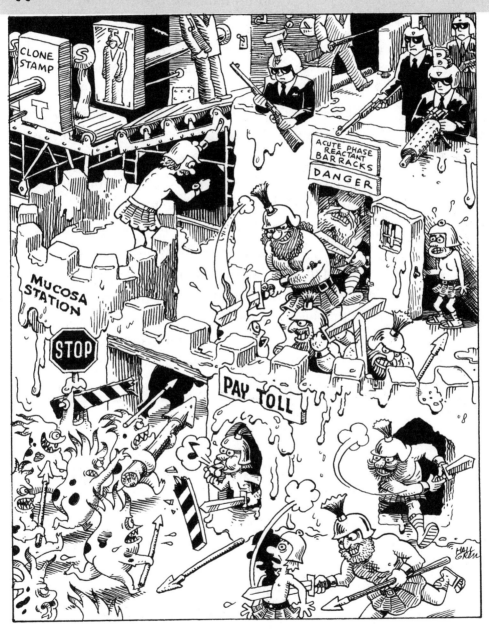

that this infection's a doozy and doesn't kick off a huge immune reaction. Luckily, we don't have to cut our own nerves to get a similar effect.

If you can do things to regulate your vagus nerve, you can block some of the bad stuff that you're feeling, whether it's caused by stress, infection, or sun-hot coals. Those fire walkers, for instance, figured out a way of meditating to change how the vagus and other nerves interpret the world around them to block not just the pain but also the blisters and other bad stuff that would happen if we mere mortals attempted the same thing.

Now, we're not suggesting that you can will away strep throat or think good thoughts to banish pink-eye. But we are suggesting that manipulating this very powerful—repeat, *very* powerful—connection between the gut and the brain may be one of the ways you can quiet the high-level inflammation and immunity challenges that can have a detrimental effect on your health. The vagus remains a mysterious nerve in your body, but thanks to new insights about it and data that seem to indicate its power, we're starting to understand not only that meditation (or, as we prefer to call it, training your vagus) might work, but *how* it works to influence your immune system and aging.

Your Immune Cells: Fighting the Good Fight

We all have images in our heads of the way bouncers are supposed to look: snarling faces, shaved heads, biceps worthy of their own mountain range. Their job: to keep the riffraff from entering the club and gently engulf and escort the fight-starting, women-harassing hooligans out without anyone noticing. In your body, you have biological bouncers called macrophages. These cells don't have shirt-ripping pecs, but they perform the same kind of job. They're always on guard to detect those who don't belong, patrolling the body and searching for potential troublemakers trying to sneak in without proper ID. The intruders? Could be proteins, parasites, a splinter, a cancer cell, spoiled shrimp, a kitchen knife lodged in your thigh, or bacteria.

When macrophages spot a potential invader, they get on their headsets and call for assistance—in this case, helper T cells, which stimulate other white blood cells known as B cells to make a surface protein (called an antibody) that binds to a molecule on the surface of the intruder (an antigen). What's tricky about this binding is that white blood cells come in ten million different types, each making its own unique antibody, just waiting for the specific intruder it recognizes to show up.

Your body can't afford to have all of these white blood cells patrolling every part of your body ready to attack at any time, so they're kept in reserve at a central place. Like a SWAT team, these reserves will be called when they're needed. Most of the symptoms of an illness are actually collateral damage from a raging immune response against a stealth infection attack, be it from food poisoning or the flu or some other kind of infection. After that, you feel the direct effects plus the effects of your body's response to the infection.

It may help to think of the antibody as a kind of molecular lock that needs to be unlocked if the white blood cell it's riding on is to take action. Now think of the antigen as the key. If the key fits the antibody lock, white blood cells start rapidly multiplying in an attempt to overwhelm and beat the bespeckles out of the invader.

Now, one of the key players in this security dance is your thymus—the gland located just behind your breastbone, where your helper T cells grow and mature, almost like barracks that house soldiers in training (see Figure 4.3). Some T cells directly destroy invaders, while others alert additional immune cells to join the battle.

FACTOID

Is cleanliness really next to godliness? Don't fret all infections; exposure to poor hygiene in life can strengthen your immunity. When you're infected, your body turns down its allergic immune system (it's frivolous when you're dealing with a life-threatening infection). That may explain why city dwellers have more asthma than nature dwellers.

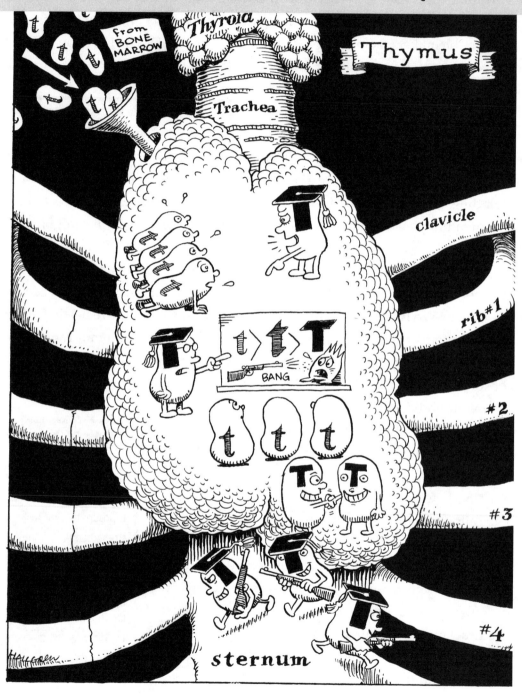

Now, when you were little, your thymus was fairly large. But as you age, your thymus shrinks to the point where it's barely noticeable. Presumably, that's because we need a much stronger immune system as children, but not so much by middle age, since by then we've been exposed to lots of stuff and are thus resistant to it. As we live into our seventies, eighties, and nineties—long after the storage house of those helper T cells has been depleted—we become increasingly vulnerable to infection. Couple that with the fact that other immune responses, like mucus production, decrease with age, and you can see how our responses become much weaker as we get older.

Another major player in the immune process is one of the markers of inflammation, C-reactive protein (CRP), which is a protein produced in the liver. Levels of CRP rise substantially when there's inflammation or acute or chronic infection, with things like gingivitis, prostatitis, or vaginal infections. It's also an important predictor of cardiovascular risk because you're more prone to plaque rupture and clotting. A primitive immune system that's more like a shark's than a sophisticated one like a mammal's, CRP doesn't pinpoint exactly where inflammation is, but it does indicate whether inflammation or some type of infection is present.

Immune Dysfunction: Friendly Fire

Like any weapon, the immune system can backfire and become dangerous to the owner. Immune system backfire happens when cells either underkill (failing to attack when they should) or overkill (attacking something when they shouldn't). Underkill results from an inadequate response, so that an infection that should have been nipped in the bud becomes serious. You've heard of people affected by flesh-eating bacteria. These are examples of underkill. Overkill results from mounting too aggressive a response to a relatively minor threat. Autoimmune diseases such as lupus and rheumatoid arthritis are the results of an overly aggressive immune system.

Till (Cell) Death Do Us Part

Biological bouncers have to do what the human ones do: guard every possible entrance. You have legions of macrophages on alert along the parts of your body that interact with the outside world: in your skin, your lungs, and your gut wall. But

The Nose Hose

You may clean your nose with tissues; kids, to our dismay, may do it with their fingers. A better option: a Neti Pot device. Sold over the counter, these devices are based on the ancient Indian technique of *jala neti*—literally meaning water cleansing—where the practitioner rinses out the nasal cavity with water using this little pot. Often used in India and Southeast Asia, it's gaining more acceptance in Western cultures (under the phrasing nasal irrigation) and can be done as routinely as brushing your teeth.

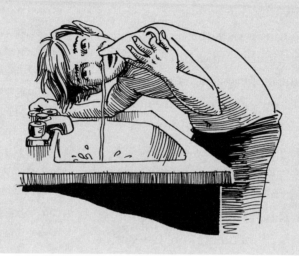

there are downsides to having your army on high alert; you have to feed it, and you increase the likelihood that segments will revolt. So your body essentially keeps a national reserve system, always on backup but ready to go.

One of its main duties is to recognize previous infections: B cells and T cells recognize the intruder and instruct the specific disease-fighting cells to go get it. But besides having an old guard, your body also needs some open-minded young ones that can figure out a new threat, make an antidote to it, replicate like a high-end copy machine, and find a way to beat the aggressor.

Once the B and T cells are done with their jobs, however, these cells are no longer needed, so they start to clump, pop a hole in their own nuclei, shrivel like a raisin, and die. Win or lose, these cells will die. It's cell suicide—a programmed cell death called apoptosis (see Figure 4.4). The individual cells die to allow the body to conserve enough energy to be able to fight the next fight. It's really an ex-

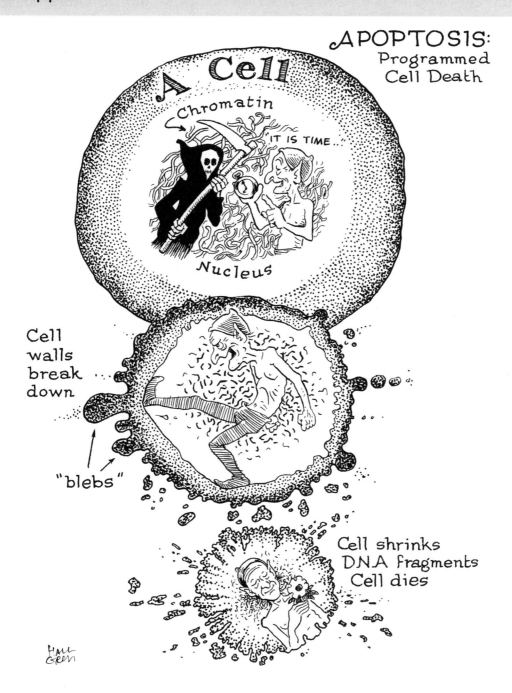

ample of how our cells have the machinery to commit suicide before they sap too much of your energy on a long-term basis. Most cells turn off their apoptosis genes for the sake of the survival of the species. But immune cells are different. In an action movie, the people who die are the bit players; they may serve a role to move the plot, but their survival isn't essential to the main story line. Same here. Your body uses these bit players to fight the infection, then kills them off so that your brain and heart and liver and all of your other organs can be supplied with the energy needed to take center stage. (Quick side note: This process of apoptosis is responsible for some of our growth from the fetus stage. For example, the reason why we don't have webbed feet is because cell death allowed us to hollow out the space between our toes.) Apoptosis is also how injured or imperfect cells are removed. When our quality control isn't working at its best, this can cause aging either because we do not make our cells quite perfect enough or because we are too strict. This is great when we're young, but it can age us as we get older (you'll read more about this process on page 120).

Apoptosis is one of the fundamental processes that could be the key to treating certain diseases. If you know that cells can commit suicide, wouldn't there be a time when you'd want to trick cells into doing so, as in the case of cancer? And maybe there's a time when you'd take dying cells and turn off apoptosis, so that the cells could become immortal and you could revitalize damaged tissues, as in your knee cartilage?

YOU TIPS!

The nice thing about modern medicine is that we have an arsenal of antibiotics that's able to wipe out bacteria with a wallop. Pop this pill, banish this bacterium. And that's a good thing. But it doesn't mean you should rely on medicine to address your chronic immunity issues, especially because there are plenty of foreign invaders (some we know and some we have no way of predicting) that won't respond to medicinal attacks. That's why we recommend you add other weapons to your security team.

YOU Tip: Train Your Vagus. You may be used to working out your muscles with dumbbells, working out your heart with a good swim, and working out your kinks with a massage. We also want you to get used to exercising your vagus nerve. By learning to modulate messages going to and from the brain, you'll better protect yourself against overreactions to inflammation caused by infections and stress. The mechanism appears to be controlled by how the vagus nerve releases its main chemical, acetylcholine, and deactivates the king of white blood cells, macrophages, so our immune system isn't in a continual state of war. Here's one elegant way (besides putting an electronic stimulator around your vagus): a form of movement we discussed in the memory chapter, called chi-gong. This exercise combines meditation and movement to soothe the vagus. See how to do it in our YOU Toolbox on page 377. Another bonus: It also seems to help ward off and decrease the severity of such immune issues as herpes zoster, or shingles. Both increase with age (because of declined immunity and the cellular damage that comes from the stress and depression prevalent in older adults). Relaxation techniques like chi-gong appear to improve immunity in these two diseases, and likely in other infections as well. If chi-gong isn't your cup of tea, just meditate nightly, as we describe in the YOU Toolbox.

YOU Tip: Fuel Your Fighters. One of the best ways to pump up your immune system is by eating the foods and getting the nutrients that have been shown to improve your natural defenses. The chart on page 110 shows you foods and supplements that have immune-boosting power.

YOU Tip: Get More 3s. Since we're eating more grains and foods with omega-6 fatty acids, you likely need more sources of omega-3 in your diet to strike the best nutritional ratio—not only to boost your immunity but for all other health benefits associated with omega-3s. Plus, the right ratio reduces the inflammatory stimulus in the liver, so the appropriate inflammation caused when our immune system defends us against an invader does not age us as much. Some fats, like flaxseed oil, have a good balance between 3s and 6s, but you should also add more 3s in the form of purselain and fish such as cod, halibut, and trout. Other ideas: Buy omega-3-enriched eggs, or eat walnuts or the pure DHA form of omega-3 from the same place that the fish get it—plankton.

Foods	Nutrients	Spices	Supplements	Avoid These
Shiitake mushrooms (may increase your natural killer T cells) Vegetables, especially cruciferous ones like cabbage, broccoli, and brussels sprouts Cocoa and coffee (because of the antioxidants) Alcohol (in moderation) Probiotics (in yogurt and digestive aids)	Omega-3 fatty acids (found in olive oil, avocado, fish oils, nuts; also can be taken as supplement) Resveratrol (found in red wine, grapes, and knotweed plants) Catechins (found in green tea) Quercetin (found in onions, tomatoes, garlic, and apples) Lycopene (found in tomatoes and red grapefruit)	Curcumin Ginger	Biotin (300 milligrams per day) B_6 (4 milligrams per day) and B_{12} (800 micrograms per day) Strontium (340 milligrams per day)	Simple sugars Syrups Enriched/non–whole grains Saturated fats Trans fats Alcohol (in excess) Nonorganic meats Fish with mercury

YOU Tip: Prevent the Onset. The popular Canadian supplement Cold-FX is said to ward off infection because the active ingredient—ginseng—helps activate your natural killer cells and other components of your immune system (many hockey players credit the product for giving them freedom from colds despite constant travel). The product seems to be effective because it activates those toll-like receptors that serve as a smoke alarm to a pending immunity invasion.

YOU Tip: Feed Your Gut Immunity. Our gut instinct is all about the gut being the first responder to outside invaders. Resuscitating the gut with key nutrients including glutamine (25 grams) and N-acetyl-cysteine (600 milligrams) restores levels of your own powerful antioxidant glutathione and rebuilds the gut's resilience to the stresses of life, including infection and inflammation. Eating extra whole grains and beans helps too.

YOU Tip: Repopulate. Not the world, but your gut. Lactic acid–producing bacteria can be taken as oral supplements to help repopulate your gut with the good kinds of bacteria. (These bacteria are short lived, so you have to re-dose often.) They help with ailments ranging from too much gas to irritable bowel syndrome to a weakened immune system that tolerates gingivitis. Lactobacilli, for example, have been used in the food industry for many years because they are able to convert sugars (including lactose) and other carbohydrates into lactic acid. This not only provides the characteristic sour taste of fermented dairy foods such as yogurt but acts as a preservative by lowering the food's pH and creating fewer opportunities for spoilage organisms to grow. Add these to your diet: yogurt, kefir, sauerkraut, and kimchi (a Korean dish of pickled vegetables).

YOU Tip: Get Your Prebiotics. *Pro*biotic bacteria are not normally found in the human intestine, so they often don't colonize well when they're introduced. Therefore, *pre*biotic foods are vital to encourage probiotic organisms to survive and thrive in the human gut. Prebiotics are nondigestible food fibers that stimulate the growth and activity of healthy bacteria in the intestines. Prebiotic carbohydrates are found naturally in such fruit and vegetables as bananas, berries, asparagus, garlic, wheat, oatmeal, barley (and other whole grains), flaxseed, tomatoes, Jerusalem artichokes, onions, chicory, greens, and legumes.

YOU Tip: Try Eastern. Acupuncture causes measurable increases in vagus nerve activity, so it is at least theoretically possible that these electrical circuits can reduce the inflammatory response by calming down aggressive white blood cells and the cytokine chemicals they release. Meditation, hypnosis, biofeedback, and relaxation therapies, which have been advocated for treatment of inflammation, may calm you by stimulating vagus nerve activity as well.

Major Ager

Toxins

Keep Sludge from Seeping into Your Body

Unpleasant as it is, we all can remember the times we've spent with our knees on the bathroom floor and our heads so far down in the bowl that we could see the city's sewer system. Perhaps the episode of vomiting was induced by bad fish, or too much booze, or a flu that ripped through your guts like a viral tornado. But, really, we should be thankful for our propensity to puke. Thankful? Yes.

Throwing up, though hell on our nerves and the person stuck with cleaning the grout, is nature's way of clearing toxins from our body. Take, for example, one of life's most frustratingly nauseating events, morning sickness, which is actually designed to protect your genes. In our Stone Age years, nausea evolved during pregnancy as a fail-safe mechanism to help women minimize their exposure to toxins, since even mild toxins can be devastating to a developing fetus, especially during the first trimester.

As we've evolved, our bodies have developed a variety of ways to combat the natural toxins we may run into. If, say, you overdose on apricot pits, which are high in cyanide, your body has a way of protecting you in the form of an enzyme called rhodanase, which helps neutralize toxins. The problem—as surely you've guessed—is that we live in a world where the prevention of apricot-pit overdoses doesn't exactly drum up federal funding. Historically, our liver and immune system spent their entire time removing simple toxins. Now we are exposed to hundreds daily, which stress our systems and tax them as we age.

We live in a world where all kinds of chemicals surround us. They come from cars and factories, they're in our foods and shampoos, and they're in our homes and offices. All of these potentially toxic substances act as pollution to our biological city (see Figure E.1). Some of the toxins we may encounter have their own warning systems so we know not to ingest them or use them (you know by the smell of bleach or gasoline that you're not going to be serving either in a wine goblet). But many of today's toxins are odorless and colorless, so you may not have such an overt warning. In a way, what we lack in minerals, we make up in heavy metals.

Now, that doesn't mean you should fear every chemical that you come into contact with. Chemicals aren't out to get us. Instead, they're really intended to make our lives better. Take shampoo, for example. There are specific ingredients in shampoo that are included to make sure that it lathers up foamier than a cumulus cloud—something that many of us like. But in some people, those very chemicals may also cause a skin irritation.

Some of the toxins that we encounter are potentially very harmful and can cause cancer, asthma, or allergies, and they can also reduce your quality of life in more subtle ways. They may cause minor irritations or fatigue or a general feeling of blahness. And all of those effects—as subtle or subconscious as they may be—can chip away at our overall health so that we're much more prone to feeling the effects of aging. That's why we recommend that you at least be aware of some of

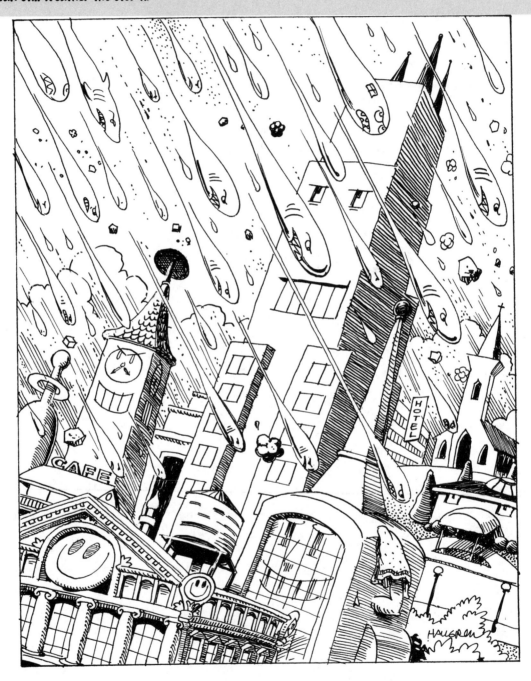

the more prevalent toxins that exist in the world (and your home), so if you are feeling off-kilter, you can experiment with small changes in your life that may actually have a big effect on how you feel. See more details in our Toolbox beginning on page 334. And sometimes the toxins force your body to replace injured cells repeatedly, which means you have more chance of developing errors, especially if the toxins affect how our cells reproduce. The mistakes result in poorly functioning organs or, worse, cancer. And that's our next stop.

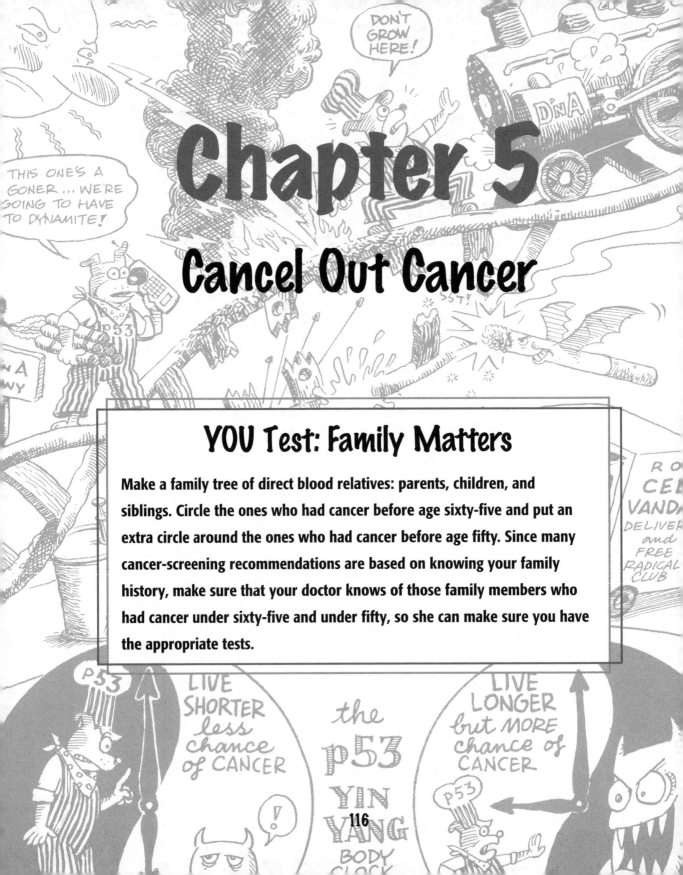

Chapter 5
Cancel Out Cancer

DON'T GROW HERE!

THIS ONE'S A GONER ... WE'RE GOING TO HAVE TO DYNAMITE!

YOU Test: Family Matters

Make a family tree of direct blood relatives: parents, children, and siblings. Circle the ones who had cancer before age sixty-five and put an extra circle around the ones who had cancer before age fifty. Since many cancer-screening recommendations are based on knowing your family history, make sure that your doctor knows of those family members who had cancer under sixty-five and under fifty, so she can make sure you have the appropriate tests.

LIVE SHORTER *less* *chance* *of* CANCER

the **p53** YIN YANG BODY CLOCK

LIVE LONGER *but MORE chance of* CANCER

We don't care about how macho or brave or unafraid of knife-throwing vigilantes you are. At some point in your life, you need protection to prolong your survival. For rock stars, it's a bodyguard. For SWAT teams, it may be bulletproof vests. For a teenage girl going on a first date, it may be a menacing father with ready-to-go knuckles. When you think about it, much of what we do and use for our health really boils down to protection: helmets to protect us from an accidental brain smoosh, running shoes to protect us from shards of glass, aspirin to protect us from clotting, fluoride to protect against cavities, and Trojans to protect us from STDs. Perhaps the greatest protector of all is the one that you can't buy in any store or order from any online discount warehouse (though *there's* an idea): It's the p53 tumor suppressor gene, which has the job of recognizing when your cells are at risk of developing into cancer and doing what it can to put a stop to it. Its job—that of biological guard dog and computer spell-checker rolled into one mean gene—is to protect your body.

Though it may seem like more of an oxymoron than jumbo shrimp, cancer is really about living forever. Why? Because that's what cancer cells want to do: live forever. Unfortunately, that comes at the expense of our cells—meaning that inside one of our biggest scourges lies the potential of infinite life. Now, the reason why cancer affects us as we age has to do with that p53 system; the p53 system regulates all our cells and causes premature aging, which we'll explain in a moment. As our immune systems weaken from aging, that also means those holes are lining up in our Swiss cheese, making us much more vulnerable to cancer, the second leading killer. Combine those factors with the fact that you may have a weakened immune system unable to fight off the Major Ager of toxins, and you've got a perfect storm of cancer-forming factors.

Without question, of all the aches, pains, conditions, and diseases we cover in this book, cancer is the one that rattles us like no other. And for good reason. While cancer's a nasty and ugly disease, our goal isn't to scare you or shock you; it's to take you inside your cells, so you can see the biological processes that cause cancer—and understand how much control you do have in fending off the disease.

Your Cells: The Cancer Chance

And you thought that the administrative assistant in your office spent a lot of time at the copy machine. Inside every human being, about seventy million cell replications occur each day. That replication process is what makes us prone to developing cancer cells. Here's how it works: Each strand of DNA has four letters in its code: A, G, C, and T. When a cell replicates, there are a certain number of typographical errors—meaning the cell miscopies the code (it's like when a piece of paper gets stuck or is only partially copied). That error is just a random error that occurs, given the astronomical amount of copying that's going on. No matter how many ground balls you field or words you type, and no matter how good you are at your job, you're simply going to make some errors along the way because of the volume of work that you're doing. Now, if the letter that gets messed up is in an important part of a specific type of gene, that can convert a normal cell into a cancerous cell.

What do we mean by a specific type of gene? There are really two types of genes that, when mutated, predispose a cell to become cancerous. One type of gene is a proto-oncogene. Normally, it regulates cell growth and differentiation. When it is mutated in a way that's always "on" instead of being on in response to a growth factor, it's as if you've pressed the accelerator on cell growth and division. And because the cells are dividing so fast, they don't mature normally—that is, they don't differentiate into the types of cells they are supposed to. And because they divide so fast, more errors are made in copying the DNA, eventually causing cancer.

The second kind are genes like p53, which normally put the brakes on growth (see Figure 5.1). When they mutate in a way that's always "off," the same results

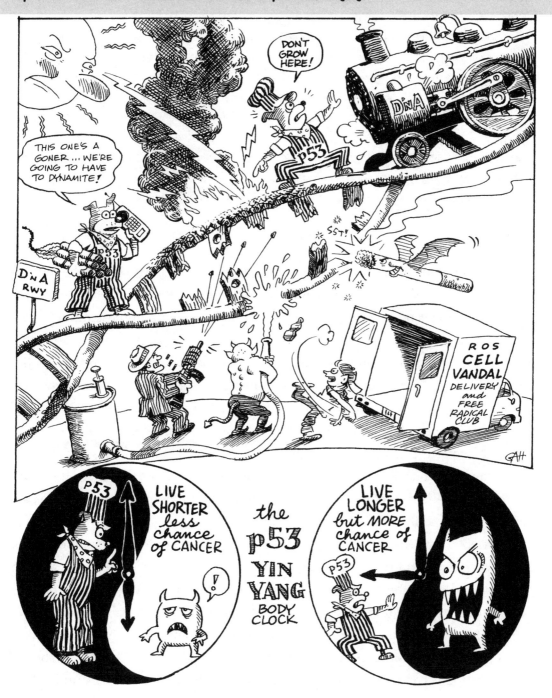

The Chore of Iron

Healthy adults usually have between 3 and 4 grams of iron in their bodies, mostly in the bloodstream. We're most vulnerable to infection at sites where germs can enter our bodies. In an adult without broken skin, that means the mouth, eyes, ears, and genitals. And because infectious agents need iron to survive, all those openings have been declared iron no-fly zones by our bodies. On top of that, those openings are patrolled by chelators—proteins that lock up iron molecules and prevent them from being used. Everything from tears to saliva to mucus—all the fluids in those bodily entry points—is rich with chelators. When we have illnesses like cancer, our immune system kicks into high gear and fights back with what is called the acute phase response. The bloodstream is flooded with illness-fighting proteins, and, at the same time, iron is locked away to prevent biological invaders from using it against us. We actually become anemic from chronic disease; not even our blood cells can gain access to this treasure of iron. It's the biological equivalent of a prison lockdown, and it's one of the reasons why people recovering from cancer may want to avoid iron, unless they are seriously anemic.

occur: accelerated cell growth and division, and increased errors in DNA replication. The importance: Over 50 percent of cancers have defective p53.

For a cell to become cancerous, it must usually have both of these mutations (a car won't move if it only has the brake released or if it only has the gas pedal pressed with the brake down). Unfortunately, having one of these mutations (in, say, p53) actually increases a cell's risk of having the second kind of mutation.

One of the ways we keep potential cancer cells in check is through that guard dog, the p53 gene, which works primarily to protect healthy cells when they're dividing. Normally, protein made by the p53 gene exists at low levels and lives in your cytoplasm, but it moves into the nucleus when it knows that the cell is coming under serious risk—kind of like the guard dog moving from the back of the police cruiser and into a ready-for-anything position.

If the p53 protein senses something suspicious is going down—like one of those typographical errors—it takes a time-out and stops the cell reproduction process. That gives the DNA a chance to be repaired. If, however, it can't be repaired, then the cell commits suicide (apoptosis). Call it extra-value biology. You either get the damaged cell repaired or you kill off the little bugger, so your body doesn't waste any more precious energy on it. The effect: That repair-or-die process prevents cancer by not allowing defective cells to reproduce. Sounds like a perfect system—fix the problem or kill it off, and have your cells live as happy as a bird with a bowl of worms.

Not so fast.

Just as an overaggressive guard dog or a guard dog too tempted by nearby peanut-butter treats can go bad, so can your p53 protein. It can be too aggressive, even though on the surface it's doing the right thing. In your body, the p53 gets too aggressive by killing off perfectly good cells and inducing the state of gradual organ wear and tear that contributes to aging and frailty. In strokes, much of the damage is actually done not by the deprivation of oxygen due to an artery's being cut off, but by the restoration of blood flow once it opens up. This restoration causes a misactivation of p53 and kills cells that are essentially normal. (One thing that happens when you go to an aggressive hospital within the first hour after a stroke: After they open up your artery, they'll inject a substance to temporarily turn off your p53, so you'll have your brain function preserved.)

Sometimes p53 can become overstimulated and halt replication in your progenitor cells (another name, you'll remember, for your adult stem cells), which is a bad thing—especially when you're older and don't have as many progenitor cells to help revitalize your organs. By stopping reproduction of progenitor cells, you reduce the ability of your body to repopulate organs, meaning you may end up without enough cells in your lungs or liver or kidney or anywhere else, for that matter. Lack of these progenitor cells equals less repaired organs.

That's especially important as you age, because progenitor cells are also prone to oxidative stress—making your p53 even more dangerous. In rats with elevated p53 action, for example, life expectancy is 20 percent shorter, and it also comes with a side order of old-age symptoms like muscle atrophy, thin skin, and hunched backs.

In a perfect world, you'd be able to train the perfect guard dog; kill the cancers and let the progenitor cells through. Chomp on the calves of the cancer cells and nicely sniff the stem cells on their way to their job. But p53 doesn't always follow our ideal model. Sometimes it's not active enough (increasing your risk of cancer), and sometimes it's more aggressive than a German shepherd with its crosshairs on a drug smuggler (increasing your risk of dying from frailty).

Skin Savers

Serving as our biological suit of armor, our skin is certainly vulnerable to its share of cancerous chinks. The majority of skin cancer, which originates from the Major Ager of UV radiation (see more on how UV radiation damages our skin and eyes on page 252), comes in the form of basal cell or squamous cell cancers. Related to excessive sun exposure (which is why most of us will never get them on our buttocks), these cancers are rarely fatal and can be simply removed as long as you catch them early. The other kind of cancer, melanoma, is related to sunburns, as opposed to long-term exposure, and it's much more dangerous.

   Interesting note: The majority of skin cancers occur on the left side of the face. Why? Driving. The trend these days is to have bigger windows and moon roofs. Makes sense, especially when you consider that driver's side windows aren't tinted. (UV protection with tinting occurred only in the last five years.) You should try to keep your window up while driving (it's energy saving as well), and make sure to wear sunblock even if you're in the car. The windows block only one kind of UV ray: the UVA kind, not UVB rays. It's smart to have a yearly checkup by a dermatologist so she can look for spots and blemishes that could be cancerous. But don't simply rely on professionals. Monitor your own body, looking for any changes in your skin. It's not a bad idea to take digital photos of your various marks, so that you and your doc can detect changes and compare marks from year to year.

One example of how this works is in people with what's called Li-Fraumeni syndrome. People with this rare syndrome have a mutant p53 gene—it's like having their guard dog asleep at the gate. Half the people with this syndrome develop cancer by age thirty, compared to 1 percent of the regular population. On the other extreme, having the perfect model of p53 (in other words, an aggressive one) means that you increase the risk of death from frailty. Most of us know the basic things we can do to prevent cancer, like stopping smoking and using sunscreen. We actually have the ability to reduce the risk of cancer ourselves, so that we may not have to rely on p53 as much.

In the grand scheme of aging, our ultimate goal may be to strike a balance so that we can turn down our p53s a notch or two; just enough to reduce the risks of frailty that come with an overactive one, but not so much as to leave us at an increased risk of developing cancer.

YOU TIPS!

While a wide-open frontier of medicine is finding cures for cancers, our job in the meantime is to avoid getting them in the first place. Of course, genetics plays a large role, but that doesn't mean that you're simply a card in a game of cancerous blackjack. Luck doesn't determine everything; in fact, we'd argue that you have enough control to make sure it doesn't. The main thing you can do to decrease your chances of cancer is reduce the repetitive injury to your normal cells—so that there's less chance that p53 will make a mistake and allow cancer to kill off a weakened but necessary cell, and then grow and spread. How do you do that? By being aware and taking steps to protect yourself against many of the Major Agers that we have already discussed, such as toxins, infections, mitochondrial damage from oxygen free radicals, and genetic defects. In addition, take these steps to help prevent the birth (and spread) of cancer cells.

YOU Tip: Get the Aspirin Advantage. One of the greatest things you can do for your health takes literally a half second. If that's not incentive, we don't know what is. A half second a day can translate into extra years of life. Taking 162 milligrams of aspirin a day (that's two baby aspirins or half a regular, taken with a half glass of warm water before and after) can decrease the risk of getting colon cancer, esophageal cancer, prostate cancer, ovarian cancer, and breast cancer—all by 40 percent. And it probably decreases the risk of stomach, throat, and several other cancers as well. Aspirin provides this through the reduction of inflammation throughout the body, although other cell repair mechanisms may be active as well. We know aspirin has side effects, but the benefits—a younger arterial system and a decreased risk of at least four big cancers—often outweigh the risks. So discuss with your doc whether it's worth it to you.

YOU Tip: Fortify Yourself with D. Vitamin D decreases the risk of cancer, perhaps because it's toxic to cancer cells. The other theory is that D bolsters the ability of the guard dog p53 gene to spot cancerous cells and kill them. Most Americans don't get enough D because we're indoors most of the time, and when we're outdoors, we're wearing sunscreen. We recommend getting 800 IU a day if you're younger than sixty and 1,000 IU if you're over sixty. You can do it through supplements or food (though you probably won't get more than 300 or so IUs through food alone, so supplementation is smart). Getting some sunlight, ideally around twenty minutes daily of direct exposure, is also protective. You cannot get enough sun in most of the U.S. and all of Canada between October 1 and April 15 to turn inactive vitamin D into active vitamin D. So we recommend you get insurance D in foods supplemented with vitamin D_3 or in supplements. Don't get more than 2,000 IUs a day.

YOU Tip: Protect Your Liver. Since your liver is your main detox organ, you're smart to keep it performing at its best. Certain foods and supplements can help improve liver function and have anticancer properties.

Liver detox systems are enhanced by broccoli sprouts, seaweed, and dark greens, and are proven to reduce the risk of cancer at various sites, including the prostate, lung, breast, and colon. How? These cruciferous vegetables rev up detoxifying enzymes at the genetic level. Other things that have been shown to improve liver health include choline (which can be found in these cruciferous vegetables), as well as N-acetyl-cysteine (600 milligrams per day), milk thistle (200 milligrams per day), lecithin (1 tablespoon daily), and rosemary extract (150 milligrams per day).

YOU Tip: B Protected. Research shows that a deficiency of folate, part of the B complex of vitamins, is linked to cancer. Folate supplementation decreases colon cancer rates by 20 percent to 50 percent, but more than 50 percent of Americans don't even get the recommended amount, and 90 percent don't get the amount that seems to reduce colon cancer (800 micrograms a day). Lots of foods—like spinach, tomatoes, and orange juice—contain folate, but it's absorbed less well than folic acid from supplements. The average intake of folate through food is 275 to 375 micrograms, so you need a supplement of about 400 micrograms to reduce your risk of cancer. That's especially important if you're allowing sun exposure to deplete your folate levels, which happens when you get more than twenty minutes of sun exposure a day. Be sure to add B_6 and crystalline B_{12} (see the YOU Extended Warranty Plan on page 313).

YOU Tip: Get Sauced. As if your grandmother's spaghetti sauce recipe weren't enough incentive. Studies show that the risk of developing certain cancers decreases when you eat ten or more tablespoons a week of tomato sauce. Many believe that the active ingredient responsible is lycopene, a carotenoid known for its antioxidant properties. All tomato products contains lots of lycopene, but it's more available to your body when it's cooked. While you're at it, add some cruciferous vegetables like broccoli to your sauce. They contain chemicals that prevent cancer.

YOU Tip: Oil On. In a test of olive oils, researchers found anticarcinogenic properties in monounsaturated fat. That would mean that olive oil, rich in monounsaturated fat, is not only a heart helper but may also deter cancer. That helps explain why, compared to northern Europeans, southern Europeans, whose diets tend to overflow with the oil, have lower rates of both heart disease and cancer.

YOU Tip: Tea It Up. Green tea has been shown to have the highest content of polyphenols, which are chemicals with potent antioxidant properties (believed to be greater than even vitamin C). They give tea its bitter flavor. Because green tea leaves are young and have not been oxidized, green tea has up to 40 percent polyphenols, while black tea contains only about 10 percent. Another interesting note: Green tea has one-third the caffeine of black tea. Even better, it's been shown to yield the same level of excitement and attentiveness, but in more even levels than the ups and downs associated with other caffeinated drinks. Just don't drink milk with it; the casein in milk has been shown to inhibit the beneficial effects of tea.

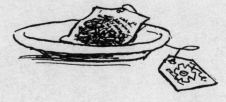

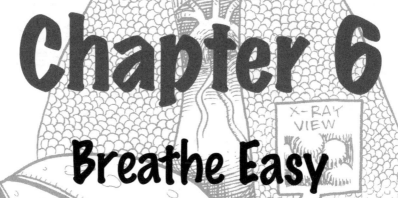

Chapter 6
Breathe Easy

X-RAY VIEW

YOU Test: Young Lungs

How fit are your lungs? Run briskly up two flights of stairs or walk six blocks. If you can do either of those without pausing to rest, your lungs are probably in pretty good shape. If you experience extreme shortness of breath or have to stop, it's a sign that your lungs are suffering at least some distress, even if it's the heart's fault. We recommend that you do this test every month (check with your doc first), as a way of periodically checking your lung function. That's important, because one of the major warning signs of decreased lung function is seeing even slight changes in your ability to complete the test. When you exercise, shortness of breath means that all your organs are not acting their best.

Ravioli

CO_2

ood Ce

Walls One Cell Thic

HALL
OREH

You don't have to be a phone-sex operator to know that there are times when heavy breathing feels pretty darn good. Like when you're playing a sport that you love or fooling around with someone you love. Those are the times when we appreciate all the sensations that go with a racing heart and tingling nerve endings. But when it comes to heavy breathing, the question really is how to differentiate between the sensation that goes with exercise, sex, and normal avoidance of an attacker, and one that's associated with a chronic medical problem. Sometimes that distinction can be tough to interpret. Like pain, breathlessness can be difficult to describe, but we certainly know the extreme example. No breath, no life. Somewhere in the middle, between having no air and breathing in clear, rich, and wonderful air, you can live in a respiratory world of coughing, wheezing, and struggling to get the oxygen you need. While your lungs may often play third fiddle to your heart and arterial system in the cardiorespiratory orchestra, it's also clear that having healthy lungs means more than just being able to shout "Sox Stink!" so everyone in three counties can hear you.

The reason why lung disease is one of the top six causes of aging, according to our government, is that we are continually renewing the very thin and sensitive cells in the lungs so that we can exchange oxygen and carbon dioxide. As the stem cells that regenerate these cells start to slow down, the renewal process lags, and the lungs scar (a process called fibrosis) and become resistant to air exchange. The Major Ager of shortened telomeres also slows down our stem cells, so the damage is compounded. The process of breathing is kind of like taking sandpaper to your lungs. But with fibrosis, the lungs are rough like cement. You can get the smoother, varnish-like lining you want by eliminating some of the risk factors, like smoking, high blood pressure, and diabetes.

Now, one of the most common complaints with aging is shortness of breath; much of this is caused by

> **FACTOID**
>
> Don't underestimate the power of treating seemingly trivial problems like sinus conditions, allergies, and acid reflux disease, which can all cause the symptom of shortness of breath. Treating them with over-the-counter medications can greatly improve your overall quality of breathing.

changes in the elasticity of the lung (so it takes more effort to bring in air) and by physiological changes in your lungs that make breathing harder. Much of this happens because of the Major Ager of toxins in our environment, like secondhand smoke and pollution, which pass into us most easily in the air we breathe (several liters per minute).

The rate of aging of the lungs is, in fact, greater than the aging of the heart. So while some shortness of breath is associated with cardiac troubles, that's not always the case—and breathing problems can indeed originate from the lungs.

Your Lungs: Breathing Easy

One of the best ways to understand lungs and breathlessness is by understanding the relationship between what comes in (oxygen) and what goes out (carbon dioxide) and how your lungs handle each. To see how that relationship works, let's look at exercise.

Muscles working hard during exercise need more oxygen, and they also produce more carbon dioxide. Special cells in the main arteries and brain stem detect those levels of oxygen and carbon dioxide, and these send signals to the brain and heart to increase breathing and pulse rates. This means that more blood is pumped throughout the body, picking up more carbon dioxide from the muscles, to be released in the lungs to be breathed out, and picking up more oxygen there to deliver to the muscles.

In a healthy person, physical fitness determines the point at which you experience breathlessness. The more regular physical exercise your body is used to, the more efficient your muscles are. They'll use oxygen better and create less carbon dioxide, and the lungs and heart will end up being more efficient too. This is why a fit person can do more exercise without getting breathless than an unfit person can.

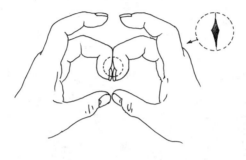
How does that relate to lung disease? Well, certain illnesses can mimic the effects of being unfit, but, unfortunately, at much lower levels of exertion than simple exercise, so that even crossing a room, getting the mail, or doing a lap around the coffee table can lead to major huffing and puffing.

To understand all of the ways that damage to your lungs can keep you from having a good air-exchange rate, it will help to think about the structure of lungs (see Figure 6.1). Functioning like sponges, your lungs are light and fluffy when filled with air, but when they get wet (as they do with some diseases), they get bogged down and don't exchange air very well. Imagine your respiratory system as an upside-down tree. When air enters the body, it goes down your windpipe, or trachea, the trunk of the tree. The trachea quickly divides into two airways to feed into the lungs; those are the bronchi. Then, like tree branches, those airways break off into four, then eight, then hundreds of thousands of little airways in each lung. Those air-

Figure 6.1 **Puff Stuff** Healthy lungs have hundreds of millions of alveoli; they're covered with a thin layer of fluid that helps you breathe by keeping the alveoli open so that oxygen is absorbed into the blood in the capillary and carbon dioxide is excreted. As you get older, that covering gets thicker—making it harder for you to breathe.

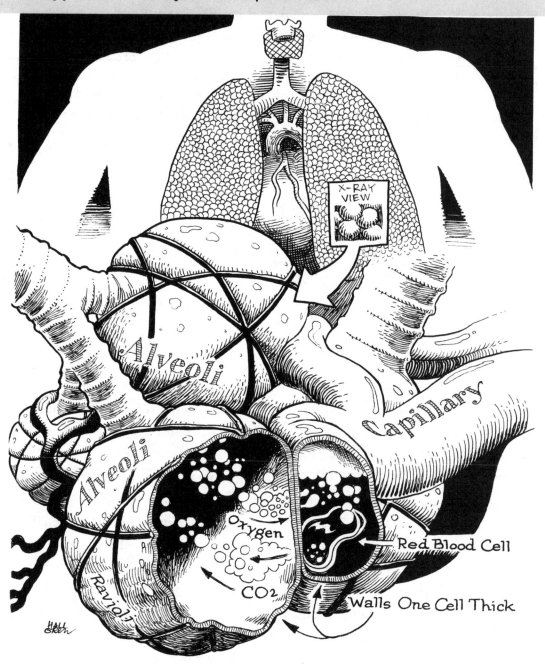

ways are your bronchial tubes, and at the end of each airway are tiny sacs called alveoli—they're like the leaves at the end of the branches, except they are small, open sacs. Healthy lungs have hundreds of millions of alveoli and are covered with a thin layer of fluid that helps you breathe by keeping the alveoli open so oxygen can be absorbed and carbon dioxide excreted.

At the bottom of your chest cavity—between your lung and your abdomen—is a large muscle, the diaphragm, which acts like a vacuum motor to pull air down into your lungs. In addition, the smooth muscle in the bronchial wall aids breathing. When you inhale, the bronchial tubes (air passages) dilate. When you exhale, they constrict.

For the perfect breathing process to happen, all of those structures should be clean and free of such air stoppers as smoke and other toxins. Your bronchial tubes are generally coated with mucus, which traps germs and dirt. Your lungs also have millions of tiny hairs called cilia, which act like little brooms that sweep up the stuff that's caught in the mucus. You then cough it out. One of the hazards of smoke, especially from cigars, cigarettes, or joints, is that it kills cilia, essentially destroying the very mechanism that's meant to protect your lungs from toxins. Restoring those cilia is one of the reasons that cigarette quitters cough more when they first stop; they're starting to sweep out all the junk in their lungs.

Unfortunately, as we age, structural changes occur in the lungs and other components of the respiratory system: They lose some of their elasticity, the chest wall stiffens, the alveoli's surface area decreases, and your respiratory muscles weaken. The result: a measurable decrease in airflow. Add on the fact that lung problems like asthma or bronchitis can restrict airflow by making the bronchial passages functionally narrower, and you can soon find yourself with more breathing problems.

One of the key players in lung health is the vagus nerve. When the lung ex-

Stop Panic Attacks

People panic for all kinds of reasons: driving in snow, taking a test, leaving a purse on the subway. One of the big causes of panic attacks is, rightly, having trouble breathing—and that triggers a vicious cycle in which anxiety aggravates breathlessness and breathlessness in turn creates further anxiety. Some patients experience such a severe case that they're convinced they're about to die. The strategy for these people is to slow down and regain control: Stop, purse your lips, and drop your shoulders.

pands during normal shallow breathing, that stimulates the vagus nerve. The vagus nerve then sends a message to the brain to constrict the bronchi, making breathing more difficult. That's really one of the reasons why deep breathing helps, uh, deep breathing. Meditation functionally serves to physiologically cut the vagus, so it disrupts the feedback loop of bronchial constriction, allowing you to breathe easier.

And that's crucial. Deep breathing may seem like a froufrou exercise, or like something you do only if you're in tights and carrying a yoga mat. But deep nasal breathing isn't just for yoga rooms and massage tables. *Dee-ee-ee-ee-ee-ee-ee-p brea-ea-ea-ea-ea-ea-ea-ea-thing* helps transport nitric oxide (see page 228)—a very potent lung and blood vessel dilator that resides in your nasal passages—to your lungs. And since it's located in the highest concentration in the back of your nose, deep breathing is also the best way to increase NO to help your lungs and blood vessels open up better and function more efficiently. Essentially, taking deep breaths helps your lungs go from 97 percent saturation of oxygen to 100 percent saturation of oxygen, and that little 3 percent can sometimes make a difference in how you feel.

While we're certainly concerned about *how* you breathe in, we're also concerned about *what* you breathe in. As one of only three ways the inside of your body interacts with the outside world (skin and intestines are the others), your lungs can be exposed to a great deal of nasty toxins. The outdoor pollutants that mostly affect your lung health appear to be ozone, carbon monoxide, nitrogen dioxide, sulfur dioxide, and lead. Others include dioxins, asbestos, and particulate matter (those are the particles produced by the combustion of diesel, gasoline, and other fuels, and tobacco smoke). Air pollution caused by particulate matter so small that it can't be seen is what aggravates and leads to respiratory (and cardiovascular) problems—and even death. How? Particles from the polluted air that are too small to be filtered out by the cilia travel deep into the lungs. Though the immune system responds to those foreign particles, those particles do a number on immune function, allowing infections to occur and asthma to develop.

One of the reasons we know this happens: Due to a labor dispute, the single largest pollution source in a Utah valley, an old integrated steel mill, operated intermittently. When the mill was operating, pollutants contributed to increased asthma and other severe respiratory problems, and increased deaths. When the mill stopped working, the number of problems and deaths dropped, and not by a little, but by more than 50 percent in a three-month period. And, of course, when the strike was settled and the pollution resumed, the respiratory illnesses and the deaths increased by over 50 percent.

Many people are rats in someone else's experiment if they live close to a freeway, where small particles roam the air and increase lung problems, especially for young children and their stay-at-home mothers, who don't escape to the safety of the workplace. You should also note that a similar damaging effect can happen when you're exposed to indoor pollutants like radon, asbestos, mite dust, and mold. Molds, for instance, produce mycotoxins, which weaken or kill the things they live on or compete with. Short-term exposure can cause breathing problems, and the research indicates that long-term exposure may also be linked to cancer.

YOU Tool: Quit Smoking

1. Start walking thirty minutes every day—no excuses, every day. Start this on day one: one month before quitting.
2. Talk to your doctor about getting prescriptions for bupropion* 100-milligram tablets and nicotine patches (21- or 22-milligram patches if you have a one-pack-a-day habit). Ask your doctor for adjustments if you smoke more than one pack a day. Fill prescriptions.
3. On day thirty (two days before you plan to stop smoking), take one bupropion.
4. Next two days, take one bupropion each morning.
5. On day thirty-two (stop day), place one patch on your arm, chest, or thigh (do so daily), in addition to your morning bupropion. (Take it off every day, bucko.)
6. On all subsequent days, take one bupropion each morning and evening, and place one patch on your arm, chest, or thigh.
7. Continue walking thirty to forty-five minutes each day; feel free to drink as much coffee or water as you wish.
8. List your daily activities.
9. Phone or e-mail a support person daily to discuss your progress.
10. Begin weight lifting on day sixty-two. Do not increase your physical activities by more than 10 percent a week.
11. Decrease patch size by one-third every two months until at six months you are patch free.
12. Decrease to one bupropion in the evening after six months, and eliminate that one at twelve months.
13. Carry one bupropion tablet with you at all times to take if you feel a craving. If the craving hits, take the bupropion, wait thirty minutes before you light up, and call your support person.

Our goal here is for you to take the steps necessary to keep your lungs clear and fluffy, so that any heavy breathing you do is associated with having fun—not slowing you down.

* The drug Chantix (varenicline) blocks the nicotine receptors. So smokers who use Chantix to help quit don't get the euphoria from the nicotine and just end up stopping. Chantix should not be taken with nicotine.

YOU TIPS!

Of course, you know the cardinal rule for protecting your lungs: no smoking. We're not going to spend much time talking about the danger of cigarette smoke because that would be like talking about the danger of swimming in a shark cage with a bloody nose; it's obvious. (See our YOU Tool on the opposite page for details about how to quit.) But we do want to give you steps you can take to improve your lung health and your breathing.

YOU Tip: Take Ten. Lie on your back flat on the floor, with one hand on your belly and one hand on your chest. Take a deep breath in—slowly. Lying on the floor at first when you practice is important, because if you stand up, you're more likely to fake a deep breath by doing an exaggerated chest extension, rather than letting it fill up naturally. Imagine your lungs filling up with air; it should take about five seconds to inhale. As your diaphragm pulls down your chest cavity, your belly button should move away from your spine as you fill with air. Your chest will also widen and maybe rise ever so slightly as you inhale. When your lungs feel full, exhale slowly—taking about seven seconds to let all the air out. Our recommendation: Take ten deep breaths in the morning, ten at night, and as many as you need in between to help relieve stress.

YOU Tip: Get Away from the Road. That is, if you live too close to a freeway or major road. One of the strongest toxins in the air—PM2.5—nearly doubles the risk of death stemming from respiratory causes. The biggest factor for PM2.5 other than mites inside your home: traffic density. That's why we recommend that you live at least one hundred meters and preferably three hundred meters from a major road (three hundred meters is about the size of three football fields). At the same time, encourage tougher government standards on pollution by writing the Environmental Protection Agency (EPA), your senator, and your representative. More stringent guidelines for certain pollution (particles in the 2.5-to-10-micron range, often produced by coal plants and diesel fuel) provide reasonable goals for most urban environments.

YOU Tip: Take Supplements. Magnesium, a mineral that relaxes the bronchial tubes, can help with asthma. Take 400 milligrams a day. If you routinely produce mucus from your lungs (you cough it up, rather than mucus coming out when you blow your nose, which is usually from a sinus condition), consider N-acetyl-cysteine. It's a substance that loosens mucus and boosts production of one of your natural antioxidant scavengers called glutathione, which helps prevent damage in lung tissue. We recommend 600 milligrams daily. Even caffeine can help people with asthma; it seems to stabilize and shrink the lining of the airways and dilate bronchial tubes to help make breathing easier.

YOU Tip: Get Fruit Looped. A diet rich in fruits, vegetables, fish, and whole-grain foods offers protection against chronic lung disease, as well as a lot of other aging-related diseases. But unlike lots of other examples, we're not exactly sure why. Nevertheless, the difference in lung disease rates between folks on the highest- versus lowest-quality diets was almost fivefold. So even if you are gasping, go for the nutritious goodies.

Glycosylation

How Excess Glucose Can Age You

Most of us can spot the obvious signs of aging: hair that's thinner than a super-model's waist, body parts that give in to gravity, and joints that creak louder than old farmhouse floors. While all those changes may be as obvious as they are painful, you should have learned by now that outward signs of aging are really symptoms of changes that occur at a molecular level deep inside your body.

While it sounds like something you order up at Jiffy Lube for $39.95, glycosy-lation is one of the best examples of a biochemical process that has dramatic phys-ical effects.

Simply, glycosylation occurs when sugar molecules (glucose) floating around in our blood attach to protein molecules, diminishing their effectiveness and causing inflammation. This process, which increases as we age, happens so readily that it doesn't even require a specific enzyme to push it ahead. That's also why glycosy-lation is so dangerous (see Figure F.1). Normally, glucose is what gives our cells energy, but when we develop insulin resistance (from having a genetic predispo-sition such as a family history of type 2 diabetes or from being overweight), the

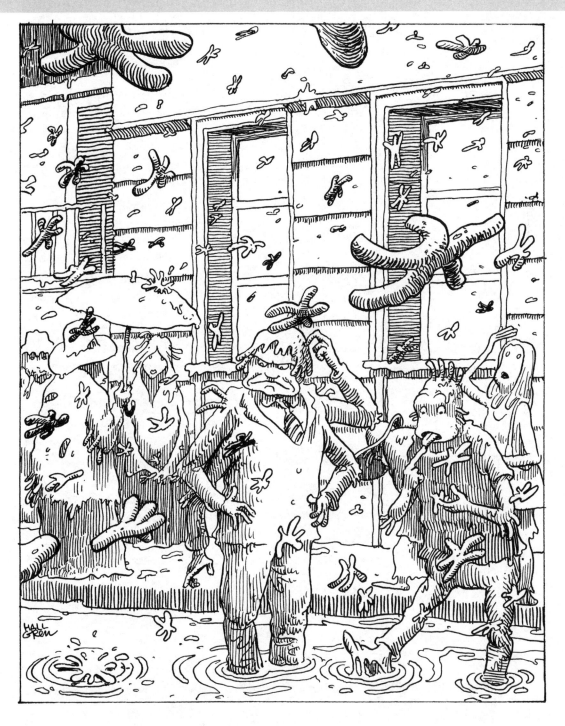

Major Ager: Glycosylation 137

insulin can't effectively get all the glucose into our cells. If glucose can't get into a cell, it stays in the blood and gunks up the proteins in our body. It's a little bit like acid rain—it damages the things it touches and makes them leaky.

When extra glucose latches onto another molecule on the outside of a cell, the extra glucose handcuffs that molecule and prevents it from doing its job well (see Figure F.2). Even science nicknames the effects of glucose on protein "aging": These glucose-modified proteins are termed advanced glycosylation end products (AGE is an appropriate acronym, because they actually age us). The receptors for glycosylated proteins (called RAGE) are major targets for new drugs to slow down the complications of diabetes, including blindness, kidney damage, nerve damage, and heart disease (see Figure F.3).

Glycosylation Is the Source of Many Aging-Related Problems

Depending on where glycosylation occurs, it can have a variety of effects on your body. When that glucose attaches to a protein, the altered molecular structure creates these changes:

In the blood: Normally, you have a very tight junction between the endothelial cells in your arterial wall, so that, like a happily married couple, nothing can get between them. But glycosylation weakens that junction between cells and makes them leaky and vulnerable to tears. The body repairs those tears by plugging them with cholesterol, which causes plaque in your arterial walls.

In the lens of the eye: When glucose attaches to proteins in the lens of the eye, it changes the lens cells from crystal clear to a little cloudy. A lot of that cloudiness leads to vision impairment that we call cataract formation. When glycosylation occurs in the tiny blood vessels in the back of the eye, they become fragile and leaky, and bleeding can occur in a condition called diabetic retinopathy, a leading cause of blindness.

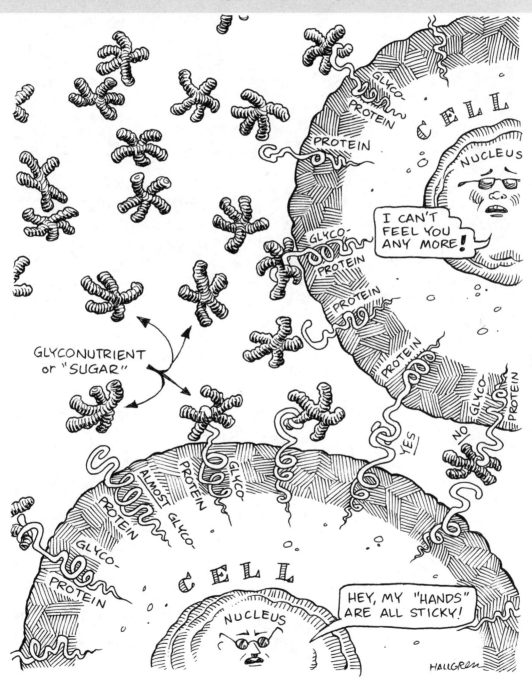

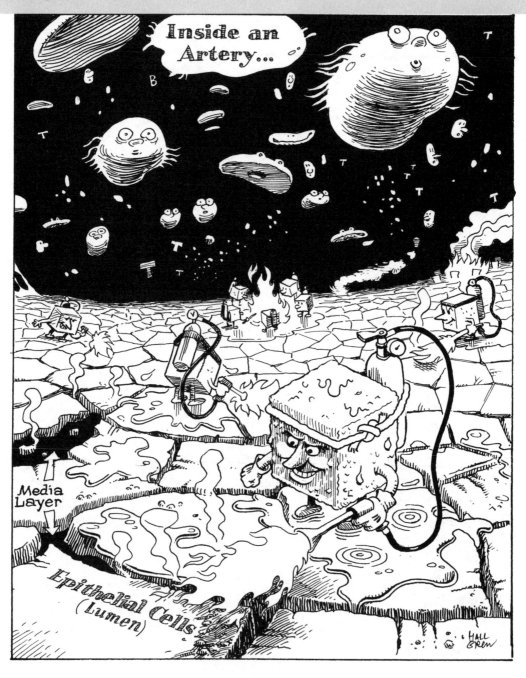

In the skin: With the glycosylation of collagen, the collagen in your skin becomes less elastic and stiffer than a happy-hour martini.

In your connective tissues: When glucose attaches to collagen in your connective tissues, you end up with less elasticity. You need collagen for the smooth functioning of joints. High blood sugar magnifies all aches and pains and can lead to impaired joint movement—and eventually arthritis.

In your lungs: The glycosylation of collagen results in abnormal recoil of the elastic tissue, so you have trouble getting the air out as well as in. This occurs slowly in lung connective tissue, but forty years of high glucose levels often lead to respiratory failure—the inability to get enough oxygen into your blood without the use of an oxygen tank.

Glycosylation Messes with Your BP

Your body has a way of self-regulating your blood pressure to deal with fluctuations throughout the day. For example, when you exercise, your body knows to dilate certain blood vessels to get more blood to your muscles. When you think, the arteries open up (a little) to your brain. If you get really upset about something (that the dog stained the carpet, the boss piled on more work, or the Dodgers blew a big lead), your blood pressure goes up (it might go from 115/75 to 220/130). But while that pressure of blood flow may be up in one area of your body (say, near your heart), other parts of your body (say, near the kidney) open up the arteries to ease the flow of blood there and keep your overall blood pressure from going bonkers. So instead of 220/130, it goes only to 125/82. That balancing act is called autoregulation and keeps your blood pressure relatively normal. But excess blood glucose negates and destroys this autoregulation system, thus taxing your arteries more heavily.

Glycosylation Causes Nerve Injury

When glucose gets inside your nerve cells, that causes big molecules to be built (sorbitol is one, for you crossword whizzes). Not only can't these get out of cells easily, but they attract water to those cells, causing them to get bigger. Big cells may be good for prisoners, but not for your body. Why? Those big nerve cells get compressed by the tight myelin sheath that surrounds them (kind of like trying to put more tomatoes in that little bitty can—the tomatoes break apart), eventually damaging those nerves. That's the long-nerve dysfunction that diabetics often get, when they aren't able to sense their feet normally. This is called stocking-glove nerve dysfunction; you lose sensation in all areas covered by a stocking or glove. Peripheral neuropathy is a major cause of foot ulcers that can lead to amputation in some people with poorly controlled diabetes. (If you can't feel your feet, you're more likely to injure them and then get infections in the injury.)

Like pollution in our metaphorical aging city, glycosylation—resulting from the diabetes we'll discuss in the next chapter—affects our proudest organs, our most critical thoroughfares, and our most beautiful traits. Its insidious nature makes it that much more dangerous.

Chapter 7
Don't Be Pickled by Diabetes

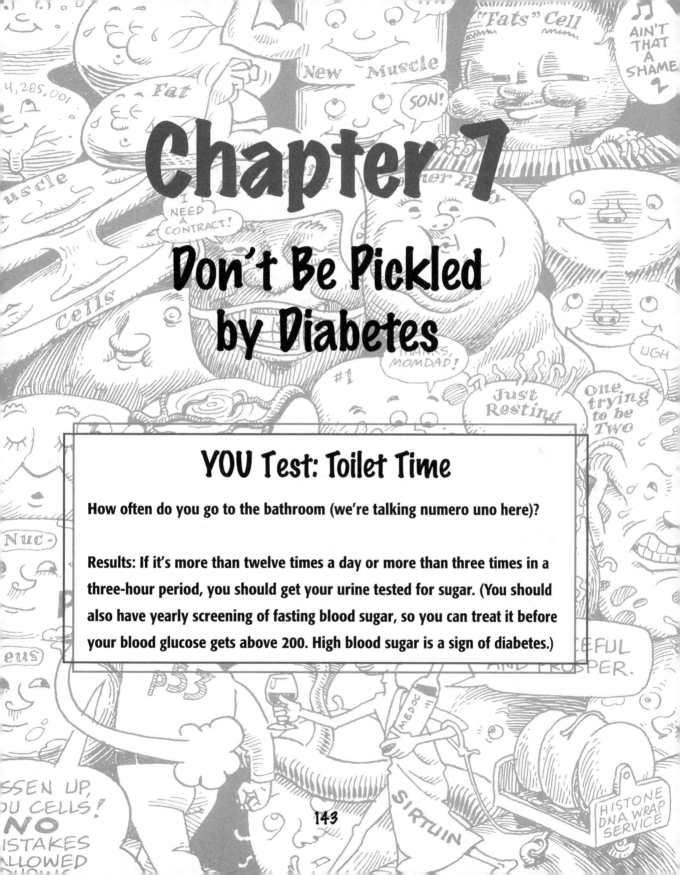

YOU Test: Toilet Time

How often do you go to the bathroom (we're talking numero uno here)?

Results: If it's more than twelve times a day or more than three times in a three-hour period, you should get your urine tested for sugar. (You should also have yearly screening of fasting blood sugar, so you can treat it before your blood glucose gets above 200. High blood sugar is a sign of diabetes.)

Plenty of people, from canoodling celebrities to crooked politicians, have found themselves in some pretty public pickles. When it comes to their health, however, millions of Americans are finding themselves in their own pickles, as they wrestle with the disease of diabetes. That's because when you have diabetes—the disease that's associated with blood sugar and insulin malfunction in overweight people—you're essentially pickling yourself, basting yourself in fluid that has a high concentration of sugar. The difference is that your diabetic pickle doesn't exactly go all that well with a sandwich and some chips.

Diabetes serves as a microcosm of the aging process. In people with poorly controlled diabetes, a variety of degenerative diseases—such as arterial disease, heart disease, premature loss of teeth, and many other conditions—occur earlier and with greater severity than in nondiabetics. How did we get ourselves in this pickle?

In the Stone Age, sugar, fat, and salt were in short supply; our bodies had to store them when we came across them. To help ourselves survive, we adapted to hunger for sugars—literally, we craved them. When our ancestors were fortunate enough to find a batch of juicy berries, they couldn't afford *not* to eat every one in sight, since it might be weeks or months before they stumbled across the next batch.

That worked fine back when there were no grocery stores, fast-food restaurants, and pie-baking grandmothers. Now? Our energy-processing machinery is still geared to life in the Stone Age while our energy supply system is twenty-first century. Because sugar (glucose) was always scarce, we developed a very efficient metabolism that could process small amounts of food and extract the maximum amount of energy. Today diabetes is the result of a fundamental mismatch between our ancestral insides and our modern world outside.

Why is that such a problem? Because the excess sugar we consume today coalesces into a syrupy mixture that coats our organs and creates glasslike shards that can cut up the blood vessels and tissues of our body. The constant wounds of these sugar surges lead to chronic inflammation, which wastes our ability to defend ourselves with false alarms. As a result, we're prone to infections and arterial damage and less able to cope with common stresses we could normally fend off—like hypertension or high cholesterol, or even cigarette smoke.

For a disease like diabetes to develop in the first place, it must have had a selective advantage for those who had it. In the Ice Age, it's theorized, blood sugar actually helped us. High levels of glucose were thought to prevent cells and tissues from forming ice crystals in them (sugar is a natural antifreeze)—meaning that diabetes actually would have prevented those who had it from freezing to death. Since life expectancy was low anyway, these people never had to worry about the long-term complications from diabetes that we have to deal with; it was simply a biological advantage because it protected them long enough to survive the ice, reproduce, and ensure the longevity of the species.

Because our bodies are designed to run on a relatively low level of glucose, when we overeat and indulge in a sedentary lifestyle, we're unable to process the extra glucose—thus pickling ourselves in all the excess—and our metabolic system malfunctions. When one of our systems, called the cannabinoid system (described on page 161), is turned on, hormones in the body block the ability of insulin to get muscle to use sugar, and we accumulate sugar in our bloodstream as our metabolism actually becomes less efficient. Eventually, especially in people with family histories of type 2 diabetes (evidence of a genetic predisposition to the disease), our pancreatic

FACTOID

The diabetes drug metformin (Glucophage and others) helps control and prevent diabetes by helping your muscles use more glucose and getting your liver to stop producing too much glucose (side effects include intestinal problems). The ideal treatment is to get your eating and activity in line and use the drug as a complement until the lifestyle changes kick in. Other promising drugs work through a biological pathway called the cannabinoid system, which we'll discuss in chapter 8.

beta cells, cells that produce insulin, can't keep up because of exhaustion after years of working against the relentless insulin resistance. And that's how we become diabetic.

Your Pancreas: Function and Malfunction

People with diabetes have high blood sugar either because their pancreas doesn't make enough insulin or because their muscles, fat, liver, and other cells close the door on insulin—not allowing it to deliver glucose to them. Type 1 diabetes, which is usually diagnosed in childhood but may be diagnosed at any age, occurs when the pancreas makes no insulin because of an autoimmune assault on the insulin-producing cells. People with type 1 diabetes have to replace their body's production with injections of insulin. Type 2 (formerly known as adult-onset diabetes and the focus of this chapter) is much more common, affecting more than twenty-two million Americans and projected to double by the year 2025. It typically occurs when your cells resist the insulin that comes knocking at their doors, leaving glucose to circulate in your bloodstream instead of being used to fuel your cells.

Essentially, diabetes is a lot like a celebrity look-alike; it is often mistaken for something it's not. A lot of us tend to think that diabetes happens because you eat too much sugar, but the truth is that diabetes happens when you eat too much. Period. Here's how:

All food—no matter whether it's a protein, fat, or carbohydrate—gets broken down into glucose. When you have insulin resistance and you overeat, be it too much meat, potato, or coconut cream pie, the cells in your body are unable to absorb the extra glucose. That causes blood glucose levels to rise higher than a helium-filled balloon. Your blood glucose level is monitored by cells in your pancreas that are the lone producers of insulin, the hormone that transports glucose from the outside to the inside of your cells so your body can transform that glucose into usable energy (see Figure 7.1).

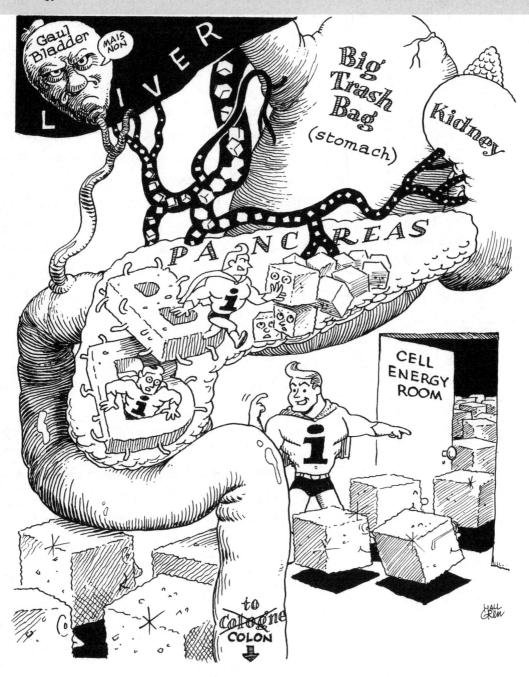

Stop kidding yourself. Research suggests that obese adults with diabetes often say they eat less than they actually do—a problem that can make it hard to manage the disease. On average, diabetic adults reported a calorie intake that was nearly one-quarter lower than they would need even for their most basic bodily functions. Many obese people have inherited abnormalities in the complex pathways that help signal them that they are satiated: They lack the cues to stop eating when they're full. It can help to take small portions and/or to eat only half of what's being served to try to work around this problem with satiety signals. Reducing your food intake a little bit every day (100 calories), which can be done without the insatiable hunger that usually sabotages most diets, will help reduce weight gain and promote weight loss.

When the alarm sounds to make more insulin to help transport the extra blood glucose, the body acts like a chubby runner at the front of a marathon; it just can't keep up. Oh, it huffs and puffs and makes more insulin, but the demand is just too great. A person with type 2 diabetes has lost this glucose-insulin struggle. And so an ugly, vicious cycle begins: It made sense for us to store fat to survive when we were likely to have famines periodically or failed bison hunts, but today that fat causes insulin resistance, which makes us eat more, which causes more fat, which is associated with eating more, so we accumulate more fat, which causes more insulin resistance, and so on.

In the modern world, elevated blood sugars get you frequent-flier miles with your local doctor. Frequent urination and fatigue are symptoms but not important problems like the other effects, such as arthritis, infections, kidney failure, accelerated arterial aging (that's heart attack, strokes, memory problems, and impotence), damage to the peripheral nerves, and the development of vision problems that can cause blindness.

Here's the big surprise for this Major Ager. For most people, grounding your hospital-home type 2 diabetes shuttle is in your control. Just beginning to lose weight will immediately shift your body's response to insulin and melt away the glycosylation. That's why this group of YOU Tips is particularly useful.

YOU TIPS!

It's clear that diabetes is as destructive to our health as hot dog–eating champ Kobayashi is to a plate of frankfurters. In fact, diabetes and its effects can steal one-third of your life. Luckily, if you can do three major things—control your blood pressure, walk thirty minutes a day, and keep your blood sugar within a narrow range—you'll practically eliminate the cardiovascular risk associated with diabetes. And that makes diabetes, though one of the scariest diseases of all, one of the most controllable. You can often manage it yourself without oral medication, and without having to shoot yourself with insulin, if you know the steps to take.

YOU Tip: Get Your Life Under Control. The most important things you can do to lower your risk of diabetes are to keep your waist thin, exercise (thirty minutes daily), and keep your blood pressure under control. High blood pressure can really magnify the effects of diabetes by aging your arteries; both high blood pressure and high blood sugar cause nicks or holes in the arteries' walls that trigger the destructive process of inflammation and result in atherosclerosis. Clogged arteries lack the ability to deliver blood to certain key areas, like the heart, brain, penis, and clitoris, which leads to heart attack, stroke, impotence, and decline of orgasm quality. A little physical activity can dramatically improve the ability of insulin to get glucose into many cells, especially muscle. See the YOU2 Workout on page 366.

YOU Tip: Add These Ingredients. Of course, to prevent diabetes, you have to do the big things right: avoid the buffet and stop planting yourself on the couch for six hours every evening. But little things count too. Ginseng, cinnamon, and tea have been shown to help increase insulin receptivity, which can help lower the risk of aging from diabetes. Some studies have shown that one of the substances in ginseng berries (not the root) and a half teaspoon of cinnamon a day can increase insulin receptivity by over 50 percent. The supplement chromium (at 200 mcg a day) has been shown to increase sensitivity to insulin as well. If you get diabetes, all is not lost. A small amount of weight loss can make the difference between elevated blood sugar and normal blood sugar. Keeping your blood sugar and your A1c level (a test that shows a three-month average blood sugar) in the normal range are among the most important things you can do. Diet, exercise, and medications can be combined to keep glucose and A1c levels normal.

YOU Tip: Drink Coffee. Research shows that coffee can decrease insulin resistance and decrease the development of diabetes by 25 percent. But watch the sugar: People who add sugar to coffee or tea don't benefit and run a higher risk of developing cancer of the pancreas. The risk of developing pancreatic cancer is related in part to the amount of sugar in the diet. Studies show that people who drink fizzy or syrup-based drinks twice a day or more run a 90 percent higher risk of getting cancer of the pancreas than those who never drink them.

YOU Tip: See the Chia. Chia pets may have no apparent purpose, but chia seed? Now, that's something to get excited about. Chia—a harvested, unprocessed, nutty-tasting, nutrient-dense whole grain with omega-3 fatty acids—has among the highest antioxidant activity of any whole food, outdistancing even fresh blueberries. One study showed that 30 grams of chia seed taken with bread decreased the sharp blood sugar spike seen an hour after eating. Another study showed that chia lowers blood pressure and the risk of heart problems. Our recommendation: two daily doses of about 20 grams of seeds each.

Calorie Consumption & Slowing Sirtuin

Understand the Ultimate Anti-Agers

The greatest year for aging Americans: 1935. That April, it was found that the lifespan of laboratory rats could be extended considerably by putting them on a serious calorie-restricted diet. Perhaps in response to this discovery, Congress inked the Social Security Act into law six months later.

You'd think the rats would have been ecstatic. Living longer, plus retirement income. But no! Although they were living longer, the rats complained that their quality of life had declined (probably because of the lack of golf courses or bingo). But since calories represent energy and energy is required to function, it wasn't surprising that the rats were tired all the time. What is surprising, though, is that their sluggishness passed.

After a few months, the rats felt their strength returning. The spring was back in their crawl. They were spending more and more time running on their little rat treadmills. This didn't seem to make any sense. Their miracle diet cut the amount of calories the rats were eating by more than 30 percent. That large a cutback not only should have caused the rodent version of chronic fatigue syndrome but should have left the rats with less energy available to fight the aging process. If anything, the rats should have been dying sooner and feeling dead the rest of the time. But this wasn't happening. The rats were living 50 percent *longer* than before and seemed to be loving every minute. Had the rodents discovered the rat chow version of the fountain of youth?

The first clue came from looking at their food plan. Instead of daydreaming about how good they were going to look in a bathing suit, the rats were focused on basic survival. Instead of "diet," the rats' bodies had interpreted the calorie cutback as a famine. And when the famine alarm was sounded, the rats shifted into survival mode.

To understand the ins and outs of the rats' survival/longevity plan, let's shift our attention from rodent to roadway. To learn how stressed-out rats pack on the years, let's take a quick look at how a stressed-out driver might respond in a similar situation. Instead of rat longevity, let's talk about car longevity.

The life span of a car can be measured not only in years but in miles. So, for argument's sake, let's assume that you get only one tank of gas during your car's lifetime, and it comes with a twenty-gallon tank. One car may "live" for 500 miles—25 miles per gallon on a twenty-gallon tank.

Now let's put your car on an energy-restricted diet. This means that instead of twenty gallons, you now get only fourteen (30 percent less). To replicate the rats' antiaging accomplishment, you have to be able to drive not just 500 miles with those fourteen gallons but 750 miles (50 percent longer life). What would you have to do to drive 50 percent farther with 30 percent less gas?

The first thing you'd probably do is get rid of any excess weight; no cargo carriers, no bike racks, no fuzzy dice. Then you might start shutting down all nonessential systems—off go the AC, the headlights, the radio; anything that isn't absolutely critical to running the car. Next you'd probably focus on making sure the engine was running at peak efficiency. You would make sure all routine maintenance had been performed, all filters replaced, belts tightened, oil changed. If the car has a meltdown, all bets are off. Now that you've cut back everything to the bare necessities, you've at least got a fighting chance. As it turns out, the things you would do to make the car drive farther are very similar to the kind of things the rats were doing to live longer. Over the millennia, rats have developed a three-pronged approach for not only surviving life's little surprises but turning them to their advantage:

- ❖ Establish priorities: As we've told you, reproduction is at the top of the to-do list for all species—even rats. Correctly calculating that it will be hard to produce healthy little rats during stressful times, the rats' visionary genes preprogrammed the rats to shut down all efforts to reproduce if even the slightest sign of impending stress was detected. Although the rats' energy had come back, they suddenly realized they had all but lost their interest in sex. No dating, much less mating (and sales of Yanni CDs plummeted). The rats were definitely living longer, they just weren't making any more rats. As if you didn't know already, reproduction takes a lot of energy, and during stressful times, that energy can be more productively used elsewhere, which leads us to the second prong of the longevity trident.
- ❖ Keep up routine maintenance: Energy "saved" from delayed reproduction can now be put to work ensuring that maintenance levels are optimal. Live efficiently now to ensure you can live vigorously later on.
- ❖ Focus on fuel efficiency: When a car engine is 100 percent fuel efficient, all of the energy produced by the combustion of the gasoline goes directly into making the car go. Nothing is wasted; everything is used. The only things left over, carbon dioxide and water, are expelled through the exhaust pipe. Not exactly major pollution threats. In the current real world, our car engines are only around

20 percent efficient. So for five gallons of gas, only one gallon (20 percent) is actually used to power the car. The rest creates a lot of heat and combines to make a lot of nasties that end up as air pollution. If combustion is 100 percent efficient, there are no free radicals and no air pollution. As combustion becomes less efficient, free-radical levels increase proportionately.

Now, inside our cells, the process of cellular respiration breaks down a molecule of glucose into carbon dioxide, water, and energy. This energy is stored as ATP (the adult human produces 150 pounds of ATP a day). It's your gasoline. The process of breaking down sugar is no different from the process of combustion in the car. In cellular respiration, sugars are literally burned up just as a car burns gasoline. And just as in the car, the burning of glucose is not completely efficient. About 40 percent of the energy and food is converted into ATP. Some of the unburned sugar leaks out and creates free radicals—just as in the car. These cellular pollutants cause a lot of damage.

A car has an engine, and cells have the mitochondria. As gasoline is fuel to the car, protein, fat, and carbohydrates are fuel to the body. But not all fuels are created equal. Rocket fuel has, pound for pound, about five times the energy of regular gas. And in the cell, burning fat produces two to three times as much energy as burning sugar.

When the rats' calories are cut back, they start relying more on fat stores as a fuel source.

Since fat combustion is several times as efficient at producing ATP than burning glucose, the same amount of energy can be created with much lower levels of free radicals. Fewer free radicals mean lower levels of free-radical damage, particularly to the mitochondria. Recent studies have shown that a calorie restriction of 40 percent leads to a 45 percent decrease in the rate of mitochondrial free-radical generation and a 30 percent reduction in the level of oxidative damage to mitochondrial DNA. The net effect of these changes decreases the rate of aging by about 50 percent. Unfortunately, humans can't live reasonably by cutting 40 percent of their calorie intake, because all they would think about is food. Fortunately, just cutting back by 15 percent gets you almost as much of an antiaging benefit. This is why you can incorporate this approach instead of the tougher 25 percent reduction that is often used by calorie restriction zealots.

Sirt Yourself

As you know by now, we don't give you the *Dragnet* approach of "just the facts." We want you to have a deeper understanding of human biology so you can know how changes in your behaviors influence your body. When it comes to calorie restriction, the mechanism that slows aging comes in the form of a protein called sirtuin.

Sirtuin seems to change the chemistry in your body to help neutralize aging. In animal models, we see that sirtuin is really a magic molecule, because it allows primates to have an even longer life expectancy than *Full House* reruns. Not everyone's sirtuin protein-manufacturing gene is activated. Researchers have found that calorie restriction helps activate sirtuin (see Figure G.1). That is, eating fewer calories acts as the light switch that turns on sirtuin.

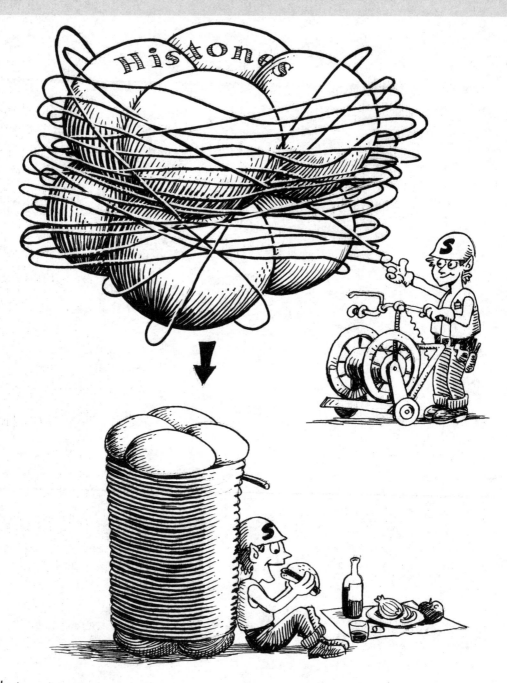

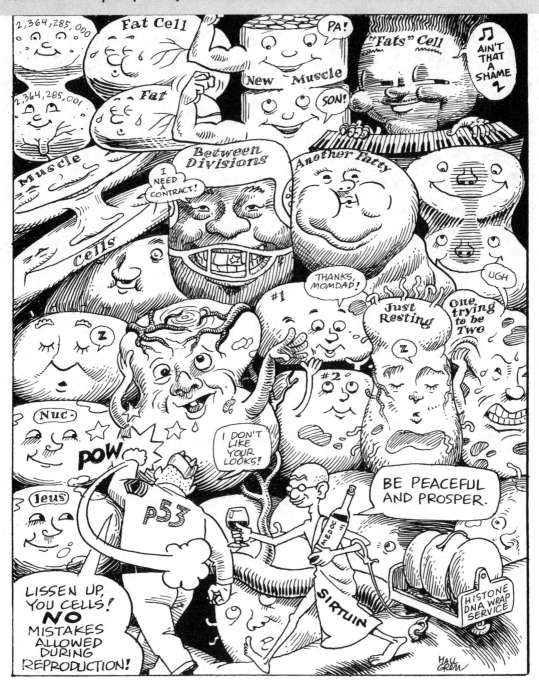

The way sirtuin works is by influencing the way DNA is made. DNA is encased in proteins called histones, which stabilize the structure of the DNA. But when the sirtuin gene is activated (through the starvation stimulus), the resulting increased activity of sirtuin protein compresses the DNA on the histones—and thus slows the way that the chromosomes are reproduced and reduces errors during the process. The main way sirtuin is activated is through restricting calories, but it's also done through the heat-shock mechanism we talked about on page 84—as a survival mechanism. When animals are exposed to extremely hot water, sirtuin kicks in to help them survive the shock and live on. Sirtuin production can also be turned on by other things—resveratrol in wine being a biggie, as well as quercetin in apples and onions, and physical activity—and may end up being the ultimate anti-ager of them all (see Figure G.2).

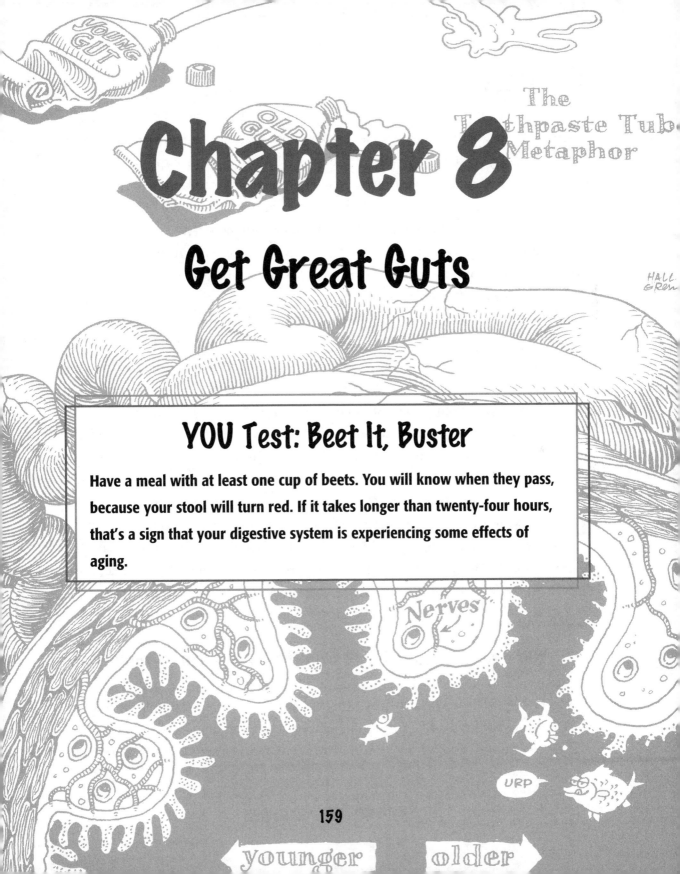

Chapter 8

Get Great Guts

HALL GREN

YOU Test: Beet It, Buster

Have a meal with at least one cup of beets. You will know when they pass, because your stool will turn red. If it takes longer than twenty-four hours, that's a sign that your digestive system is experiencing some effects of aging.

Nerves

URP

younger   older

Though it may not seem like it, holding beer cans and selling magazines aren't the only things that stomachs are used for these days. Beneath it all—whether it's hair, abdominal muscles, or key-lime fat cells—exists an underworld of cells and organs that serve one of the most vital functions in your body: They process your fuel and deliver nutrients (and toxins) all throughout your body.

Considering all the other life-threatening health problems we tend to worry about, it may seem that digestive distress ranks somewhere between canker sores and bunions in the pecking order of age-related problems. But the truth is that there's a whole world inside your gut (quite literally, depending on what you eat) that influences how you age. When you eat too much and engage in the Major Ager of excessive calorie consumption, you don't allow the ultimate antiager—calorie restriction—to give you the benefits of longevity. (Interestingly, as we'll show you in a moment, a big part of being able to restrict your calories and control your hunger is actually out of your control—as you may be at the mercy of a chemical system that cunningly influences how much you eat.) Plus, perhaps no other system influences how you feel as much as your digestive system, especially when conditions such as reflux disease and constipation are as common today as reality TV. Serving as your body's second brain because of similar body chemistry (your intestines house the majority of your body's feel-good neurotransmitter, serotonin), your gut is where swings in food lead to swings in mood.

And that's why getting a good handle on the area between your love handles is important. Understand the range of digestive issues, some of which actually start in the brain, and you'll take a major step in slowing down the aging process.

You Can't Avoid It: The Stealth System of Hunger

Anybody who's ever tried to lose weight—especially a significant amount of weight—knows that it's like trying to swim upstream against a strong current. If you just let go and do nothing, you'll drift away and get zero accomplished. But you also know that there are only two ways to make it back upstream: You have to either change the rate at which you swim or change the rate of the current. People who make changes in their lifestyle are, in effect, changing the rate at which they swim. Some people are able to successfully navigate the waters and break through the strong currents with their eating and exercising habits. But others, no matter how hard they swim, can't fight that current. So physics would dictate that the only way those swimmers can win is to change the rate of the current. That is, to change their biology so that it's easier for them to swim upstream.

In this case, the rate of the current comes in the form of a system that helps explain why some people have more problems with obesity than others. It's called the cannabinoid system. But we like to call it the "can't avoid" system, because once the system is turned on, food becomes something that you simply can't avoid.

Cannabinoids are like traffic lights; when they are always green and don't restrict traffic into an area, then it gets too crowded, and inefficiencies start, like cars circling the block looking for parking spots and double parking, which worsens traffic (see Figure 8.1). A more efficient system is one in which there's a steady alternation of red and green lights to efficiently manage all the traffic that's coming from different directions.

Research into cannabinoids, hormones made from omega-6 fatty acids primarily in the liver and kidney, started when scientists wanted to know why marijuana caused the munchies (marijuana being the cannabis plant; hence the name). What they found: The cannabinoid system has receptors that can be produced and destroyed quickly. The ones in the brain make you stalk the fridge at midnight. But the more dangerous receptors are produced in omental fat—that's the fat around your belly.

Essentially, cannabinoids hinder the ability of insulin to push sugar into cells,

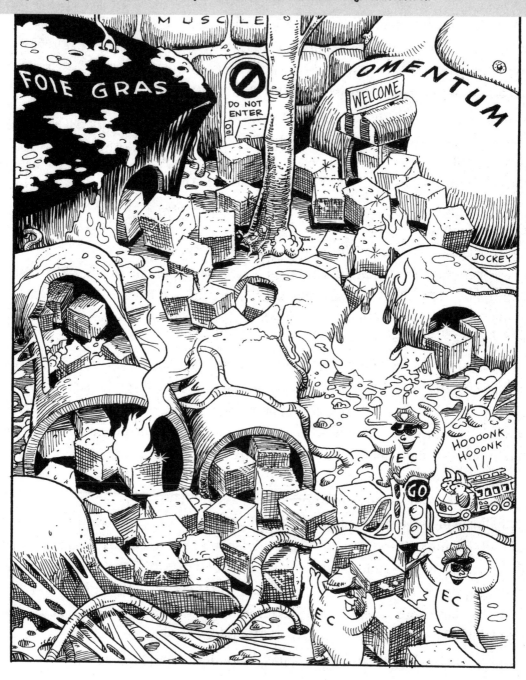

so we don't burn the sugar, and we end up insulin resistant. Cannabinoids do this by blocking a substance called adiponectin, produced by fat cells, which normally allows muscle to use carbs and fats effectively. This probably explains why some people gain weight and others burn calories more readily—and probably also explains why some are often hungrier when they get fatter, since a brain that doesn't have sugar pushed into it still senses hunger.

Cannabinoids also bias you toward fatty foods and sugars—meaning that your can't-avoid system pushes you to eat hedonistically. That type of binge doesn't simply happen because you're stressed or because you're been working like the Tasmanian devil to finish a project, or sad because of some struggles in your relationships, or mad because your favorite Idol got kicked off. That's part of it, but the biological basis for food binges is that your cannabinoid system causes uncontrollable urges that drive you to the foods that, in effect, will make your waist protrude like a baking cake, just as malfunctioning traffic lights cause cars to jam up inefficiently.

But this is more than just an issue of crowding or obesity; it's an issue of morbidity. Cannabinoids also stimulate the liver to make more fat—so our triglyceride and LDL levels become elevated, another risk factor for things like high blood pressure, diabetes, and heart disease. And they stimulate the brain to increase food intake, which leads to abdominal obesity, which leads to insulin resistance and glucose intolerance.

Since it doesn't seem to do much good, why would we even need this cannabinoid system? Good question. Its purpose is to calm us after periods of stress, which in prehistoric times usually coincided with lack of food. So at the same time the cannabinoids told our brain to relax and stop pumping out steroids in response to panic, they also stimulated us to store whatever food we might have nearby. And you would never guess where. The lucky omentum—a fat-storing organ around your stomach—soaks up excess steroids released during stress, and these steroids help the omentum fat cells bulk up like mini Thanksgiving Day floats. And just in case we didn't have lots of our favorite animals nearby to eat, cannabinoids also helped our ancestors overcome aversions to new foods, so that we could get the nutrients we needed. But the system is maladaptive in today's society, because food is abundant, and we have enough temptations without our biology turning against us as well.

In a way, cannabinoids work a little bit like a middle manager of hormones that control hunger. Cannabinoids have some influence over the many different signals that your brain gets to eat—some coming from the stomach, some coming from hormonal regulators in the brain. They can influence how other hormones work and how fast you feel hungry.

But the pot-smoking munchies are only the tip of the iceberg when it comes to the potential insight we can gain from studying cannabinoids. If we can understand how certain chemicals turn hunger signals on and off, we can understand how people can *stop* being hungry and lose weight.

Back to our swimming analogy, if you can train yourself to swim upstream or slow the current, you're going to have much better success in managing your waist long term. You have a couple of options, including strenuous exercise, which trains your muscles to use energy and restrict calories, especially unhealthy amounts of omega-6 fatty acids that give rise to these cannabinoids. However, about 20 percent of obese people will fail even when they try the correct steps, and they may benefit from making the can't-avoid receptors avoidable, with cannabinoid receptor–blocking drugs that are in development. This has decreased weight more than twice as much as just restricting calories alone—meaning it actually increases your metabolism (the energy used by muscle). Plus, this receptor-blocking substance decreases the morbidities from obesity twice as much as could be expected from weight loss alone. It's like the traffic moving twice as fast when the broken traffic signals are fixed.

The Food Freeway: Your Gut

We tend to think of digestion as an easy math equation with three different answers. When you add food to your body, it can go in one of three directions: (1) burned up and used as energy for your body, (2) stored up and turned into fat

Makes Sense: Smell and Taste

While it may seem that smell and taste are there solely to allow us to enjoy the aesthetics of eating, they're actually there for a life-or-death reason. Historically—before the Food and Drug Administration, before chemists, before lab rats—smell and taste helped us decide whether foods were safe to eat. Working together, smell and taste now don't have as crucial a function, but they too play a part in the aging process.

Taste: When you age, you're usually less sensitive to taste and also to textures like oiliness. A decrease in taste can be caused by a decrease in nerves that determine taste or because of things like dry mouth (naturally or as a side effect of medicine), which makes food taste less appealing. So you crave the stronger tastes of more salt and sugar. Remedy: Try more herbs and pepper.

Smell: As you age, you're more likely to lose smell than taste. The smell process—in which odors combine with one thousand different receptors in your nostrils—can be damaged by certain diseases, drugs, or even environmental exposures. And the reasons we worry are the same as for taste: Without your smell and taste barometers, you're more likely to overeat the foods that make your RealAge older and undereat the foods that make you younger.

on your body, or (3) churned up and eliminated out of your body. Now let's take a look inside to see how we get to those three possible endpoints.

When food enters your mouth, your glands secrete saliva to start the digestion process. Saliva also helps protect the teeth and gums from bacterial infection by inhibiting bacterial growth, and it spreads the taste all around your mouth (important for satisfaction). As you get older, that saliva tends to dry up—leading to the dry-mouth, lip-smacking, *myaw-myaw-myaw* that you may hear when older people talk (see Figure 8.2). It's one of the reasons why drinking plenty of fluid can help combat the effects of aging. During this process of salivation, and as food travels down the esophagus, calories and nutrients start to come out of food into you.

How does it travel? Not through gravity or little food-carrying gremlins but through a process called peristalsis—a rhythmic contraction of smooth muscle in your gut that moves the lump of food (the bolus) down through the esophagus and into the intestines. (The gut, by the way, is what docs term the totality of tubes from your mouth through your esophagus, stomach, small intestines, large intestines, and rectum.) For up to 75 percent of people, peristalsis slows with age. The reason

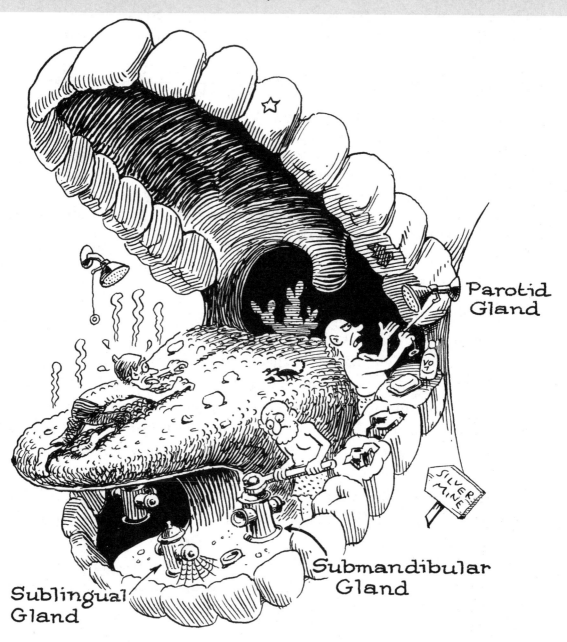

is that the number of neurons in our gut drops by half. When you don't have the normal nerve-firing sequences to control peristalsis, food doesn't move through the system smoothly, leading to indigestion and constipation (see Figure 8.3). In a good system, the food moves like toothpaste through a tube if you're squeezing from the very end (see Figure 8.4). In people with slowed peristalsis, it's like you're pushing the paste out from the middle of the tube, so the pattern becomes irregular, choppy, and unpredictable. And we certainly don't have to tell you what irregular, choppy, and unpredictable movements in your gut feel like.

Digestion is regulated by many chemicals, including one called 5-HT. A precursor to the feel-good chemical serotonin, it can be controlled by drugs that stimulate the serotonin system. When they're working correctly, these aid digestion by stimulating more neurons, releasing nitric oxide (which aids anal relaxation), and releasing a substance called acetylcholine, which helps stimulate colon contractions so you can go to the bathroom. It also allows you to move gas through the intestines without sensing discomfort.

As food enters your stomach from your esophagus, your stomach mixes it up. Your stomach serves as your body's washing machine—mixing foods with acids, breaking apart foods into different nutrients. As you age, you not only have less digestive fluid in your stomach, but the fluid you do have has less acidity. That may seem like a good thing, but it means your body has a weakened ability to jackhammer out the proteins it needs for normal functioning. That's one of the reasons why pharmaceuticals have very different effects as you age.

Think of your twenty-three-foot-long small intestines as an underwater cave with coral—the coral being the finger-shaped villi that line the inner walls of your intestines and act like little sponges, sucking up nutrients. As you get older, those villi become rocky and ragged and dulled, so they're less able to absorb nutrients (although they are still great at absorbing calories). And you can imagine what that does. A decreased ability to absorb calcium means an increased chance that you'll experience bone loss. A decreased ability to absorb vitamin B_{12} or folate or niacin or vitamins C or E may mean an increased risk of neurological deficit or damage from free radicals.

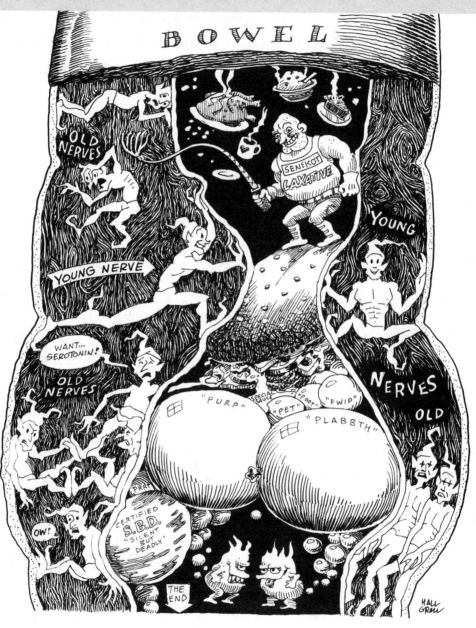

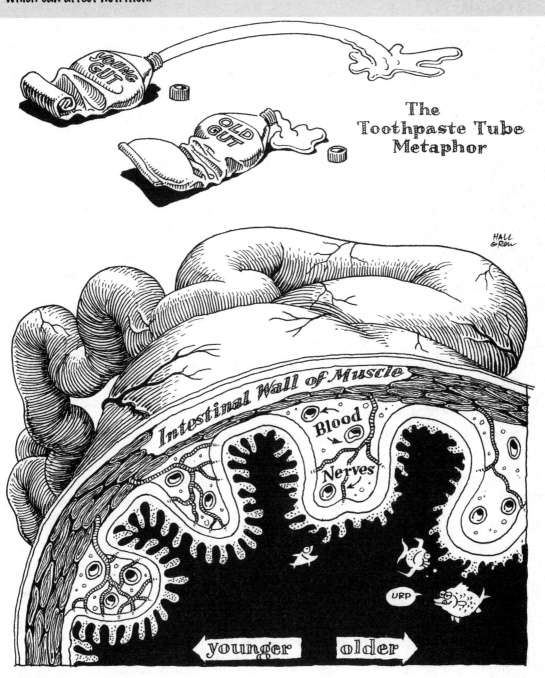

Other common GI problems associated with age include:

Swallowing disorders: Because peristalsis slows down with age, you're more likely to get reflux—making swallowing more difficult. It's important not only to limit your portions but to slow down when you eat, and as Mom said, stop talking with your mouth full. By the way, swallowing problems are often the first sign of dementia, because they can indicate a loss of nerves in your gut.

Diverticulitis: Small pouches in the intestinal wall form when you have too little fiber and water, and your intestines are forced to squeeze too hard (and so are you) when you're going to the bathroom. Feces can then get stuck in these pouches, creating GI discomfort. The answer? You got it: More fiber plus more water equals less straining.

H. pylori: These bacterial infections are a leading cause of gastrointestinal injury, and the prevalence increases with acid loss in the stomach as you age. Some say that 80 percent of the elderly are affected by it. The presence of *H. pylori* can create an inflammatory response, more reflux, or ulcers.

Urinary incontinence: Though technically not part of the GI system, we've included it here because it's awfully close—and often associated with aging. What happens is that as a woman ages and experiences a decline in muscle strength, she actually loses the ability to control her bladder. That's because the muscles around your bladder, typically suspended from the pelvic floor, are supposed to constrict the urethra tube that goes from the bladder to the outside world. But if these muscles become flaccid, meaning you don't have as much control of the kink, then laughing or coughing can build up pressure on the bladder and force out urine (see Figure 8.5). Weakness often happens due to the stretch that pregnancy causes. Doing Kegel exercises—working the muscles that you tense as if you were pulling on a tight pair of jeans—can help strengthen those muscles. By the way, the same

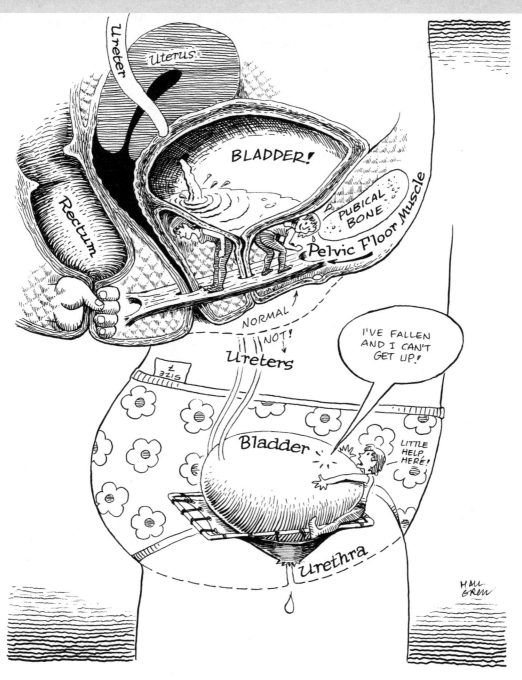

mechanism is at work with bowel incontinence, only the muscle tone comes from the rectum as well as surrounding muscles. Kegel exercises don't help here, but rectal tampons have been developed by some entrepreneurial sufferers. Aging of our intestines can sabotage our antiaging crusade by simultaneously causing malnourishment and obesity. What a combo. But by forming a healthy alliance with nutrient-rich foods, the gut also holds some of our greatest opportunities to halt our Major Agers.

YOU TIPS!

Of course, being kind to your stomach means more than just avoiding drinking hot sauce by the six-pack. Deciding what to put in your mouth (and what not to) greatly influences how well or how quickly your digestive system ages. By taking these steps, you'll keep your innards running smoothly, so you can too.

YOU Tip: Add Bulk. The food duo with the most muscle: fiber and water. Together they keep your food bulky and soft so it can move easily through your system without putting too much pressure on your intestines. Remember, without water, fiber often turns to cement. Containing no calories but still making you feel full, fiber combined with water helps your digestive system and your overall health because it helps keep you from eating the other things that are more likely to lead to problems associated with obesity, like heart disease and diabetes. Fiber is found in fruits, vegetables, whole grains, oats, beans, and some cereals. Your goal: 35 grams a day for women and 25 grams a day for men.

YOU Tip: Shower Your Insides. You hear the advice about drinking eight 8-ounce glasses of water almost as much as you hear "the tribe has spoken." There's no magic to this number, and the right amount varies according to your activity level and size, so if you want, just drink enough water so that your urine is clear. Or 8×8 ounces might be easier. Of all the reasons H_2O (preferably filtered) is oh-so-good, the work it does for your guts is one of the best. For starters, it helps lubricate everything so food can slide through more easily. Plus, it helps quell hunger, fights bad breath, and helps you avoid dry mouth. Your mechanism for detecting thirst doesn't work as well when you're older as it does when you're young, which makes it that much more important to remind yourself to drink regularly throughout the day—before your body even tells you it's time.

YOU Tip: Play the Elimination Game. The best way to experiment with foods that may be causing you general digestive irritation is to do the food elimination test. For three days in a row, eliminate certain groups of food from your diet—dairy products, wheat products, and sugars being the top three to try. Write down how you feel during those days, and notice any changes in digestive feelings as well as things like your energy level. The test will give you insight not into allergies specifically but into food irritabilities—symptoms that can make you feel like you have a touch of the flu. Another bonus: Learning to eliminate certain groups (sugars and refined carbohydrates, especially) can also help you lose weight.

YOU Tip: Choose Your Fats. You may know that there are good fats and bad fats. The good fats (omega-3 fats) come in the form of fatty fish, great greens, and supplements of fish oil, fresh flaxseed oil, or DHA, and walnuts, while the bad fats (like saturated and trans fats) come in the form of brownies and burgers. But there's a reason why one fat leads directly to fat on your waist, while the other helps clear your arteries. Trans fats are rigid, so they make your arteries spasm and cause dangerous inflammation, while omega-3s relax your arteries and quell inflammation (see Figure 8.6).

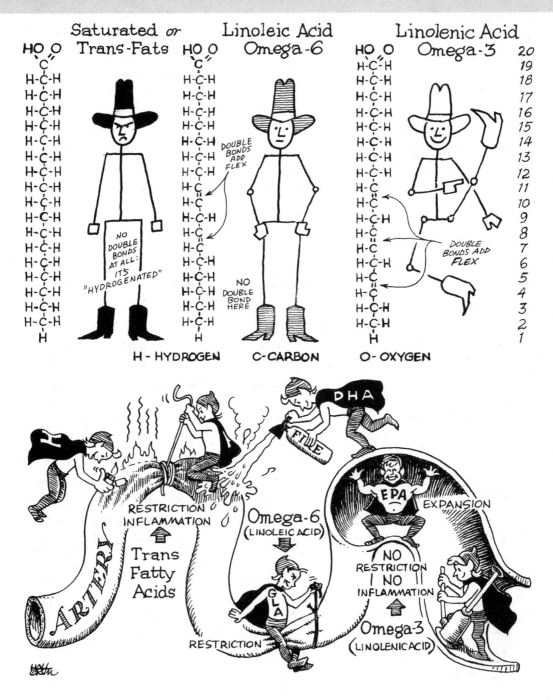

Figure 8.6 Fat Attack Omega-3 fatty acids are more beneficial than the rigid trans fats because they have double bonds. Rigid fats cause inflammation and spasm of our arteries; omega-3 fatty acids put out these fires and relax our arteries. DHA and EPA are omega-3s.

Neurotransmitter Imbalance

How the Chemical Message System in Your Brain Can Age You

All of us get messages on the phone and computer. Some of us get messages in bottles. And the lucky ones get messages on steamed-up bathroom mirrors telling them that someone's waiting for them in the bedroom.

In a society that sends and receives messages at an Indy 500 pace, we're all well aware of the advantages and disadvantages of the communication process. Sometimes we get messages instantaneously. Sometimes it takes longer. Sometimes we get too many messages. Sometimes messages are like socks in the laundry—they can get lost in some other world.

Now take the same concept and apply it to your brain. Amid all the moosh and goosh and squoosh that's jellied up under your skull, there's the ultimate communications company. It's in the business of sending and receiving messages that help dictate how you act, how you feel, whether you want to be asleep, or whether you're craving a triple-chocolate, deep-fried, Hades-worthy dessert.

How? Well, the nerves of your body communicate through spaces called synapses—they're the gaps between the end of one nerve cell and the beginning of another. Your body has about 2×10^{14} synapses (that's one hundred times greater than our national debt measured in dollars). Most of the communications between nerves use substances called neurotransmitters, which are chemicals that help send a signal across a synapse. Think of these neurotransmitters as a one-way electrical impulse between nerves. When one nerve wants to communicate to a neighboring nerve, it releases neurotransmitters.

These neurotransmitters have keys to your neurological mailboxes, which are called neuron receptors. And only the messages with the right keys will fit into the receptors (see Figure H.1). Once the key is in the lock, a lot of things can happen; it can allow glucose in or out, or it can cause a muscle to contract, or it can make you want to go to sleep. So some messages may make nerves excited, while other neurotransmitters may slow, or depress, neuron activity. It depends on what messages are being sent and how (and even if) they're being received.

While the message-transport system is important, so is the receiver system. The receptors determine where the keys fit and can even determine whether or not you're getting too much of a neurotransmitter. Your neuron receptors—and this is where it all comes together—can be modified by the drugs you take or the foods you eat, making them more or less effective in the long run. In addition, prolonged exposure to a certain neurotransmitter, even if it's bad for you, can cause receptors to be unresponsive.

The entire neurological system is protected by something called the blood-brain barrier, a set of tightly packed cells that acts as kind of a filter system, protecting the brain. One of the reasons why many supplements are useless is because they can't get to the brain to have an effect. As you age, your brain actually shrinks (don't worry, it's normal), and you lose a little bit of brainpower. You also lose some of the neurotransmitters you produce. Average levels of serotonin and dopamine each decline about 5 percent every ten years—and that's been linked to emotional issues like depression as well as other cognitive abilities, like how well you sleep, which is the subject of our next chapter. Aging of the brain

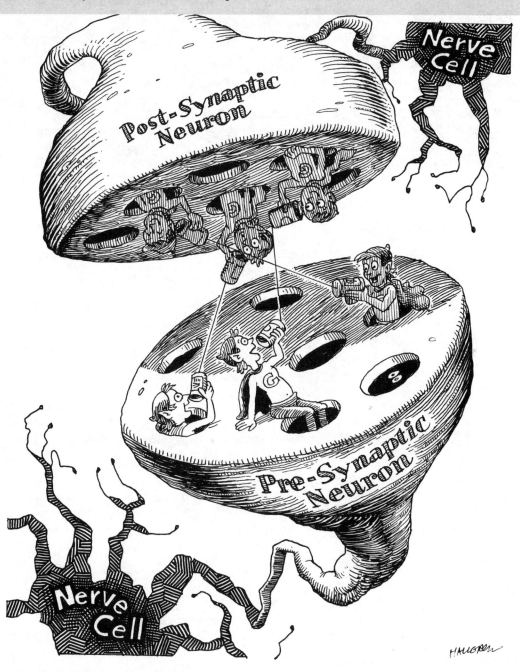

has also been linked to problems with Major Ager toxins influencing the message system of neurotransmitters (through such things as industrial-size doses of MSG, for example). See Figure H.2.

The good part, however, is that food and exercise and sleep work as dials on your neurotransmitter radio, regulating how you feel from day to day and hour to hour, and thus can have a profound impact on the emotional side of aging. Events controlled by neurotransmitters, like insomnia, also affect longevity, not just the quality of life.

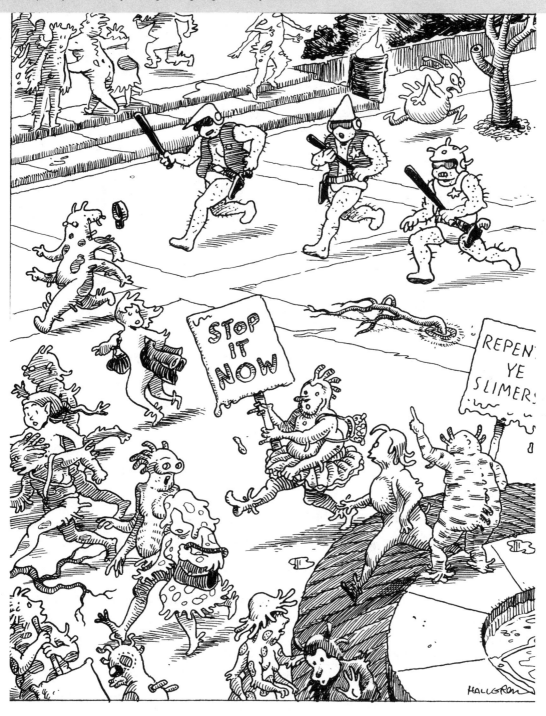

Major Ager: Neurotransmitter Imbalance 179

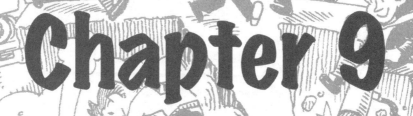

Chapter 9
Sleep Your Way to the Top

YOU Test: A Real Snoozer

Rate your likelihood of falling asleep in the following places on a scale of 0 to 3 (with 0 being no chance of dozing and 3 being a high chance). Then add up your total points.

- ☐ Sitting and reading
- ☐ Watching TV
- ☐ Inactively sitting in a public place, like a theater or meeting
- ☐ As a passenger in a car for about an hour without a break
- ☐ Lying down in the afternoon to rest
- ☐ Sitting and talking to someone (regardless of whether you like them)
- ☐ Sitting quietly after lunch
- ☐ In a car stopped in traffic for a few minutes

With all due respect to your favorite recliner or antique armoire, is there a finer piece of furniture than your bed? Really. Your kids bounce on it. Your dog hides under it. You probably started your family in it. And you're very likely reading these very words in it.

In a way, your bed is one of life's few sanctuaries. It's a place where you can retreat with your own thoughts, or where you can be naked with the love of your life, or where you can be entertained and inspired by a dream that includes a dentist, a tornado, and a three-legged black unicorn that speaks Croatian.

Why, then, is it that we have so little regard for this sanctuary of solitude?

It's not as if we don't love sleep. In fact, despite a few key differences, sleep is like another popular bedroom activity in more ways than one: We all want more of it. We can't wait for it to start and hate to see it end. And we're none too happy being interrupted in the middle of it.

But the truth is that most of us don't get enough sleep, and that plays a significant role in our aging. In fact, people who sleep fewer than six hours a night have a 50 percent increased risk of viral infections and an increased risk of heart disease and stroke. Plus, lack of sleep is associated with mental decline and overeating (which leads to major aging conditions). Even worse, we don't care enough that we don't get enough sleep, even though it's one of the major things that make us feel old. Most of us think that a lack of sleep—be it for a night, or a week, or a lifetime—is no big deal. We go on our way, trudging through our daily lives and responsibilities tired, defeated, sluggish, caffeine infused, and longing to sledge-hammer the alarm clock at 6:07 every morning.

Simply, few of us are losing sleep about losing sleep.

Not sleeping is not merely making you more agitated than an out-of-balance washing machine. It could be killing you.

Sensing Sleep: Your Third Eye

Moms may have back-of-their-head eyes, arrested celebrities may get black eyes, and adulterers may have wandering eyes. But we all have another kind of eye that plays a role in how we age. It's our "third eye." And it's located deep inside the middle of our brain—in the exact center of our brain, actually (see Figure 9.1).

Our pineal gland, which is the only endocrine gland that is in contact with the outside world, senses when we're exposed to light, much in the way that a security-type light sensor does. The pineal gland has cells that resemble the back of the retina, but it is nestled deep in our brain, far away from any direct access to light. In some animals—for instance, chameleons—it senses light directly through the skull. In human beings, it likely senses light through special receptors in the backs of our eyes that don't actually provide vision but do dictate our circadian rhythms. Even the blind have this rhythm, indicating that our pineals along with other neurological inputs can substitute for these special cells in our eye.

We know that the pineal gland plays a role in aging because research has shown that putting young pineal glands in old animals helps reverse aging. The old animals' hair grew thicker and lusher when the new pineals were inserted. By contrast, putting old pineal glands in

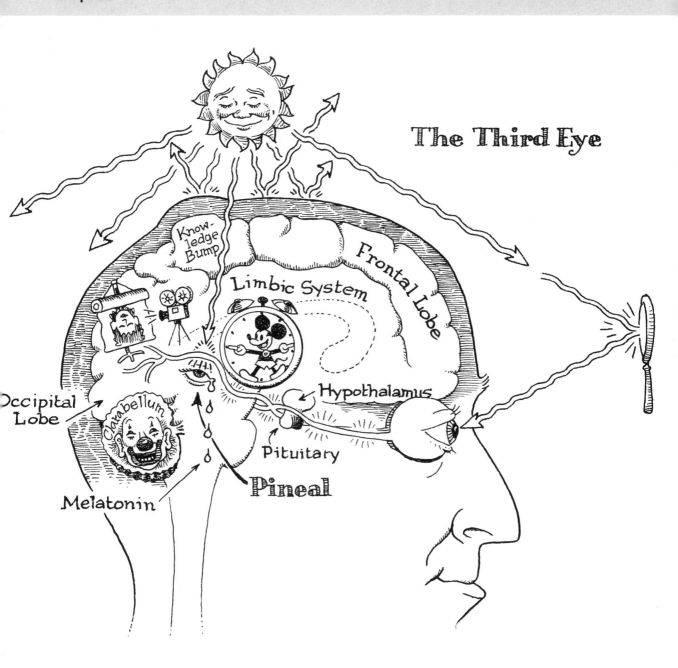

The Third Eye

Knowledge Bump

Frontal Lobe

Limbic System

Hypothalamus

Occipital Lobe

Cerebellum

Pituitary

Pineal

Melatonin

young animals quickens the aging process. Mice with new pineals lived 25 percent longer, but we're yet unable to determine if the same statistics would be true for humans. So don't plan on sacrificing any younger friends anytime soon.

To live longer and healthier, you need to know about the pineal gland not because of an upcoming *Jeopardy* appearance, but because it produces a substance called melatonin, which conducts the symphony of your hormones. Melatonin modulates menstruation, helps control desire for mating, helps lower heart rate and blood pressure, increases immune function, and helps decrease stress by blocking the body's stress response. Plus, it helps regulate sleep.

If you're a trivia expert, you may remember melatonin as the neurotransmitter that helps bears hibernate. Its levels peak at night and during winter months. (Serotonin, which converts to melatonin, helps regulate our daytime activity.) When the lights go out, your pineal senses that and starts producing melatonin.

When you lose melatonin (which is also found in the gut, by the way), you lose your normal sleep pattern, which then cascades into a whole host of health problems.

The reason why we're concerned about it here: Our own melatonin loses some of its potency as we age—our receptors for that neurotransmitter (you knew we'd link it with a Major Ager, didn't you?) don't create the same power from the dose of melatonin they receive. As you get older, you also lose some of the *oomph* you get from melatonin, which may explain why so many of us suffer aging-related sleep and health problems. In fact, melatonin production peaks around age five and starts a downhill slide from there. Unfortunately, we lose up to 80 percent of those original levels by the time we reach sixty. And that's likely one of the reasons we don't sleep as well when we get older and why Great-aunt Theresa is up at four-thirty every morning. When you're twenty and can easily sleep until noon, your levels of melatonin average about 80 picograms per milliliter; at sixty, those levels drop down to 10. At age twenty you might have had a level of 10 in the late afternoon. You slept through that late-afternoon class. We know that 10 is less effective at age sixty than it was in the afternoon at age twenty.

Melatonin evolved for us to sense light and dark, as well as changes in season, because our circadian rhythms help regulate our reproductive rhythms. Originally, nature tried to schedule the occurrence of births at a time of year when the odds of survival for mother and baby were the greatest—that is, when the days are long and the nights are short (and the food supply is the greatest). So melatonin cycles meant more babies were conceived to be born in spring.

Now, you probably also know the word *melatonin* because in supplement form it's often used as a sleep aid, and for good reason. As a supplement, it helps get our body clocks adjusted to sleep better. We can also find natural ways to make our sleep patterns more predictable. One way, which we explain in detail on page 350, is through meditation. Meditation seems to cause the release of melatonin to soothe your body and protect your own tissue-friendly stem cells. It makes the only tossing and turning in bed you ever do the va-va-voom kind. So now you know why our sleep action plan (that's not an oxymoron) includes meditation before bed.

> **FACTOID**
>
> Are we supposed to sleep for eight hours straight? Good question—and the answer seems obvious. Not so fast. You may know about the nooner, but there used to be such a thing as the medieval midnighter. In those times, people would go to bed when it was dark in the early evening; wake up in the middle of the night for a few hours and have a meal, go to the bathroom, have sex; then go back to sleep for a few hours. Most mammals, in fact, don't sleep eight hours in a row.

Night Plight: Your Need for Sleep

Sleep doesn't exist just to pass the time during an anthropology lecture or to keep you from working twenty-two hours a day. Our bodies make us sleep because our brains need sleep the way trains need tracks—they don't work without it. Sleep exercises the part of your brain that you don't normally use. What do we mean by that? Think back to our cavemen. They spent each day focusing on the tasks that

YOU Tool: Deep-Sleep Program

We talk about personal hygiene for our teeth or job interviews, but most people don't talk about sleep hygiene—that is, creating the perfect sleep environment. Much in the way you'd put candles on the table for a romantic dinner or Luther Vandross on the stereo for a romantic night, you also need to set the mood for sleeping. The perfect environment for sleep:

❖ A cool, dark room: The temperature and darkness are signals to the pineal gland to kick up melatonin production and knock you out.

❖ No laptops, no TV: Ideally, the bed is used for two things and two things only. If you have any other type of stimulus, like work or a TV, you're not sending your body the right message that it's time for sleep. Need more incentive to kick Leno to the living room? People who don't have a TV in the bedroom have 50 percent more sex than those who do.

❖ Add white noise. Use a fan for background noise, or one of those machines that lets you pick sounds, from the rain forest to the ocean. This drowns out the couple fighting next door and the drag races outside so your subconscious stays pristine as you count sheep.

❖ Dress appropriately. The best clothing should be nonrestricting and nonallergenic (both the fabric and how it's washed). Your body is better at keeping itself hot than keeping itself cool, so you'll make it easier on yourself the fewer and looser clothes you wear.

❖ Establish a standard wake-up time, including on weekends. This helps reset your circadian rhythm and trains you to stay on schedule if your rhythm happens to wander, as during traveling.

❖ Get the best mattress. We believe there are four things in life you should overpay for. The first three: pillows, mattresses, and their coverings. The fourth thing? A good kitchen knife (not to be used in the bed). While there's no one standard mattress that works for everyone, you have to pick what feels right for you (and try it out with your partner if you sleep with one). But you can't judge that in thirty seconds in a store. Tell the salesperson to back off and give you fifteen minutes to get the feel for a mattress before you pick it. Judge it for comfort, support, and heat (you don't want heat dissipated too quickly, but a mattress pad may help). One good option: a memory foam mattress, which bounces back to the original flat plane after you get out of bed, rather than forming an indentation. They can be costly (up to $2,500). Instead, you can take a standard mattress and flip it every couple months to avoid body indentations that will disrupt your sleep. And get a 1-micron cover that blocks allergens from floating from the pillow or mattress to your nose and body.

would keep them alive: hunting, cooking, caring for the tribe. During the day, other parts of the brain—say, the creative parts that would allow cavemen to come up with solutions and ideas for stronger weapons or shelter—didn't get used because the cavemen were so caught up with living and surviving in the moment. That is, except during sleep, which is what allows those creative parts to strengthen and grow so that they'll be fully developed when the situation arises to use them.

As we started to take on more cognitive abilities in our evolutionary history, we needed the restorative process of sleep even more. That's because vision is extremely expensive cognitively, meaning that when you're seeing things and processing the world visually, your brain can do little else except that. You need nonvision time (sleep, or to a lesser extent, meditation-type activities) to process information and store it in your memory. In a way, sleep allows your brain to lay down the code that your mind will use in the future so that you can reset and reboot your system each and every night. It gives your brain the chance to work and consolidate your memories so you can use them in the future.

As a citylike organization, your body needs that downtime to repair and refresh its systems; after all, highways are repaved at night, when there's no traffic or street cleaning. If the city never had any downtime, you'd never be able to perform the maintenance that allows your city to run smoothly, or you'd be inefficient when you tried to do it during high-peak times (ever been stuck on a highway that goes from four lanes to one?).

As we said, sleep is a serious deal. Still don't buy it? Think about what happens in the extreme situation. When people don't sleep for three or more days on end, they become psychotic; that's why so many forms of torture involve sleep deprivation. With no sleep, you're vulnerable, weak, and more whacked out than a 'shroom-scarfing hippie. Sleep problems and sleep deprivation are self-imposed torture. And the stakes are high: a weakened immune system, increased risk of heart disease, and a brain that works about as fast as a Commodore 64 computer.

Now, you may think that your occasional restless night or your shift from a good eight hours a night to lucky-if-you-get-six isn't much to worry over, since you're still managing to live OK, albeit a tad tired. The truth is that sleep problems affect 70 percent of Americans, up from 60 percent in 1990. A sleep disorder is defined as having a problem sleeping or not feeling rested at least a few nights per week. And that's enough to chip away at your health—and longevity. The good thing, however, is that 50 percent of people with sleep disorders can be helped by simple behavioral changes that you make by yourself—to your bed, to your body, and to your life.

Interestingly, sleep is your body's default state; you're supposed to be in a sleep state all the time (see Figure 9.2). The way you fall asleep is through the activation of the neurotransmitter gamma-aminobutyric acid, or GABA. Now, the reason you're not asleep is that your hypothalamus secretes a chemical called acetylcholine to wake you up. When you're asleep for a long time, you experience a buildup of chemicals, and the acetylcholine wins. (That's how caffeine seems to work, by influencing levels of acetylcholine.) In contrast, a chemical called adenosine builds up with activity and hinders acetylcholine, so we get tired.

As the day wears on, your sleep drive builds as acetylcholine and other chemicals that induce wakefulness decline. Meanwhile, your melatonin rises several hours before bedtime, eventually overpowering what's left of your acetylcholine. So if you have trouble sleeping, then it's actually your preparation for your default state that's broken, indicating you have a very fundamental biological defect that needs some examining.

The evidence is clear that a good night's sleep (night after night, not once every couple of weeks) is fundamental to both your health and your longevity. But what exactly is a good night's sleep? While the length of sleep is important,

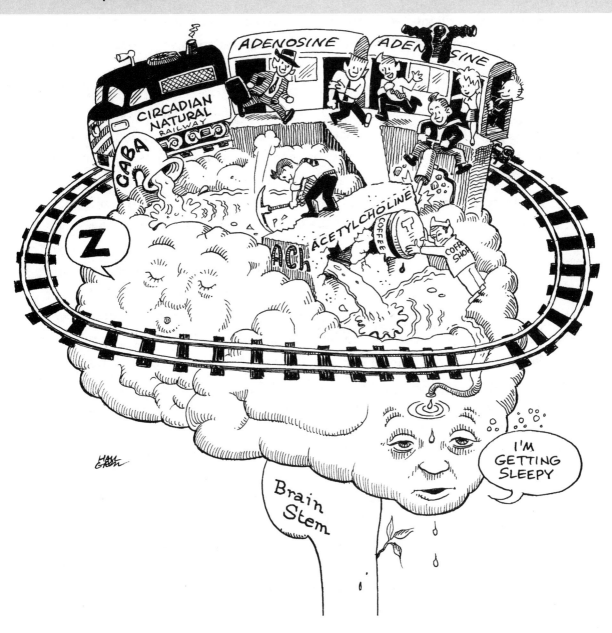

Figure 9.2 **Losing Snooze** Sleep is stimulated by the neurotransmitter GABA. We stay awake because the hypothalamus secretes a chemical called acetylcholine that dams up the onslaught of GABA. When we're awake for a long time, we experience a buildup of adenosine, which disrupts the acetylcholine and enables GABA to triumph. Coffee works by plugging the holes in the acetylcholine dam.

equally vital is getting through the sleep cycle several times. The cycle comprises the following stages:

Sleep latency: This is the time it takes for you to fall asleep from the time you go to bed.

Stages 1 and 2: light sleep. Drowsiness as your brain is just getting into sleep. In stage 2, your brain waves start to slow down noticeably, resting those parts you use while awake.

Stages 3 and 4: deeper sleep, which you get less of as you age because of frequent awakenings. These stages are both restorative. Both REM sleep and sleep stages 3 and 4 are homeostatically driven—that is, if a human is selectively deprived of one of these, it rebounds once the person is allowed to sleep. This suggests that both are essential in the sleep process and its many functions.

REM (rapid eye movement): the deepest sleep. Your eyes are moving fast, but the rest of your body is paralyzed. It's the stage where some sleep-related disorders take place, like sleepwalking.

Each one of these cycles lasts about ninety minutes, and you go through four to six of them a night. But the important part is that you have to get to REM sleep to feel rested. People who have sleep problems often don't make it to REM sleep because it takes up to sixty minutes to make it to REM. If you're having frequent awakenings before you make it to REM, then you're never getting that restorative, healthy sleep.

Now, complex changes occur in your body and mind as you awaken. Your melatonin levels have peaked, the stress hormone cortisol is on the rise, your body temperature has bottomed out, and your psyche is immersed in your dreams. Increased levels of melatonin associated with deep sleep promote immune system activity, protect you from viruses, and have remarkable anticancer properties. Deep sleep also increases human growth hormone naturally, so the levels oscillate as they are supposed to, and you start to feel like a puppy. Growth hormone also plays a critical role in fostering optimal body weight.

As we mentioned, sleep problems that develop with age can be attributed to a decrease in REM caused by frequent awakenings. Why does that happen? Historically, a lack of sleep served as a warning signal of sorts; insomnia actually helped us survive. We're restless when something's on our mind, like a predator (you'd do your tribe no good if you were off snoozing in stage 5 while a woolly mammoth trampled through the village). Today, that lack of sleep—harmful to your health and generally unnecessary as a protective mechanism—serves as a different kind of warning signal: that you're experiencing some kind of bodily system malfunction.

While there are literally dozens of clinically diagnosed sleep disorders, we'll concentrate on the ones that are most disruptive.

Insomnia: You know it as toss-and-turn disease. No matter what you do or try, you lie in bed, stewing like a Crock-Pot of Swedish meatballs. Technically, insomnia is defined as either not being able to get to sleep in the first place or not being able to get back to sleep after waking up. Unbelievably, people over the age of sixty-five have an average of twenty-five awakenings a night, and that number increases with age. And one-third of all of us wake up repeatedly during the night, while a quarter of us wake up early in the morning and can't get back to sleep. The big problem for most of us is an increase in sleep latency—as you worry about your job, bills, and why Junior came home with a purple Mohawk. The likely chemical culprit in insomnia: melatonin. Normally, melatonin levels rise about two hours before bedtime and peak when your body temperature is the lowest, to help induce sleep. But without adequate melatonin, your body is unable to transition from sleep latency to stage 1.

Sleep apnea: You know it as the honey-shut-up disease. While we often associate sleep apnea with snoring, the truth is that sleep apnea is actually signaled by silence (often preceded or followed by power-tool sounds), where you're not breathing for up to ten seconds at a time. And that's what actually rustles you awake. You can have as many as two hundred episodes a night (two hundred!),

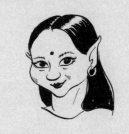

Do You Need Sleep Drugs?

Your first line of sleep therapy should be trying the hygiene strategies we outline on page 195, but for some people, medications or herbal supplements can be the answer—if you know the right one. Despite the fact that thirty-five million prescriptions for sleep medicine were written in the United States in 2005 (twice as many as in 2000), many docs don't prescribe medications that are intended to get at the source of the problem. This guide will help you and your doctor make the decision that's right for you.

Is This You?	Try	Why
You're just beginning to experience some mild sleep problems.	Benadryl	The nonaddictive OTC option contains an ingredient that makes you groggy (it's also the ingredient in OTC sleep medications). If you don't have pains or other symptoms, stick to straight Benadryl. But if you do, you can add an OTC medication with a pain-killing element. Downside: You may feel groggy in the morning and suffer memory problems. If so, stop it.
You're jet-lagged or work shift work.	Melatonin	Available in health-food stores, this supplement helps reset your body clock and is a first-line therapy for travel-related sleep issues. The dose varies between 0.5 and 5 milligrams, so you'll have to experiment with dosing to see what works best for you.
You've had sleep issues over an extended period of time.	Ambien or Ambien CR or Lunesta or Rozerem	This long-acting prescription will give you less of a hangover than other drugs may, but some docs feel it is addictive. The controlled-release (CR) version will give you a boost after four hours to avoid middle-of-the-night awakening. Lunesta works like Ambien but is thought to be nonaddictive. Rozerem works like melatonin in our opinion, and it is nonaddictive.
You wake up in the middle of the night.	Sonata	This fast-acting prescription hypnotic drug is good if you wake up in the middle of the night, because its effect is quick and won't last all night. It works to initiate your going back to sleep, but it will not keep you asleep.
You can't get to sleep because you're worried or depressed.	Desyrel (trazodone)	This antidepressant is less expensive than some of the popular sleep drugs, and it's actually one of the most popular drugs prescribed for sleep, because it's effective and nonaddictive. It works even if you're depressed, as the doses are much lower than for treating depression. One side effect: priapism (which is maintaining erections for a lot longer than you want). Amitriptyline, an older antidepressant, may also be effective, but has caused constipation in our patients.
You kick so much that you're considering trying out for the Chicago Bears.	Requip	This drug helps with restless legs syndrome. But a first option is just drinking a little diet tonic water at dinner. It contains quinine—an ingredient that helps quiet muscle cramps.

CHI-GONG SLEEP AID

Next time you find yourself squirming like a toddler in church as you're trying to get to sleep, try this relaxation and sleep-promoting move taken from the practices of chi-gong (featured in the next chapter).

❖ Rub your hands together to warm them (and gather chi). Place each palm over the respective eye.
❖ Press the center bone that sticks out on top of each eye with each index finger.
❖ Press the outside corner of your eye at the bone.
❖ Press the bottom center of the eye on the inside of the bone.
❖ Press the inside of each eye.
❖ Use your thumbs to push where the jaw and cheekbone meet at the temporomandibular junction.
❖ Pinch the ears around the pinna from the top to the bottom.
❖ End the sequence with the move called "Beating the Heavenly Drum," by tapping the back of your head nine times with your hands; the thumbs rest on the neck as an axis as shown below.

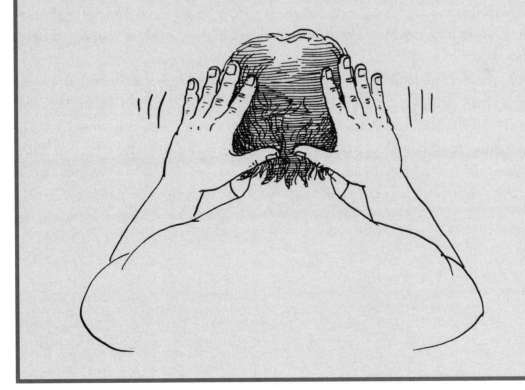

though it's more typical to have about five episodes an hour. They act like a series of rear-end collisions—one might not necessarily be damaging, but time after time after time after time, eventually you're going to damage your infrastructure. In fact, sleep apnea leads to hypertension, heart trouble, lack of energy, and a decrease in the all-important growth hormone. What's the primary cause of it? Fat. (Those with a neck size larger than seventeen inches are at increased risk.) When your heavy jaw naturally moves backward while you're sleeping, it meets the fatty tissue in the back of your mouth in the throat area. That's what blocks the airway and stops air from getting to your lungs.

Other sleep problems: As we age, we can experience a variety of problems that either mess with our sleep or are sleep-related themselves, like depression (where you sleep too much) and anxiety (which can keep you awake). Circadian rhythm problems are frequent in shift workers, and up to 30 percent of people over fifty have restless legs syndrome—the periodic movement of limbs during deep sleep. This inability to stay asleep serves as the source of many sleep difficulties, but, as you'll see, many can be treated with shifts in your sleep "hygiene," as well as with other tactics.

At the risk of sounding like a broken MP3 file, we'll repeat: Of all the strategies we outline in this book, getting the right sleep is one of the most vital things you can do. Sleep should serve as a major health barometer. Not only does a lack of sleep cause health problems, but health problems also cause a lack of sleep. Plus, we need sleep so we can dream. You can't live your best life unless you can dream. So if you're not sleeping, it's a clue that something besides your sheets isn't working the way it should be.

YOU TIPS!

Sleep seems as if it should be easy and automatic: Change into PJs, brush teeth, crawl into bed, shut eyes, see you in seven. But sometimes we just can't tear ourselves away from the TV until Jon Stewart, David Letterman, or that Stephen Colbert fellow have finished making us laugh. As everyone with sleep problems knows, sleep is about easy as making the final twelve in *American Idol.* We believe that's because many of us don't know the tricks and solutions that can help put our mind—and body—at rest.

YOU Tip: Plan for It. We're big on planning, so decide when you want to wake up and count backward about seven hours. Now take about a fifteen-minute period before that to start your slowdown process. That means taking five minutes to finish up must-do chores, followed by five minutes of hygiene stuff (flossing, washing face, and so on) and five minutes of relaxing into your sleep state, through things like meditation and saying "I love you" as you lie in bed.

YOU Tip: Use the Night. Most of us do things at night that are counterproductive to sleeping. Instead, make slight changes in your rituals to prepare your body for rest:

* Dim your lights several hours before bed to avoid the stimulation caused by artificial light pollution—which is all around us through TV, computers, and indoor lighting—and serves to stimulate us.
* Come up with a regular, rhythmic evening ritual that allows you to embrace anxieties that are released when you slow down. Meditation, prayer, and deep breathing are all good methods.
* Surrender to sleep. After all, you *go* to the movies; you shouldn't *go* to sleep. There is nothing you have to do to sleep—except let go of waking. Practice "dying" into sleep, rather than forcing yourself to sleep, and cultivate awareness of your personal twilight zone.

YOU Tip: Attack Insomnia. Tossing and turning works for salads, not sleep problems. If you can't fall asleep within fifteen minutes, the answer is not to keep trying. Don't force yourself to stay in bed, because the wait will be interminable. Instead, get out of bed and do some light activity. Getting your mind off sleep resets and reboots your system. Try a yoga pose, meditation, or a short walk. To get back to sleep, music and meditation seem to work best.

YOU Tip: Know the Nos. Generally, we don't like telling you not to do something unless it's smoking, slurping trans fats, or spending sixteen hours in front of the tube. But for optimum sleep preparation, there are a few things you should avoid to increase your chance of falling—and staying—asleep.

❖ No alcohol or nicotine for one and a half hours before bed.

❖ No exercise that makes you sweat for one and a half hours before bed (doing things that make you sweat *in* bed are OK).

❖ No caffeine, caffeinated beverages or food, or caffeine in pills for at least three hours before bed, or as long as your body dictates.

❖ No eating for three hours before bed, so you can avoid reflux issues that can disturb sleep.

YOU Tip: Find Your Pain. Some sleep problems don't arise because of worry or melatonin problems. Some are caused because your back hurts like the dickens. Truth is, some people get through general back pain or knee pain during the day because they're so focused on other things. But when trying to get to sleep, they feel the pain and focus on it. A simple over-the-counter anti-inflammatory medication can help—not specifically to get you to sleep but to help alleviate the pain that's preventing you from sleeping. Take aspirin with a glass of water at least one hour before bedtime so that the acid doesn't have as much chance of refluxing up from your stomach to your esophagus.

YOU Tip: Treat Allergies. Allergies can make sleeping trouble worse because of the congestion they cause. About 40 percent of people with allergic rhinitis have trouble sleeping. Over-the-counter nasal strips and sprays help open up everything and clear up symptoms like headaches, watery eyes, runny nose, or new-onset snoring. If you experience those symptoms and aren't aware of any allergies, search for the source in unexpected places. Some people have allergies to gluten (wheat, barley, oats), which can lead to congestion and increase insomnia, as can allergies to detergents and the cleaning products you use on your clothes or sheets. One note: Decongestant nasal sprays are addictive and raise your blood pressure. Saline or antihistamine sprays (or a prescription steroid spray) are better options.

YOU Tip: Think Opposite. You'd think that the way to treat a lack of sleep is to get more of it, but one way that sleep docs treat insomnia is by making their patients sleep *less*. For instance, they'll take a patient getting five hours a night and force her to get only four a night, and then gradually increase by ten or fifteen minutes a night once a week. The sleep deprivation approach can work as a way to force your body to reset back into a regular sleeping pattern.

YOU Tip: Consider Herbals. Several supplements have been shown to decrease sleep problems. These are the ones we recommend:

Valerian root: It contains ingredients with sedative properties and is generally considered one of the more effective herbal therapies for sleep. Our recommendation: 300 milligrams.

Ginseng: Studies have shown that the ingredients in ginseng help decrease the amount of wakefulness in a twelve-hour period and increase the amount of slow-wave sleep. Try 200 to 600 milligrams of the extract.

Major Ager

Wacky Hormones

The Natural Fluctuations in Hormonal Levels Aren't All Bad

When we were growing up, we may have blamed our hormones for sprouting hair in new places. When we went to college, we may have blamed our hormones for having a sexual appetite satisfied only by the buffet of bodies in the next dormitory. Now that we're adults, we blame our hormones for foul moods, for sex drives that can be more like crawls, for hot flashes that keep us up all night, or for the ability to spend thirteen hours on the couch watching football.

Unlike a bone that can break, or blood that can clot, or even a neuron that can occasionally fail to fire to give you the numbers of your combination lock, hormones are enigmatic and intangible. But that doesn't mean that your hormones are any less important than the other systems in your body, or that you should simply accept hormonal decline as a fact of aging.

From an evolutionary perspective, hormones may be considered the most important system in your body. Testosterone and estrogen (and their derivatives and relatives), the major sex hormones in men and women, respectively, give us the urge and ability to try to reproduce and continue the survival of the species.

Biologically, it don't get bigger than that.

We need adequate (not necessarily high) levels of sex hormones to complete the equation of male + female = the next generation of the tribe. But once we're past our reproductive prime, our hormone levels drop. Men lose their testosterone, while women lose their estrogen and experience menopause. The tangible outcomes: lack of sex drive, insomnia, impotence, weight gain, and countless other potential health problems that can chip away at the quality of your life.

But instead of cursing our hormones for not having the stamina to keep up with our lives, what we ought to do is figure out *why* our hormone levels dip and drop. Thinking about that reason from an anthropological perspective will help us think about aging not as inevitably bad, but rather as inevitably, well, *inevitable.* That's the way nature is *supposed* to work.

Try considering your waning hormone levels as a way to benefit society. Men needed testosterone to give them the strength (and guts) to fight for land, to compete against warring tribes, to woo mates, and to protect the offspring that resulted. But as they grew older, they didn't need the reproductive effect of testosterone, because the next generation was already in place. And—here's where it gets interesting—they also didn't need testosterone's aggressive effect. If mature tribesmen spent all their time fighting neighboring tribes, they'd jeopardize their own survival and wouldn't live long enough to help the community in another way: through mentoring, through passing along wisdom, through helping to develop the intellect of future generations. In essence, that hormone surge in our youth and the hormone drop as we age isn't bad per se; it's actually quite advantageous.

Similarly, from an anthropological perspective, women stop ovulating (and the levels of hormones needed for it drop) so they can graduate from making babies to nurturing the entire community. If you look at brain scans, postmenopausal women think more like men and play a more dominant role in society—because they're not dealing with the hormonal and physical challenges of being fertile (like PMS and pregnancy).

Yeah, we know what you're saying: All your little tribesmen stories might make good fodder for a campfire and med school reunions, but what the heck are you going to do about my hot flashes, Doc?

We hear you. We're not saying that you need to just accept a drop in hormone levels and an increase in life-altering side effects. What we want you to do is acknowledge the fact that aging occurs for a reason, and that reason may actually be good for society. When it comes to your hormones, the problems—as we'll talk about in the following chapters—happen when they fluctuate too much or decrease. If that happens, then, yes, you are going to experience side effects that no anthropological yarn is ever going to quell. Still, some of the most intriguing and enticing hormonal treatments dealing with vitality—things such as DHEA and growth hormone—offer some promise in terms of treatment. We'll explore those vitality-based hormones in chapter 12. Ultimately, we want you to make sure your hormonal and related systems are in good working order, no matter what your age (see Figure I.1).

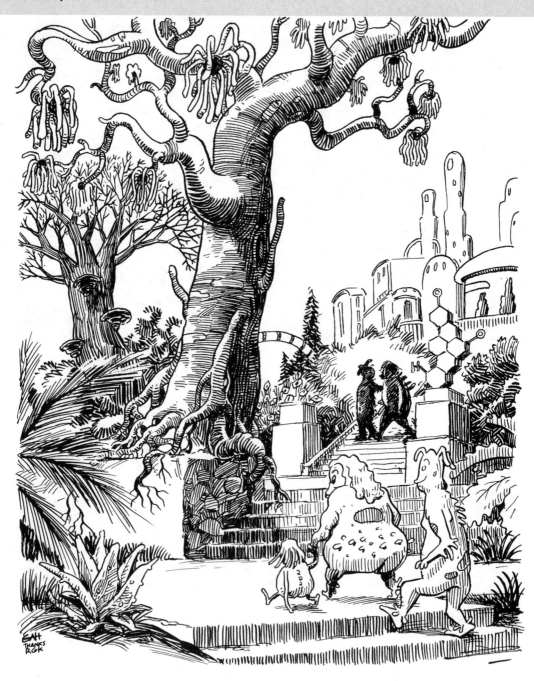

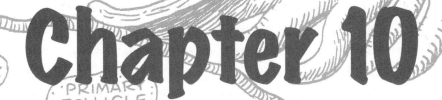

Chapter 10

Make the Most of Menopause

YOU Test: Hair Care

Women: Think of how often you had to shave your legs when you were twenty-five. How often do you have to shave them now?

A. About the same.

B. Less. Maybe a lot less.

C. Just call me gorilla legs.

If you answered B, that means you may be experiencing hormonal drops that are signs of menopause and menopausal symptoms.

Nobody would disagree that today's medical world is pretty darn advanced. We can replace bad hearts with good ones, we can make artificial limbs and ligaments, we can prevent seasickness and the flu, and we can do everything from scan the innermost parts of your body to cosmetically alter the outermost. But one of the many things we haven't been able to do—yet—is get a real handle on your hormones. (No, that's not a pickup line.) It's not that we haven't tried. (Nor is that.) Ever since the scientific world recognized that men's and women's lives were being adversely affected by dropping estrogen and testosterone levels, the question has been clear: Can we safely and effectively replace hormone levels so that you can live young at any age?

In this chapter, we'll discuss how hormonal and sexual issues are Major Agers for women. That's because declining estrogen is associated not only with such life draggers as hot flashes and insomnia but with sexuality—a key quality-of-life issue. When your hormones drop, sexual problems like loss of libido and lubrication arise. For the record, many other things can cause a drop in libido, including stress, financial problems, gain in waist size, and partners who are about as romantic as paperclips.

The treatment of symptoms related to estrogen decline has been controversial and confusing, and for good reason. This hormone replacement story has all the drama of a classic medical mystery complete with conflicting evidence: antiaging docs who vehemently defend hormone therapy, and other docs who think it's the worst thing since sliced buttered bread made with refined flour.

Here we'll clear up some of the confusion so you can decide whether restoring your hormones is right for you—and we'll tell you what we recommend to our families and patients.

Let's Pause for a Moment: Your Female Hormones

Every woman knows the cycle of reproductive life that starts and ends about when menstruation does is controlled by hormones. But to figure out how and why those hormones work, let's look at how estrogen affects aging. From before you hear "It's a girl," women are programmed to have a predetermined number of eggs. While biology textbooks teach that throughout a woman's reproductive life, those eggs come through her body like sand through a monthly hourglass and eventually run out, recent research suggests that adult stem cells (progenitor cells) can influence a woman's total number of viable eggs. We'd expect that to be true and offer some specific therapies to increase egg numbers in the next ten years. But it's not really the eggs we're concerned about; it's the estrogen that controls those eggs, turns the dials of menopause, and determines whether you'll feel its effects.

From the onset of menstruation, every twenty-eight days or so, one of the thousands of eggs that have been sitting in the ovaries since before birth tells the brain it's ready to be stimulated. The brain responds by telling the ovary to start maturing that dominant egg (see Figure 10.1). The follicle from that dominant maturing egg also secretes estrogens, some of which are metabolized to androgens (relatives of testosterone and similar to the ones that allow baseball players to break home run records). A woman's sex drive is partially dependent on her level of these testosterone-like androgens. When women enter menopause and cease to ovulate, 50 percent of their androgens disappear, leaving only the androgens produced by their adrenal glands to stimulate their sex drive. But adrenal production can decrease with age or medications, too. And after menopause, adrenal glands produce even less testosterone. Because androgens promote lean muscle production, and lean muscle mass increases metabolism, decreased ovarian and adrenal production can contribute to a woman's loss of muscle mass and to weight gain—especially the stomach pooch.

FACTOID

A group of people of northern European descent have an abnormal clotting factor called factor V Leidin. The most common clotting disorder, affecting 5 percent of the population, it predisposes them to clotting. Often, this goes along with a family history of deep vein thromboses and clots going to the lungs (called pulmonary emboli). If you have this factor V Leidin, a simple but expensive blood test and a family history will confirm the diagnosis. You want to take 162 milligrams of aspirin daily regardless of whether you pursue HT. It's worth noting that estrogen skin patches or transvaginal suppositories seem to decrease the risk of clotting, perhaps because estrogen avoids going immediately to your liver, where it stimulates the production of clotting factors.

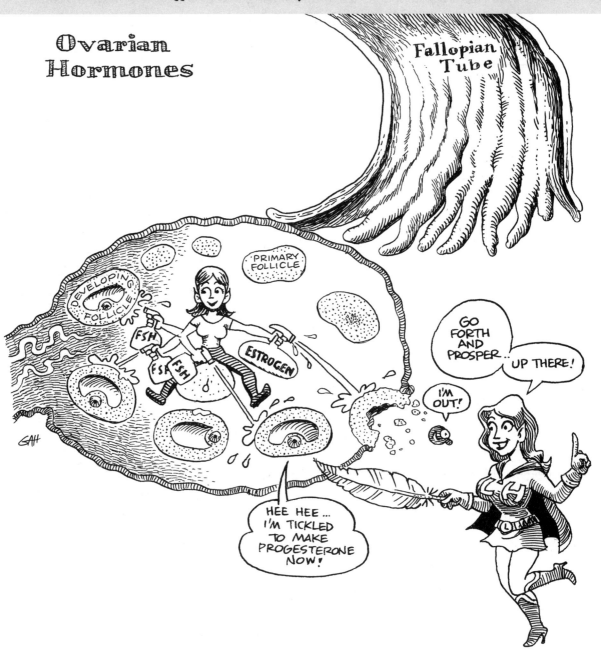

Back to reproduction and the life of the ovaries before menopause. Each month, the chosen egg produces a substance that prevents other eggs from developing. A combination of other hormones matures that one egg and pops a hole in its sac in the ovary (corpus luteum) so that it can escape to the uterus. The corpus luteum then produces progesterone to plump up the uterus and prepare it for pregnancy. If the egg isn't fertilized, the corpus luteum stops producing progesterone and women experience a period (what a great term for the end of a cycle).

Somehow nature got it just right. Typically, your body produces the perfect amount of hormones at the appropriate time, so that you have only one egg available for fertilization and implantation each month. Too little of these hormones can result in infertility or miscarriage. Too much—which often happens when women take fertility drugs—can have the opposite effect, leading to twins, triplets, quadruplets, and septuplets.

Essentially, menopause signals the end of the hormonal symphony that produces ovulation: Your ovaries run out of viable eggs, interrupting your cycle of hormones and monthly periods. It may take a while for your body to settle into a new hormone equilibrium; in the interim, you may suffer menopausal symptoms: hot flashes, insomnia, loss of libido and lubrication, itchy skin, dry hair and nails, achy joints, mood swings, memory lapses, even heart palpitations and an increased risk of seizures.

In spite of all these symptoms, estrogen decline is not totally a bad thing. You don't want to be in reproductive mode for your entire life, because you're meant to serve other purposes as you grow older. But that doesn't mean you have to suffer the side effects that occur during the process.

A half century ago, researchers came up with an idea: If you could restore estrogen to the levels at reproductive age, then you might avoid menopausal symptoms altogether. Now, if you've spent any time at all with your

FACTOID

The hormone oxytocin is naturally released in the brain after a twenty-second hug from a partner, triggering the brain's trust circuits. A side note: Men need to be touched two to three times more than women to maintain the same levels of oxytocin.

nose in a newspaper or fingers on a mouse, then you know that estrogen therapy is a highly controversial health issue. Some docs say it's a true miracle treatment, while others say they wouldn't touch estrogen with a ten-foot rubber glove. Estrogen therapy is not one extreme (it's surely going to kill you) or the other (it's 100 percent without risks). Your decision should be based on what shade of gray you're comfortable with. Deal? Good. Then let's start from the beginning and explain a little bit about how estrogen works and why there's been such a deep crevasse between the two sides of the issue.

The Three-Headed Hormone: Why Estrogen Is So Powerful

A lot of us like to fling around the word *estrogen* the way a pizza maker flings around dough, but the truth is that estrogen is a lot more complicated than that. With regard to *hormone replacement therapy* (HRT), or as it's now called, *hormone therapy* (HT), there are three important estrogen pathways to consider. In each case, the hormone works by locking onto a specific estrogen receptor in the body (we'll name them 1, 2, and 3, for simplicity):

❖ **Estrogen receptor 1:** located in breast and uterine tissue, and associated with female traits such as breast growth and menstruation. Estrogen that attaches to receptor 1 is thought to be linked to certain cancers because it promotes growth of breast and uterine tissue.
❖ **Estrogen receptor 2:** linked to the cardiovascular system and estrogen's apparent protective effect on the heart and arteries.
❖ **Estrogen receptor 3:** linked to the bones, allowing estrogen to strengthen bones.

These three receptors make estrogen therapy tricky. You get benefits by increasing the levels of estrogens that bind to receptors 2 and 3, but risks when too much estrogen binds to receptor 1. That's why we're seeing, and will be seeing, an

Should You Have Hormone Therapy if You've Had Breast Cancer?

Almost all breast cancers are classified as to whether they're estrogen-receptor positive or negative—meaning whether or not they're stimulated to grow in the presence of estrogens. About half are and half aren't. If you're estrogen-receptor positive, most docs would advise you to stay away from all estrogen, even bioidentical pharmaceutical-grade estrogen and soy (the exception being that in late-stage estrogen-receptor-positive cancers, high doses of estrogen can induce remission). If you're estrogen-receptor negative, taking estrogen may still be an issue; many doctors are reluctant to prescribe estrogen after breast cancer treatment. If you don't know your type, ask the physician or the hospital where your cancer was removed. Virtually all breast cancers have had receptors typed since 1992.

increase in so-called designer estrogens—estrogens that protect the heart and bones (and diminish menopausal symptoms) without increasing cancer risk. (Interestingly, men could take them too. Men don't have the same receptors associated with breast growth and high-pitched voices.) These designer estrogens (you may have heard of early ones, like Evista) may prove to be one of the most promising developments in medicine because of their potential to give what you really want when it comes to hormone therapy: the rewards without the risks. As of now, it seems that Evista does not treat menopausal symptoms and does not provide arterial protection, but it does protect bones and reduce frequency of some breast cancers. By the way, you also lose testosterone when you go through menopause, which means you lose muscle mass. Combined with inactivity, that's the true culprit in perimenopausal weight gain.

The Risks and Rewards of Estrogen Therapy

The reason why hormone therapy is controversial is this: The early studies of women who replaced estrogen were epidemiological—just collections of information on everyone who could be found. These studies compared postmenopausal women who did and did not take estrogen, but there was no attempt to select by a randomized process who took the estrogen and who did not; it was just a side-by-side comparison. These epidemiological (and not random) studies showed that women taking estrogen had a dramatic decrease in heart attacks and ischemic strokes compared to those women who weren't taking hormone therapy (not just a little decrease; up to a 75 percent decrease). And the women who took estrogen also had higher HDL (good) cholesterol, increased bone strength, and substantially decreased menopausal symptoms. Hot flashes, mood swings, and insomnia practically disappeared.

These early studies made estrogen seem truly beneficial, but with time, women on estrogen replacement also suffered a buildup of uterine tissue that led to an increase in uterine cancer, as well as a proliferation of breast tissue, associated with an increase in breast cancer.

To reduce the risk of uterine cancer, a cyclical dose of a specific progestin (nonbioidentical, synthetic progesterone) was added to the estrogen. The progestin caused the excess estrogen-stimulated uterine tissue to slough off (continued menstruation was the side effect associated with this reduction in cancer risk). Now we know that only women who have undergone hysterectomies should consider taking unopposed estrogen. By the way, obese women have an increased risk of uterine cancer because body fat is a significant source of peripheral estrogen storage.

Eventually, randomized studies were done to assess the effect of estrogen on arterial aging—preventing strokes, heart attacks, and memory loss. The largest and most publicized was the Women's Health Initiative. To many people's surprise, the studies showed an *increase* in heart attacks and strokes soon after starting therapy, mainly, in our opinion, because the estrogen and progestin had a clotting effect in leg veins and critical arteries. It turned out that there were problems with the studies, however: First, nobody was prescribed 162 milligrams of

What Are the Risks of HT?

Scary fact: Research shows that more than two-thirds of doctors overestimate the risks of hormone therapy. For example, many docs overestimate the increased risk of heart attacks, and many do not realize that estrogen decreases death from all causes in the first ten years after menopause by 30 percent. Furthermore, based on studies with the most recent data, we believe that taking aspirin decreases the risk of heart attack enough to allow an overall significant benefit. This table outlines the associated risks depending on what kind of therapy you use. One note: The final two columns have not been measured in controlled studies but are our best calculations of how the risks would look using our recommended therapy (with and without aspirin).

If you took estrogen and progestin therapy for forty years, what would be your change in risks? What is the change in absolute percentage that you will experience a problem, compared to a typical woman—i.e., 2.8 percent increase means 2.8 percent more than expected over a forty-year treatment period. We do not know how long you'd like to consider estrogen and progestin therapy, so just modify by the years divided by 40 if you think that is too long. For women without a uterus (who have undergone a hysterectomy), no progestin is needed to protect the uterus. The data of estrogen-alone therapy are similar to column one (or column four if aspirin is used).

(*continued on next page*)

aspirin to reduce the clotting effect. Second, the progestin studied in the Women's Health Initiative was one that has been shown subsequently to counter estrogen's positive cardiovascular effects. And third, the studies enrolled women who had not previously used hormone therapy, were usually more than fifteen years post-menopause, and had no symptoms that warranted starting treatment. (Women with significant menopausal symptoms were excluded from studies.)

In recent years, HT formulations have evolved and can now be obtained with new substances (we'll explain in a moment) and in much lower doses than previously available. So they're safer and better tolerated, though they still have some side effects.

Our stance when it comes to all this: If you are one of the 25 percent of women who are not miserable during menopause, don't complicate your life with pills. However, if you're one of the 25 percent of women whose hot flashes have given you a misdemeanor rap from threatening to tap fire hydrants, then don't fear putting HT on your radar screen. And what about the remaining 50 percent who

	Women's Health Initiative study with conjugated equine estrogen and a methyl progesterone acetate (example: Prempro)		Best estimate using tailored dose of bioidentical estrogen and a micronized progestin or progestin patch/cream (example: Angeliq)	
	for all times since menopause	if started within ten years of entering menopause	without aspirin	with 162.5 milligrams of aspirin
Death rate change (all causes of death)	None	30 percent reduction in first ten years after entering menopause	None overall, but 30 percent reduction if started in first ten years after entering menopause	Death delayed one to two years, due to effect of aspirin on cancer and stroke—same 30 percent reduction for first ten years
Heart attacks	2.8 percent increase over forty years	8 percent decrease (26 percent decrease from death and disability from heart attacks)	2 percent decrease	12 percent decrease (35 percent decrease from death and disability from heart attacks)
Strokes	3.2 percent increase	3.2 percent increase	4 percent increase	5 percent decrease
Deep-vein thrombosis	7 percent increase	7 percent increase	7 percent increase	1 percent increase
Breast cancer	3.2 percent increase	1 percent increase	3.2 percent increase	1 percent increase
Colorectal cancer	2.4 percent decrease	1 percent decrease	1 percent decrease	1 percent decrease
Memory loss	No change	Delay of two to three years	Delay of two to three years	Delay of four to six years
Hip/spine fracture	2 percent decrease	2.2 percent decrease	2.2 percent decrease	2.2 percent decrease
Hot flashes, vaginal dryness, insomnia	94 percent gone	94 percent gone	94 percent gone	94 percent gone
Overall changes if you count all major adverse effects as equal	4.8 percent increase	29.8 percent decrease for first ten years after entering menopause	2 percent increase	18.2 percent decrease (47.4 percent decrease in first ten years after entering menopause)

What Age Is Too Old to Start Hormone Therapy?

Since we believe that hormone therapy for women (say, aspirin plus Angeliq at a very low dose—you can split the pill in half) will eventually prove to be beneficial for overall health, the answer to this question may change. But for now, experts say that without menopausal symptoms that disturb you the risks outweigh the benefits if started ten or more years after menopause. While the data in the table are based on a projected forty years of HRT, the data are still incomplete, and we currently recommend our family members take hormones for up to ten years after the start of menopause.

are hot and bothered but could get through with some of the supportive approaches we describe below? Even in our own families, we are split, but we agree that hormone therapy with aspirin and with a micronized, not conjugated, progestin (definitions below) is not psychotic—because the potential benefits might outweigh the potential risks. Most physicians remain appropriately skeptical and will likely avoid recommending HT therapy to you until we have more studies.

But when the dust settles in twenty or so years, we believe that women who use HT (in the form of bioidentical estrogen and micronized progestin) along with aspirin to reduce clotting risks will experience a prolonged higher quality of life, including a decrease in heart disease, arterial aging, and memory loss, and an increase in bone strength. The downside: We'll see a slight increase in breast cancer. (That's because estrogen helps estrogen-sensitive breast tissue grow.) Keep this in mind as you and your doctor decide if the potential benefits (that address your personal concerns) outweigh the potential risks (considering your personal risk factors and family history).

YOU TIPS!

While there are several things you can do to increase your estrogen naturally, those strategies (exercising or deep breathing) aren't the big guns when it comes to preventing and reducing the symptoms of menopause. Hormone therapy is by far the most effective solution, but the decision to go on HT must be made on an individual basis. Figure out whether it's a good fit for you.

YOU Tip: Educate Yourself on the Replacements. If you've done any research about replacement therapy, you've probably noticed that there seem to be as many hormonal compounds as there are corner coffee shops. And the reality, as you've likely guessed, is that some of them are not all that effective. Some you get from the pharmacy, some you get from the health food store, and some you might as well be getting from a street vendor wearing a trench coat. As with anything you're going to inject, swallow, or rub on your body, you have to be aware of what you're using. Some definitions to familiarize yourself with:

Micronized progesterone: To allow absorption of progesterone from pills, it has to be protected from digestion by the acid and enzymes of the stomach and early intestine. Originally, an acetate group was attached to protect the progesterone. Unfortunately, that acetate group also seemed to change some of the beneficial effects of the progesterone. So a newer technique—putting the progesterone in minicapsules called micronized progesterone—was developed. You get the benefits of the progesterone without the side effects of the acetate protection.

Bioidentical compounds: These chemically synthesized or natural molecules of estrogen and progestin are "most like" the ones in your body. They are mixed and matched by compounding pharmacies or by pharmaceutical firms. This term has been hijacked by some who use only products from compounding pharmacies, but in truth, there are natural compounds made to the more rigorous quality-control standards of Big Pharma.

Natural compounds: Herbal supplements like soy and yam contain plant hormones that "may" resemble your hormones (according to those that market them). There are a lot of natural compounds, such as estrogen from pregnant mares' urine, but for this chapter, we're using the phrase *natural compounds* to indicate only over-the-counter herbal supplements.

YOU Tip: Choose Your Option. Hormone therapy comes in a variety of delivery methods, including pills, patches, gels, vaginal creams, and combinations of the above. In the cycle method (where you still get a monthly period), you take estrogen continuously for three weeks a month and add progestin for twelve days of the month. (Newer preparations are available that cycle every three months or even every two years, so you have less-frequent periods.) With continuous dosing, you take both hormones daily, often in one combined pill. Irregular bleeding is common when starting this—and indicates not quite enough hormone. This may seem unnatural, but remember that due to constant pregnancy and breastfeeding, our female ancestors had only about 100 menses in their lifetimes. Most women today will have 350 menses, so reducing the monthly event might be more natural than we suspect. In theory, this would also reduce the incidence of cancer of the reproductive organs.

Women who prefer not to take pills can apply patches to their thighs or abdomen or use an estrogen gel or cream; some patches contain estrogen and progestin, but many patches, as well as the gels and creams, are estrogen-only, and you will need additional progesterone pills to protect the uterus. Compounded bioidenticals are usually delivered in a cream. Some data show that gels and creams are safer and give benefits, but the research isn't solid enough to insist on this approach to our family members. Whatever the delivery method, it's best to try something that lives for a short time in your body, so that if you have negative side effects, you can stop or lessen your dose. One benefit of using a compounded product is that you can really control the dosing by starting low and moving up. Shots and implants, by contrast, aren't great to start with because once they're in your system, they can't be taken out until the cycle has ended.

YOU Tip: Make a Plan. How do you know which kind of HT to take? Well, the drug used in the Women's Health Initiative was Prempro—a combination of conjugated equine estrogen (Premarin, from pregnant mares' urine) and a methyl progesterone acetate (medroxyprogesterone, formally). This latter progestin choice proved unfortunate because it turned out in test-tube studies to antagonize the benefits of estrogen on arterial health. That's why we recommend a pharmaceutical-grade synthetic bioidentical estrogen. For the progesterone component, we recommend a micronized pill like Prometrium. (Prometrium is in a peanut-oil base, so don't try this if you or a family member has a peanut allergy. If you have an allergy to peanuts, ask your doc to prescribe an alternative progestin that is not conjugated and not peanut based.)

Most experts agree that your goal should be to be on the lowest possible dose for the shortest period of time. Blood tests are not very good at predicting estrogen's effectiveness on a cellular level. Because hormone levels can fluctuate as a woman approaches menopause, we focus on symptoms more than blood tests to determine what and how much to prescribe.

Here are the specifics:

For women with significant quality-of-life menopausal symptoms who want to consider hormone therapy, the first thing to do after you and your physician have agreed on this plan is to start taking 162 milligrams of aspirin a day at least two days before taking the hormones. For a woman near fifty with a

FACTOID

In many ways, humans are the most sexual of all species. Most other species are sexually active only when they're fertile and ovulating. Compare that to our species: With the right partner, women can have orgasms and can be sexually active throughout ninety-some years, as well as throughout the month's cycle and even during pregnancy.

Horny Supplements

While the herbal supplement horny goat weed sounds like it should boost libido, it actually doesn't seem to work for women, or even when taken orally for men. (It *has* been shown to work for male rats when injected directly into the penis—ouch!) Another herb, black cohosh, reduces hot flashes in 35 percent of cases—the same as a placebo. Because no harm is caused, and 35 percent is nothing to sneeze at, lots of women are plenty happy to keep using it. You might think that placebos are useless sugar pills for hot flashes or insomnia, but 35 percent of users get relief from them, which is an example of the power of positive thinking and your mind's control of your body. If you suffer from these symptoms, it may be worth it to see if exercise, paced respiration, black cohosh, or evening primrose oil work for you.

uterus and menopausal symptoms starting to disturb her life, we recommend an estradiol—usually Angeliq, a 17 beta estradiol (many generic preparations are available), in a small dose of about 0.3 milligram. Use the smallest amount that controls your symptoms.

❖ Increase in 0.25-milligram amounts every ten days until your symptoms are controlled. (The equivalent for patches is 0.025 milligrams patch a day).
❖ Add a micronized progestin—Prometrium at 100 milligrams (or occasionally 200 milligrams)—for twelve days a month. We like to use Angeliq, which combines estradiol with Prometrium and can be used continuously for women who don't want periods. If you wish to use a patch for the estrogen, you'll need a cream or the Prometrium pill alone for the progestin.

We think it is completely reasonable to keep this program going for its antiaging benefits while symptoms last and perhaps for up to ten years.

YOU Tip: Fix the Flash. Most hot flashes will resolve in three to five years. While we don't think you necessarily have to "deal with it," we also know that if the symptoms are minor enough, you can use non-hormone-therapy techniques to try to help control them. Estrogen is about 90 percent effective in reducing hot flashes, but other methods may also help (see Figure 10.2). Why? If you can control your central thermostat and relax your arteries, you'll avoid that roller coaster of vascular contraction and dilation that causes the sweats. That's why things like meditation and relaxation techniques may be helpful for reducing the red heat. Deep breathing, which helps counteract the Major Ager of a lack of nitric oxide, is more effective than any other therapy except estrogen. Yoga incorporates belly breathing and also offers poses that could help to lower blood pressure and heart rate. Vitamin E is anecdotally helpful, and if you are desperate, why not? And one big item that's often overlooked: the amount of saturated fat in your diet.

Figure 10.2 **Hot Hot Hot** Estrogen dilates arteries, but when it's produced erratically, arteries are unprepared for sudden spikes. So they overdilate, leading to blood surges to the skin, which can feel like a blowtorch. The roller-coaster process is well treated if you can keep the arteries relaxed permanently.

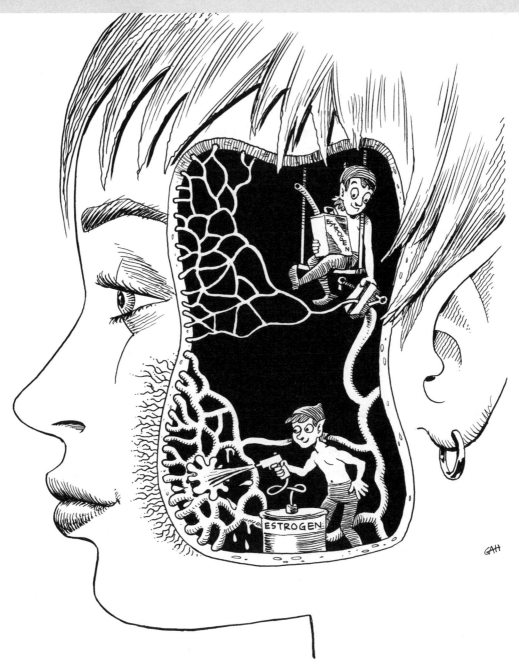

Why Not Just Take Some Soy?

It's true that soy products do contain more than fifty estrogenlike substances (phytoestrogens) that can influence the three estrogen receptors for uterine and breast health, bone strength, and artery stabilization. So it would seem to make sense: Pop a few more hunks of tofu, and you can turn back hormonal time. But here's the deal: Soy is as unpredictable as a morning DJ's mouth. That's because things such as the soil in which the product grows can influence those levels of phytoestrogens, meaning that there's really no way of knowing whether you're reaping benefits or not (or risking problems if you're a woman with an estrogen-responsive breast cancer). Many studies in which soy supplements were used to treat menopausal symptoms have proved inconclusive. But that doesn't mean you ought to toss soy to the back of the fridge for good. Soy's good for you because it contains relatively healthy fat (it has too much omega-6 fat in it to be called really healthy by our standards), its protein is healthier than that found in meat or chicken, and it contains fiber. All have nutritional benefits that may not directly eliminate those hot flashes but may still be beneficial to your overall health. Plus, studies do show lower breast cancer rates among Japanese women who eat traditional diets, which include soy, compared to those who eat a typical Western diet. (Other elements of a traditional Japanese diet may also be factors, such as a high intake of fish, vegetables, and tea and a low intake of red meat and dairy products.) The benefits of soy phytoestrogen seem best achieved by societies that have used moderate amounts of these products for generations—rather than Americans forcing down entire tofu forests in a single bound.

Saturated fats cause constriction of arteries after a meal. The fluctuation between dilation and constriction causes the flash. Fewer saturated fats equal fewer symptoms.

YOU Tip: Consider Other Meds. The epilepsy and pain relief drug gabapentin has been shown to ease both the severity and the frequency of hot flashes by almost 50 percent. It may be the new best thing other than estrogen for the flush. Also, a class of antidepressant drugs called SSRIs has been shown to reduce symptoms by 60 percent, as have alpha blockers such as clonidine (used to treat high blood pressure). All have side effects that many consider more problematic than estrogens, but some women prefer these choices. We do not recommend clonidine because of the risk of rebound hypertension if it's abruptly discontinued. Patients are supposed to taper down use of the drug to avoid the side effects, but many patients don't comply with those rules, risking the chance of developing high blood pressure when they stop taking it suddenly.

YOU Tip: Get Creamed. If you're experiencing a decrease in libido, your man's relationship with ESPN may not be the only thing to blame. You may be experiencing a drop in your own androgen levels. Your doctor can prescribe small doses of a testosterone cream or a pill called Estratest, which combines estrogen with libido-increasing testosterone. (Ask your doc to modify this if you are taking an estrogen for hormone replacement therapy.) The cream is applied around the vagina, on the skin, or as drops under the tongue because that's how the large molecules are best absorbed. (If taken orally, the enzymes in the stomach might destroy the hormone before absorption takes place.)

YOU Tip: Avoid Your Trigger. You remember the first time you suffered hot flashes. Now remember what started the symptoms? That is one of your triggers. Common culprits include stress, red wine, chocolate, coffee, and hot rooms (although it's hard to tell after the flash has started).

Low Pro

When it comes to waist gain, progesterone deficiency may be to blame. Progesterone increases basal body temperature, which burns calories. No ovulation, no progesterone, no increased temperature, fewer calories burned. Those calories can add up to several pounds a year.

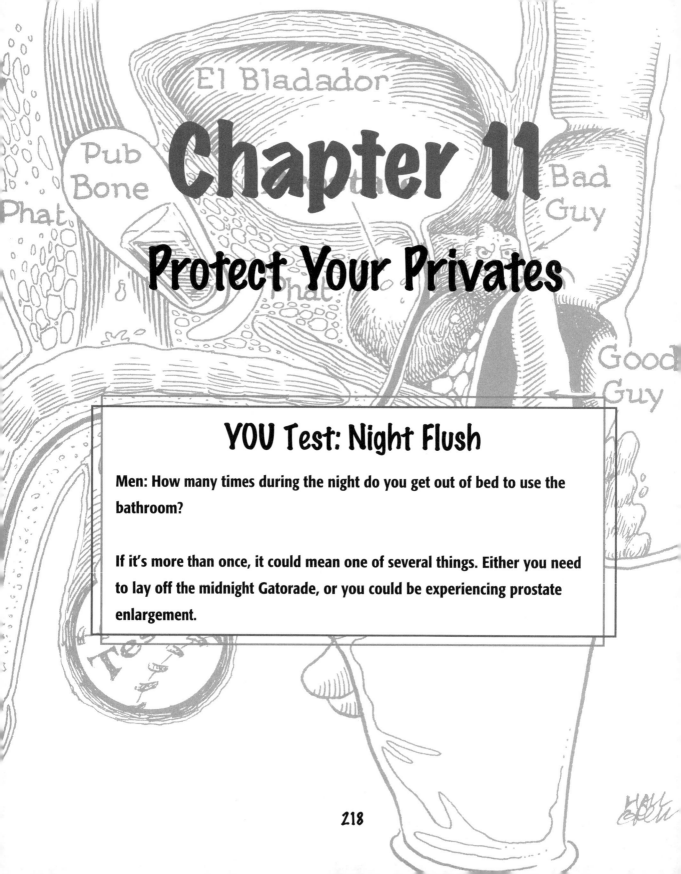

Chapter 11
Protect Your Privates

El Bladador

Pub Bone

Phat

Bad Guy

Good Guy

YOU Test: Night Flush

Men: How many times during the night do you get out of bed to use the bathroom?

If it's more than once, it could mean one of several things. Either you need to lay off the midnight Gatorade, or you could be experiencing prostate enlargement.

Though they may not admit it, men have all sorts of fears, be it public speaking, missing a field goal with time expiring, or being told by the tenth straight woman that, no, you may not buy her a drink. Though men tend to walk around with a shield of bravado and concrete-solid emotions, they sweat over one particular fear more than they sweat in a heavily populated steam room: doctor, rubber glove, bend over.

Though the digital rectal exam lasts only a few moments, many men squirm like a sun-fried worm when they think about medical happenings that occur bellow the belly button and above the thighs. When it ages, the prostate gland—which is responsible for maintaining, protecting, and enhancing the viability of the sperm in ejaculate—comes with side effects that don't exactly make for nice small talk. An aging prostate can lead to such conversation stoppers as urinary irregularity and a pelvis that burns hotter than a George Foreman Grill. (By the way, avoid some embarrassment by not confusing *prostate*, which can be inflamed enough to knock you to the floor, with the word *prostrate*, which means you are lying flat on the floor.)

But here's the thing. While you may feel embarrassed to talk about urine spots on your shorts or the fact that you've lost some propulsion in your ejaculation (not that you're looking), prostate problems affect lots of men—frankly, the majority of men, if they live long enough—making it the hormonal equivalent of female menopause. So let's take a look and see how the prostate can malfunction and what you can do to keep it healthy.

Rubber glove, please.

Your Prostate: Go with the Flow

With the exception of yoga teachers, most of us don't have that good a view of the prostate. Resting below the bladder and in front of the rectum, the prostate is around the size of a walnut (see Figure 11.1). The seminal vesicles (the ducts that

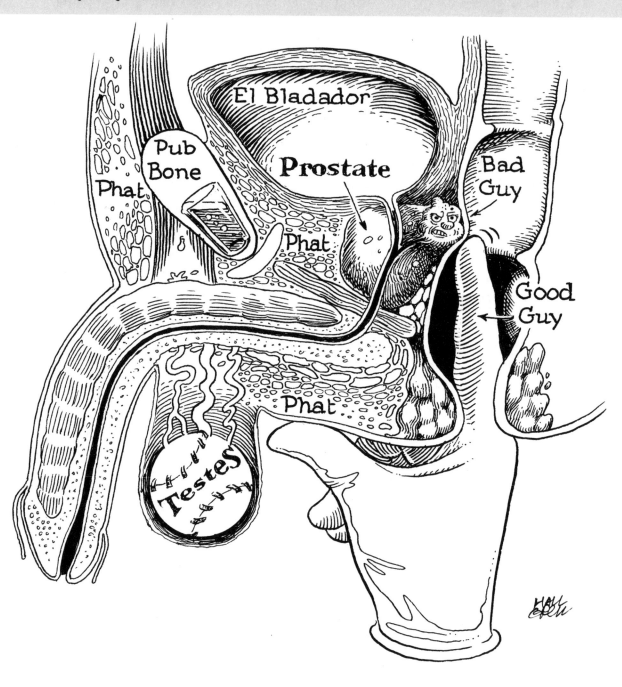

Figure 11.1 Digital Picture The walnut-sized prostate has semen-shuttling ducts that intersect with urine-carrying ones. Tumors or an enlargement can be assessed with the often maligned digital rectal exam.

shuttle semen for foreign exploration) are attached to the prostate and intersect with the urethra to take urine from the bladder.

Unlike most other organs, the prostate grows with aging. How? The Major Ager of wacky hormones sends to the prostate its representative, testosterone, which is the active steroid in nonsexual tissue like muscle. Testosterone is converted to dihydrotestosterone (DHT), the active steroid hormone in sexual tissue. DHT causes the prostate to grow (that's called hypertrophy). Yes, it is also the stuff that causes your bald spot to grow. Quick side note: If you're using those scrotal testosterone patches (we will talk about in chapter 12), they cause an increase in DHT production, because the scrotal skin has the highest concentration of the enzyme that converts testosterone to DHT.

FACTOID

Dogs get BPH in the outer areas of the prostate, so they don't get urinary obstruction (to the disappointment of fire hydrants everywhere), but, rather, rectal obstruction, which takes the pressure off curbing your dog.

But just as in urban planning, growth isn't necessarily bad—as long as you keep it under control and have the infrastructure to handle it. What's important is to determine why the prostate is growing as you age, and whether or not that growth is due to something that will kill you, change your quality of life, or do none of the above. Here are the major things that can change your walnut-sized gland into more of a coconut-sized one (or at least make it feel that way):

Prostatitis. An inflammation of the prostate, prostatitis is often caused by bacteria. Though some men don't have any symptoms even if they do have the condition, those who do can experience leg-crossing pelvic pain. The reason: The inflamed prostate swells and squeezes the urethra, causing pain. That squeeze also means that you may experience urinary problems, such as feeling the way you would if you'd had four beers in forty-five minutes: gotta go, gotta go right now. Just as gingivitis can be an indicator of general inflammation throughout the body, prostatitis is a sign that you may have dangerous inflammation throughout your body.

Benign Prostatic Hypertrophy (BPH). Occurring in the inner part of the prostate gland (called the periurethral gland), BPH is noncancerous growth that happens with age (and only if you have testicles). It's a very common condition, with 50 percent of men getting it by age sixty, and 9 out of 10 men having it by age eighty-five. This very slow and progressive growth of the prostate happens when you experience a decrease in nitric oxide and an increase in oxidative stress (which can be caused by chronic infection and nutritional deficiencies, as well as the more common cell growth). The symptoms can be similar to those of prostatitis: You feel as if you always have to go to the bathroom, you feel an incomplete emptying of the bladder, and you may feel burning when you urinate. Because you have an incomplete emptying of the bladder, you may dribble like a Harlem Globetrotter. And you may have to get up at night to pee more frequently than an on-call intern stops for coffee. (That coffee, by the way, is a diuretic, so having a cup after dinner can make you pee even more.) Contrary to popular belief, these symptoms don't (let's make that a capital DON'T) increase your risk of getting the next condition.

Prostate Cancer. Usually found in the outer zone of the prostate, prostate cancer tends to be thought of as an all-or-nothing situation. Either you remove the prostate, or you die. What we want you to know is this: Not all prostate cancer needs to be treated aggressively with surgery (the side effects of removal can be urinary incontinence and sexual dysfunction, because the nerves that control erections are next to the prostate). Certainly, prostate cancer needs to be followed more closely than a high-speed fugitive, but you should make treatment decisions taking into consideration such things as life expectancy, quality of life, potential side effects of treatment, and the aggressiveness of the cancer. Docs will use what's called the Gleason score to determine how aggressive the cells of the cancer are.

About 90 percent of men have prostate cancer by age ninety, and their life expectancy is generally not limited by this disease if they are older when diagnosed because the tumor is so slow growing—making it different from many other cancers.

The tough part about diagnosing a prostate condition is that the symptoms can be similar, usually involving some at-the-urinal issues. (Prostate problems can also be asymptomatic.)

If women have *What to Expect When You're Expecting,* men ought to have *What to Expect When You're Asked to Drop Your Drawers, Turn Around, and Bend Over.* When docs are looking to assess your prostate health, they'll start with a rectal exam to see if they can feel any inflammation or abnormal growths. They may also use an ultrasound, as well as biopsies to diagnose inflammation and/or cancer. Urologists may also do tests that measure such things as urinary flow rates and other urinary symptoms associated with prostate conditions.

Now, the primary way to measure prostate health (along with the digital rectal exam) is through a prostate-specific antigen (PSA) blood test. This test measures inflammation in the prostate. Contrary to popular belief, a high score doesn't automatically mean you have cancer; it simply means that your prostate is enlarged for some reason, be it cancer or something else. More important than learning the actual number is monitoring your change from year to year or every six months if the number is high, so you can see whether growth and inflammation are gradual or shoot up like a hot stock. A normal increase is less than 30 percent per year. That's why we recommend an annual PSA test for men, starting at age thirty-five or forty. A PSA test is not a substitute for a rectal exam; at least 20 percent of cancers don't involve elevated PSAs, so you need both the exam and the PSA to make the best starting-point diagnosis.

PSA is a little bit like cholesterol—the total number isn't as important as the breakdown of two components is. Like testosterone, your PSA test should measure "free" and "bound" PSA. The lower the free PSA, the more likelihood there is to be cancer (usually, less than 15 percent free means you should have a biopsy). The reason? Cancer cells make compounds that enhance the binding of PSA, making the number an important clue if the PSA is in the borderline range of 4 to 10 (see chart for normal levels). Another side note: PSA (which, to repeat, isn't cancer but indicates an irritation of the prostate) can be elevated by such things as urinary infection, bike riding, prostatitis, or having sex within twenty-four hours of the test.

Here's where the levels should be, remembering that an increase over time is more indicative than just a single test:

Age	PSA Levels (nanograms of PSA per milliliter of blood, or ng/ml)
40–49	0 to 0.25
50–59	0 to 3.5
60–69	0 to 4.5
70–79	0 to 6.5

Treatment Options

Various medical procedures exist for treating benign diseases such as BPH, as well as cancer if you decide that the discomfort of your symptoms or rate of the cancer's growth outweighs the risks associated with losing your prostate. In some cases, surgery may be preferable to taking drugs for the rest of your life. In fact, 30 percent of men will eventually undergo some type of prostate surgery. Following are the procedure options, but it's a fast-changing field, so you should talk to your doc about all available options.

For Cancer

❖ Radical prostatectomy. In this procedure, the gland and surrounding tissue are removed. It can "cure" the cancer if the cancer has not spread. Losing the prostate also means you'll lose some bladder control, at least temporarily. One good option: nerve-sparing radical retropubic prostatectomy, so you'll be more likely to have erections. Minimally invasive, laparoscopic, or robotic laparoscopic nerve-sparing radical prostatectomy are variations.

❖ Radiation. Radiation and radioactive seeds (which irradiate and kill cancer cells and tissues surrounding the seeds) are nonsurgical options. We favor the nerve-sparing radical retropubic prostatectomy by an experienced surgical team if you are under sixty or expect to live at least thirty years; and directed beam radiation if you expect to live fewer than twenty years. In between, you choose based on your health. No matter what, add the nutrition plan we outline below.

For Benign Prostatic Hypertrophy (BPH)

❖ Transurethral procedures. Various procedures like laser prostatectomy, microwave prostatectomy, and electrovaporization can remove some of the inside tissues of the prostate using various technologies to relieve inflammation and reduce symptoms associated with BPH. In general, these are outpatient, simple procedures, and your urologist can help you choose the one that will best alleviate your symptoms. Downside: these procedures may need to be repeated, and in case you haven't translated *transurethral* yet, then realize that an instrument's gotta go into a hole that's used to letting urine out.

YOU TIPS!

A growing prostate can be like a stage in the Tour de France—lots of ups and downs. While a number of things have been shown to prevent prostate-related diseases, understanding the various treatments and interpretations of prostate problems is especially important. You may not prevent the growth, but you can prevent the growth from shutting you down. In general, what is good for the heart is good for the prostate.

YOU Tip: Stay Relative. As we mentioned earlier, don't go into full freak-out mode if your PSA score seems high. You have to put it in the context of your previous scores. Likewise, realize that different laboratory kits give different results, so if you change doctors, an increase or decrease could be a result of the lab, not actual changes in your prostate. And that means you'll have to establish a new baseline when a new lab is used.

YOU Tip: Rock Your Guac. Food fact of the day: The avocado is known as the testicle plant—not just because it's shaped like the lovely sperm holders, but because it grows in pairs, and one side hangs lower than the other (really, we're not kidding about the plant). The other reason why it could be named after the sacred scrotum: The healthy fat in avocado has also been shown to decrease BPH. Saw palmetto has the same fat as avocados and should decrease prostate growth as well. The major benefit: smaller prostate size, less BPH, fewer nighttime awakenings for urinating.

YOU Tip: Veg Out. Prostate problems have the same risk factors as so many other health problems, like a diet high in saturated fats and being overweight. But a number of nutrients have been shown to improve prostate health, such as green tea (because of the polyphenols) and pomegranates. In a study of men who refused prostate surgery, one group of men only did watchful waiting (which is having a doc observe a patient but not intervene unless it's requested), while the other group went on an aggressive plant-based diet and stress reduction program. Their diet was low in fat and rich in selenium, lycopene (found in tomatoes), and vitamin E. The outcome: The latter group reduced their PSA levels by 40 percent, and none went on to surgery in a two-year period. Many in the control group required an operation, and their PSA levels remained elevated. After being on the healthy diet for fifty-two weeks, the men also had their blood mixed with prostate tumor cells (in a lab experiment), and the blood arrested the growth of the tumor cells. This did not happen with the normal population. Wow.

YOU Tip: Supplement Yourself. Men should consider taking zinc supplements, because men with higher zinc levels seem to have a lower risk of prostate cancer. Try a dose of about 30 milligrams a day (if you take a multivitamin, it may be in that already).

YOU Tip: Kick the Caffeine. For men with BPH, going to the bathroom can be hard. That's because the pressure on the bladder and a sphincter that spasms make it difficult to let the urine out. But once the sphincter relaxes, all flows like a rushing river. To help the sphincter relax, cut down on coffee and caffeine—which put the serious squeeze on. It may not make your prostate shrink, but it'll feel like it.

YOU Tip: Know the Meds. Prostate conditions can be tougher to treat than lovesickness—it's hard to extinguish the pain. While not full-fledged cures, many medications have been shown to have some levels of success. Your major options:

❖ Selective alpha-1 blockers: These medicines, like terazosin (Hytrin) and tamsulosin (Flomax), control the smooth muscle contraction around the prostate, relaxing the muscles to allow for easier urinary flow from the bladder. About 50 percent of men who take them see a reduction in prostate-related symptoms, while about 5 percent experience the side effect of hypotension (low blood pressure).

❖ 5-alpha-reductase inhibitors: Medicines like finasteride (Proscar) and dutasteride (Avodart) shrink prostate cells to reduce prostate volume (up to 25 percent in one year) and reduce PSA by 50 percent, though they take six months to take effect and work only about one-third of the time. One rare side effect: decreased libido.

No Nitric Oxide

How Your Levels of This Gas Can Change Your Health

Most of us have a pretty limited view of what's swirling around inside our bodies: We've got our organs, our bones, our blood and water, our chemicals, and perhaps a wheelbarrow's worth of fat all jumbled together to form a miraculous being that has the ability to swing from trapezes, solve complex math equations, or do both at the same time. Essentially, we think that our bodies are biologically constant. Besides what we put inside our bodies (and then, obviously, what comes out later), many of us assume that we're made with a set amount of chemicals, nerves, and gook that coexist finitely in our bodies. Either we have a lot or a little of chemical A or neurotransmitter B, and whatever those levels are dictate how we act and feel.

But that's hardly the case, especially when it comes to another one of our biological explanations of aging. Over a few weeks, or even days, we can modify these precious molecules to tune up our bodies.

Inside your body, you have a short-lived gas that tremendously affects your body's function. This gas—called nitric oxide—has a half-life of less than several

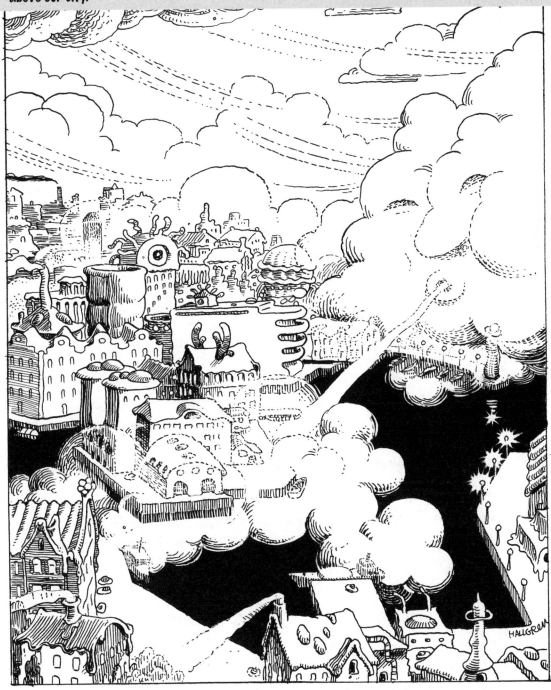

Major Ager: No Nitric Oxide 229

seconds. Like a wind that comes in and blows away pollution, nitric oxide is fleeting and exhilarating (see Figure J.1). You have nitric oxide, then you don't. (Before you start winking with sweet remembrances, nitric oxide isn't the same thing as *nitrous* oxide, the laughing gas used as an anesthetic and at some parties.)

So what? We've all got gas from time to time.

But we're not talking about gas that clears dinner parties; we're talking about the kind that's important enough to have generated a Nobel Prize in Medicine, important enough to influence whether you have a heart attack, and important enough that it powers a man's anatomical cranes. In fact, this gas—nitric oxide (NO)—was discovered to be the neurotransmitter in the nerve cells that control erections (this finding led to the development of Viagra and its friends).

And that makes the declining functioning of NO over time a key cause of erectile dysfunction and other age-related and artery-related problems. The bottom line when it comes to nitric oxide and aging is this: Nitric oxide plays a fundamental role in keeping a body healthy, and the reverse is also true. In many diseases, the production of nitric oxide is impaired, and that leads to (or contributes to) cell injury or the dysfunction of organs.

Despite its short-lived existence, nitric oxide affects many organs. In the brain, NO acts as a neurotransmitter to rapidly transmit messages. Much like the way that the brain chemicals serotonin and dopamine promote don't-worry-be-happy emotions, NO has a calming effect. Why? Nitric oxide turns on a chain reaction in our cells that allows our blood vessels to relax and dilate. People with atherosclerosis (clogging and hardening of the arteries) commonly don't make enough nitric oxide to keep their arteries open. The lack of NO helps to explain the detrimental effects we feel during periods of high stress as well as periods of low sleep. The common angina treatment nitroglycerine increases NO, dilating blood vessels and thus decreasing heart pain.

Now, you should be asking, how do you get your hands on some of this? If you want to open the valve on your own biological NO tank, you do it through your nose (without using your fingers). Nitric oxide is found in the highest levels in the nasal pharynx, and that's why nasal breathing and meditation are so important (see Figure J.2). The flow of air that happens when you breathe through your nose allows very rich sources of nitric oxide to be fuel injected into your system. The NO then helps dilate your arteries, so that your blood keeps moving as if it's on an empty country road rather than on an L.A. freeway.

Interesting side note: Marathoners breathe through their noses to stimulate nitric oxide and keep blood moving through their bodies. Sprinters, however, don't need the artery-dilating effect for a ten-second race. Instead, they need quicker access to the oxygen, and they get it through big ol' gasps through their mouths.

Specifically, here's what we know about NO and how it manifests itself in your body:

❖ Stimulating nitric oxide is one of the ways to promote wakefulness. If you're feeling sluggish, it tends to mean that you don't have good levels of NO in those areas of your brain and brain stem that keep you awake. (Narcolepsy is the ultimate example of not having enough nitric oxide, because you lose all alertness and fall asleep.)

❖ Not having enough nitric oxide promotes aging of the skin (because good circulation is essential for young-looking skin).

❖ NO enhances the action of minoxidil, which has been shown to slow hair loss.

❖ Sleep apnea, a condition in which you stop breathing during sleep, inhibits the absorption of nitric oxide into your body. Makes sense, right? When you're overweight, you tend to breathe through your mouth instead of your nose. The theory goes that because of that, you're not sucking those rich sources of nitric oxide into your lungs, so the airways are less dilated, and oxygen levels can drop. And that's

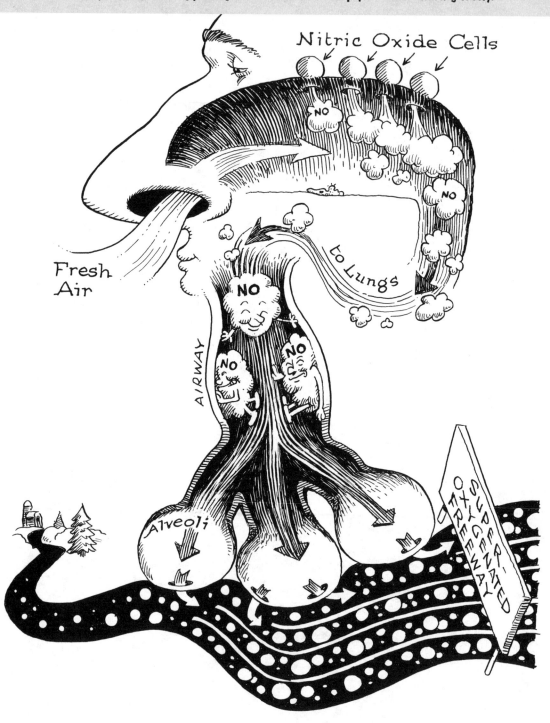

what might make you fall into one of the cascading cycles where you feel drained, tired, and stressed, which further inhibits your ability to get NO.

In fact, NO may soon become one of the clear markers that can help us diagnose (and treat) conditions before they show more outward symptoms. Research shows that you can see nitric oxide impairment months—maybe even years—before diabetes and atherosclerosis are clinically diagnosed.

Chapter 12
Live the Sexy Life

YOU Test: Deeds of Desire

Women (men, see next page), ask yourself these four questions:

A. Do you notice a change in your interest in sex (for the worse, that is)?

B. Do you have trouble becoming aroused or sufficiently lubricated?

C. Does sex feel about as pleasurable as walking on thumbtacks?

D. Do you reach orgasm about as often as the census is taken?

If you answered yes to any of these questions, it's fairly obvious that your desire and arousal are declining faster than VCR sales. Good sex isn't just about orgasm, it's about desire and interest, which often can help improve quality of life, making it an aging issue as well. Read on to follow our tips for increasing the quality of sex.

Men: Right before bed, place a strip of four to six stamps around the shaft of your penis. Overlap them and moisten the last stamp so it can seal the ring. Wear snug briefs to bed. Do this for three nights. In the morning, check the stamps. Have the stamps been broken along the perforations?

If yes on at least two of the nights: That means you're having erections during the night—a sign that you have good blood flow to your penis. If the perforations haven't broken, it could be a sign of some vascular difficulty.

YOU know how the stereotype goes. When you're young and not having sex, you can't think of anything else except sex. When you finally do have sex, you have about as much of an idea about how to have good sex as you have an idea about how to crack safes. And when you finally reach the point where you've become a master at sex (if you do say so yourself), you'd rather be knitting blankets than messing around under them. Cruel nature. Cruel, cruel, cruel nature.

By now, though, you probably know how we feel about biological generalizations—many of them belong in the infectious waste bin right next to the dirty syringes. Because you know what? As you age, you should be able to experience the best of what sex has to offer; a deepening of your emotional relationship with the pleasure of your physical relationship. The best part about great sex is that benefits extend far beyond the eighty-four-second ecstasy you may feel at the time. Having monogamous, regular sex has been proven to extend your life. The more you have it (for men) and the higher the quality (for women), the healthier you are.

While we don't care much for stereotypes, we, of course, have to acknowledge that there is a biological reality about sex. Sometimes our desire slows down, and sometimes our equipment shuts down. For men, the issue is really an intersection of two Major Agers: wacky hormones and no nitric oxide. That's because nitric oxide plays a large role in maintaining erections, as does the main male sex hormone, testosterone. For women, nitric oxide doesn't play as large a role in libido and arousal, but some of the most intriguing answers to increasing sexual desire lie in hormones that purport to restore overall vitality and sexual vibrancy. In this chapter, we'll examine not only how a man can deal with his version of *men*opause (that is, erectile dysfunction and loss of testosterone), but also whether men and women should consider the so-called miracle hormones that many claim to be the answer to better sex and more energetic lives.

What Goes Up: The Anatomy of an Erection

Yes, erections provide comedic fodder for movies. Yes, erections have more nicknames than superstar athletes. And yes, it's not exactly a word that most of us use at the dinner table ("Pass the corn, dear. How was your day? Feeling pretty good about the strength of your erections?"). But when it comes to aging, few things rival sexual dissatisfaction—and the sexual dysfunction that can cause it—as the area that makes a person's quality of life plummet faster than a deflated balloon.

Thanks to Viagra and her relatives, which increase the duration of the effect of NO, erectile dysfunction is no longer an in-the-closet, never-to-be-talked-about disorder (didn't know she was a she, did you?). Clinically defined as the consistent inability to attain an erection sufficient for sexual activity, erectile dysfunction (ED) hits about 50 percent of men ages forty to seventy and 70 percent of men older than seventy. Suffice it to say that most aging men are going to have at least some experience with losing a little pulp in their juice. We should also note that getting older isn't all bad when it

> **FACTOID**
>
> About one-quarter of men with elevated LDL cholesterol have erectile dysfunction, while half of men with depression experience it.

Mood Boosters

Women having trouble with arousal, desire, lubrication, or all of the above can see a doctor for medical or hormonal treatment methods, but don't hesitate to try your own methods too. Some options:

Go novel. Desire increases with new situations, new stimuli, new anything. So maybe it means taking a bath before sex or using the recliner for other things than watching TV. Or maybe it means the two of you take lipstick and write sexy messages on each other as a method of foreplay. Doesn't matter what you do, as long as you break up routine and drive up desire.

Add lube. We all know that there's nothing pleasurable about sex if the glide and ride feels about as smooth as a ride in a car without shock absorbers. For the smoothest results, you want oil or silicone lubricants. The only problem is that they degrade latex, so use water-based lubes if you're using condoms.

Be honest. First, with yourself. Ask yourself about your anxiety and feelings about the relationship. Then, talk with your partner. Though it's not an easy conversation, men should know what they can do to help increase your pleasure and mood—be it with more foreplay, more romance, or more everyday conversation.

comes to erection issues, since it does mean for most men that it takes a little longer to ejaculate.

As you might have guessed, a lot of research has been done on what causes ED, and, as is the case with cancer, heart disease, and so many other conditions, there isn't one single factor to blame. Rather, many things can cause the erectile rocket boosters not to fire—including hormone problems, which we'll discuss later in this chapter, trauma to the area (like that caused by poor-fitting bicycle seats, which block off the blood supply to the penis), alcohol, some prescription drugs, and obesity. But the biggest cause of erectile problems is fleeting levels of the Major Ager nitric oxide due to vascular disease. The way blood flows throughout your body (which is largely determined by the hardening of your arteries) determines your body's ability to maintain and sustain an erection (see Figure 12.1). In fact, erectile disorders are actually precursors of heart problems, so if you or

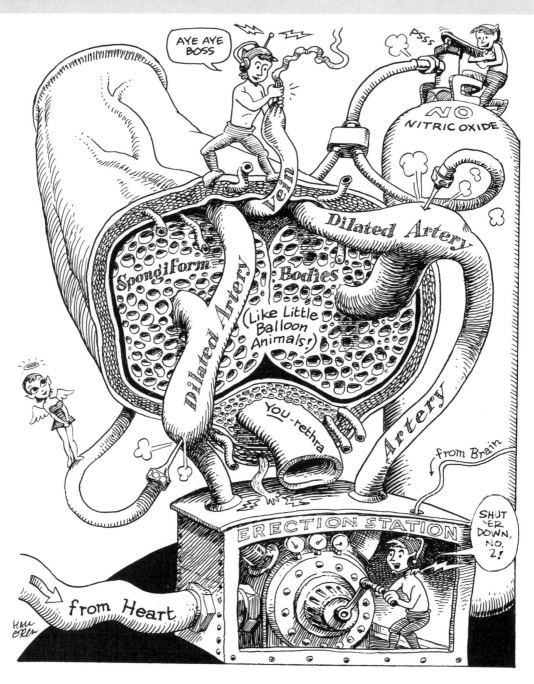

You're Going to Do What to My Huh?

Viagra-like drugs did more than make celebrity endorsers the butt of Jay Leno's jokes. They squashed many of the early treatments for ED. Just for fun, you can get a legs-crossing look at what used to be popular treatments for sexual softness. Some are still available.

Vacuums: These devices sucked on the penis (and aren't recommended to clean up crumbs) and worked by allowing blood to flow into the penis by negative pressure. Then the user put a rubber band around the base of the penis to hold the blood in to sustain the erection.

Injections: Prostaglandins (hormone-like chemicals) were injected directly into the penis with a small needle. Though it sounds about as pleasant as walking barefoot on Miami asphalt, the injections were especially popular for men with diabetes. Why? They weren't afraid of the needles.

Squirting: Docs also used to squirt hormones through the urethra, the little opening in the penis. Yeow.

Surgery: Surgeons would try bypass surgery on arteries that brought blood to the penis—because it used to be thought that veins were leaky and they needed a better arterial foundation to allow blood in. These new but small arteries didn't work well. Now we have better options.

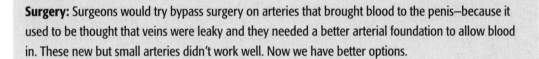

your partner is experiencing erectile problems, it's important to seek treatment, not just to improve what happens when you're lying down in bed but also to make sure that the next time you're lying down isn't on a surgeon's table.

To see how the cardiovascular and sexual systems work together, let's peek inside our illustrative trousers on page 238 and scout out the biological processes of stimulation.

Let's clear up the first misconception about erections: It's not testosterone that's the main driver of erection, though it does play a role, as we'll address in a moment. The reality is that erections happen because of many things going on in the body at once. The major way that the penis gets hard isn't through X-rated Internet sites, it's through receptors on cells lining our arteries that stimulate a chain reaction that ultimately relaxes the blood vessels that go to the penis. That reaction is mediated by nitric oxide, that short-lived gas floating around in your body. The aging link? NO is usually made by the endothelial cells that line all of our arteries. As soon as even a small amount of hardening of the walls starts with the creation of mild plaque, levels of NO plummet, so the vessel cannot dilate normally when you need a little extra blood, as when running for the bus or rummaging around in bed.

During stimulation (no matter whether it's physical or mental, lights on or lights off, with whipped cream or without), the muscles around the arteries in the penis relax. That relaxation happens so that blood can be absorbed by a spongy structure on the top of the penis called the corpus cavernosum. After the blood rushes in like a tailback breaking for the end zone, the veins in the penis clamp down to keep that blood trapped in the penis. And *voilà!* We've got liftoff, Houston.

If those arteries are inflamed and/or clogged, then you don't have proper blood flow. And that means you don't have enough nitric oxide to open up your arteries, so you can't get an erection because you can't get blood into your penis. Plus, without an engorged penis, the veins that drain the blood don't kink off, so whatever meager blood enters the organ quickly spills back out. That's why erectile problems, for the most part, aren't manhood problems or mental problems or "You don't do it for me anymore, honey" problems. They're plumbing problems that require you not only to be turned on but to have the right biological faucets turned on as well.

Gimme a *T:* The Truth About Testosterone

Hear the word *testosterone,* and we know immediately what you're thinking. You know it's what puts the moan in hormone. You think of muscle, of sex drive, of bravado. It's the vitality hormone that gives men the strength to win a fistfight (and the guts or stupidity to get into one in the first place). And it's the hormone that partly controls how much sex men want—and whether or not they're going to experience erectile dysfunction.

Most men produce 4 to 7 milligrams of testosterone a day, with the highest blood level in the morning and the lowest level in the evening (which helps explain why the first thing some men want in the morning is neither coffee nor a shower). Science has yet to explain why the levels

rise and fall at these times, but it may be related to action of the brain's pituitary gland. For practical purposes, those time frames do give some insight into why the so-called nooner can be an effective way to match a couple's sexual urges.

Just like women, middle-aged men experience male menopause (or andropause, if you prefer), a decline in sex hormones that affects their quality of life. Testosterone declines as we age. Symptoms include decreased strength, decreased libido, or decreased ability to swing the bat. One of the most outward signs of declining testosterone is a decrease in how often a man has to shave; slower beard growth equals a drop in male hormones.

While low testosterone affects two million to four million men, only 5 percent get treated for it, even considering the fact that we've recently seen a significant increase in prescriptions for testosterone (though some may be for women as well since it is an important sex hormone for them too). That increase indicates that men are becoming much more aggressive about wanting to have low testosterone treated, because they fear or are experiencing effects such as thinning bones (osteoporosis), infertility, reduction in facial and body hair, or a decrease in mood, energy, and sexual function and desire. Luckily, we can suggest who might be a candidate for testosterone replacement.

While the majority of erectile-dysfunction cases are caused by vascular issues, about 20 percent are associated with low testosterone levels. As part of a checkup to determine the root of erectile difficulties, your doc could measure your hormone levels. Though it's a simple blood test, it's unlike most others, because testosterone is not measured directly. To get an accurate assessment of your testosterone levels, you need to have two measurements. One measures the combined level of bound and free testosterone (the active kind that matters in terms of what symptoms you're experiencing) in your blood, while the other measures only the testosterone that's bound to proteins. By subtracting the second number from the first, you'll find your level of free testosterone. Because free testosterone can bind protein in a test tube, and bound testosterone can be displaced, the resulting number will be, at best, a close approximation. It's sort of like trying to get an accurate measurement of spaghetti sauce by weighing the pasta with the sauce, scraping off the sauce, and then weighing the pasta again. It's not a direct measurement of the sauce, and it's nearly impossible to separate all of the free sauce from the sauce that sticks.

Here are standard free testosterone levels for men your age. We should comment that part of the challenge is that if you want to feel thirty when you are fifty, you would theoretically want to get your testosterone level to that of a thirty-year-old, but most practitioners would rather get you to where your age predicts. Nevertheless, if you feel like sludge, then some docs will treat you even if your levels are in the low normal range for your age. Here are the typical ranges for men:

Age	Free Testosterone Level (ng/ml) (percentage free is 1.6–2.9 percent)
20–40	400–1,080
40–50	350–890
50–60	250–750
70 or above	250–650

The Ancient Aphrodisiacs

It may sound like a character in a sci-fi movie, but *Tribulus terrestris* might have some benefits for men and women experiencing a decline in libido. The fruit, which has been used since the times of ancient Greece, increases luteinizing hormone, which enhances testosterone production—possibly leading to an aphrodisiac effect (studies using an extract have found it to be effective). Formerly recommended as a treatment for female infertility, impotence, and low libido in both men and women, it was also used to aid rejuvenation after a long illness. The herb became widely known in the West when medal-winning Bulgarian Olympic athletes claimed that use of *Tribulus* had contributed to their success. High-quality studies on its use and dose are still limited, but we recommend 300 milligrams daily, since side effects are few and far between.

Another herb—red velvet bean plant—is used widely in Indian Ayurvedic medicine and contains L-dopa, which is converted to dopamine once it crosses the blood-brain barrier and might be used to treat Parkinson's disease in higher doses. However, it's also reported to stimulate the pituitary gland to release growth hormone and testosterone, and has been historically used as an aphrodisiac. Patients need to be cautious taking dopamine and should discuss a 400-milligram dose of this herb with their doctors.

Let's make one thing clear: We are not recommending testosterone therapy for men with normal testosterone levels as some kind of antiaging miracle treatment. Testosterone therapy should be used only for men diagnosed with enough of a deficiency to cause some of the problems we've already outlined. Unfortunately, blood tests are not always accurate enough—remember, the sauce on the spaghetti is difficult to measure. In the same way, total blood testosterone levels aren't a perfect measure of what's available where you need it. If your doc recommends that you boost your testosterone with supplementation, here's what you need to know about its benefits and potential side effects:

> **FACTOID**
>
> About 1 percent of testosterone is converted to estrogen, which may help explain why a small percentage of men do get breast cancer.

In Favor: Besides improvements in the areas most associated with testosterone (libido, muscle mass, bone strength), testosterone therapy has been shown to decrease levels of lousy LDL cholesterol and improve insulin sensitivity, so your chance of suffering diabetes decreases.

The Knock? The main criticism of testosterone therapy has been its reported links to prostate cancer. While there's evidence that the total size of the prostate enlarges in men who take testosterone, there's no clinical evidence that it actually influences prostate function, such as blocking urinary flow so you are up all night visiting the toilet. And there's no strong data to suggest that testosterone therapy is linked at all to prostate cancer, nor is testosterone in general, as evidenced by the fact that twenty-year-old men with the highest testosterone levels are at no more risk for developing prostate cancer later in life than men with normal or low levels. The other theoretical concern is heart disease, because men develop the disease earlier than women, but no link has been identified when men take supplements with careful monitoring. Long-term testosterone treatment has also been linked to increased baldness, fluid retention, enlarged breasts, and aggravated sleep apnea.

Testosterone is a little like chicken: You can get it prepared any way you want. You and your doctor just have to decide which way works best for your health (and your finances). Ideally, you need to work with your doctor to figure out what amount of testosterone will put you in the middle of the normal range, rather than being at the upper or lower end. If you do decide that testosterone therapy is right for you, these are your choices for delivery:

❖ Injections: It's the "wham, bam, was I supposed to pay and thank you, Doc?" method. With weekly, monthly, or even quarterly injections, you get your doses of testosterone immediately. The problem is that they can cause noticeable fluctuations in hormone levels that can affect your mood and your energy.

❖ Sublingually: Here, the testosterone is delivered through a tablet placed under the tongue, typically every twelve hours, which evens out the delivery better than the injection. The downside is that sublingual testosterone has been linked to liver abnormalities.

❖ Through the patch: It's costly, but replacement of testosterone with a patch on your skin—the testosterone is absorbed through the skin to increase the active form of testosterone—is considered safe (though some men have skin reactions to it). It is also a much better match for your body's natural cycles and rhythms. Depending on which you use, the patches can be applied to your abdomen, back, or legs, or (hold the snickers, please) directly onto the scrotum—which seems erotic, but actually works because the key enzyme (DHT), which converts testosterone to its more active form, is in the testes, which are close by.

The Vitality Hormones: Worth the Investment?

Though we think of testosterone as the major source of sex drive in men and women, we also need to look at other hormones that influence our overall energy and desires. DHEA, for example, turns into testosterone, while growth hormone is purported to have some of the same characteristics of the big T—like leading to increased muscle mass and increased bada-boom (see Figure 12.2). Here, a look at three other so-called vitality hormones:

DHEA: A steroid hormone that's similar to testosterone and estrogen and can actually be converted to these hormones, DHEA (dehydroepiandrosterone) has been considered by many to be the snake oil of medications. It's been marketed as a cure-all that improves just about every system in the body (it started back in the early 1990s, when reports came out that people taking DHEA felt really good). One big problem: DHEA is considered a food supplement, so it's

FACTOID

The herbal remedy yohimbine seems to work as an alpha blocker that prevents the arteries from spasming and shutting off blood to the penis. That means that it may be able to dilate the arteries near the penis to promote good blood flow.

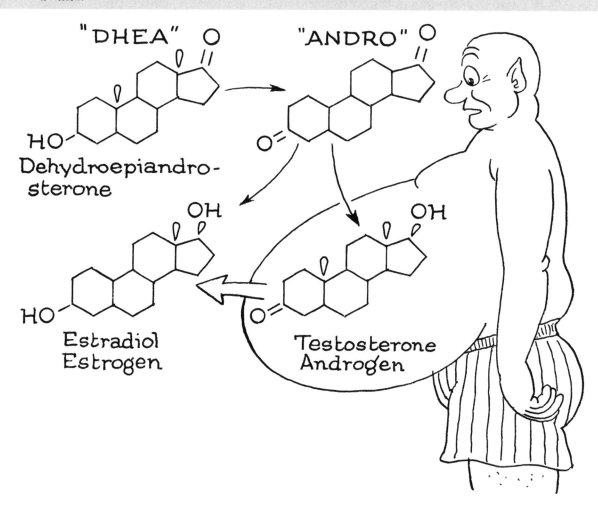

Figure 12.2 Fat Chance DHEA is only a small adjustment away from the controlled substance androstenedione ("andro"), which then becomes testosterone and estrogen. Belly fat converts testosterone to estrogen, which is why obesity predisposes to some cancers (and breasts in men).

not regulated tightly by the FDA. Another: Since it's a steroid, it has the same potential long-term side effects as other steroids, such as cancer and a weakened immune system. Just because something makes you feel good doesn't mean it's good for you (think cocaine, heroin, or pints of ice cream).

Nevertheless, we do believe that DHEA can be effective for boosting energy, stamina, and reduced sex drive. So if you are wiped out or have low libido, and you've been checked out by docs for everything else, maybe—just maybe—low doses of DHEA might help. You need to talk to your doctor about your own levels and be cautious if you have thyroid issues or a rising PSA, because DHEA is the precursor of androgens, and superhigh levels of androgens might be linked to prostate cancer; even normal levels may be a problem if you already have the disease. We don't endorse DHEA as the miracle antiaging drug that it's often purported to be but, rather, in measured doses as a way to possibly counteract general fatigue and low moods associated with aging, when the usual suspects have been rounded up and no other obvious culprits exist—and then only at the lowest dose that seems to work. Our recommendation is to try 25 to 50 milligrams and to monitor if it is working.

Growth Hormone: You may have seen a lot of it in the news because of athletes accused of taking it to improve performance, but human growth hormone also has gotten a lot of press for its purported antiaging benefits. Here's how it works. Growth hormone, naturally produced by the pituitary gland, the pea-sized organ at the base of the brain, acts on the liver and other tissues to stimulate production of insulin-like growth factor-1 (IGF-1). That IGF-1 is what's responsible for the growth-promoting effects of growth hormone, especially important in the proper development of children.

> **FACTOID**
>
> To help understand how Viagra-like drugs work, think about how nitroglycerin works in people with angina. Nitroglycerin is converted to nitric oxide, which opens the heart's arteries to allow blood to flow through, which gives you pain relief. Only nitroglycerine selectively dilates the arteries near the heart instead of the ones further south. Nitroglycerin and Viagra are dangerous together because there's too much dilation and low blood pressure. That can cause you to faint or to have heart problems.

Today's debate focuses on how much growth hormone we need as we age, since production is highest during childhood and the hormone-drenched adolescent years, then typically starts tapering off around age thirty, continuing to decline into old age and if we become obese. Many marketers want you to believe that boosting HGH blood levels can reduce body fat; build muscle; improve sex life, sleep quality, vision, and memory; restore hair growth and color; strengthen the immune system; normalize blood sugar; increase energy; and turn back your body's biological clock. But the flip side is that it causes swollen and painful joints, carpal tunnel syndrome, gynecomastia (big breasts are a big price to pay for men), and a trend toward the onset of diabetes (a big price for both genders). It also offers no benefits in clinically relevant outcomes, such as bone density, cholesterol and lipids, and maximal oxygen consumption. We think growth hormone might help with cholesterol and lean muscle mass, but the differences are so small that adopting even a few of the many non-HGH options we suggest for increased vitality will offer you equivalent results—and without the $1,000-a-month price tag of growth hormone.

Thyroid Hormone: Surprised to see thyroid hormone here? Well, so many people experience thyroid problems that we consider it a vitality hormone as well. If your thyroid slows down, you can experience things like fatigue and weight gain, but they can be reversed with thyroid medication so you can return to feeling vibrant and strong. We recommend that both men and women have their thyroid-stimulating hormone level checked every other year starting at age thirty-five. (TSH is the trigger from the brain that tells your thyroid gland to make thyroid hormone.) You can also do a prescreen yourself: Every morning, as soon as you wake up and before getting out of bed, put a thermometer under your tongue for three minutes. If your under-the-tongue temperature is less than 98 degrees Fahrenheit, you are likely hypothyroid. Repeat the test every day for two weeks.

YOU TIPS!

When you were fifteen, you probably thought that a light breeze was the only thing a man needed in order to achieve an erection. Those were the good ol' days. You only had to think the words *Charlie's Angels,* and your gun was out of its holster. Times change, and it's not so easy anymore. The real reason why you may be slow on the draw isn't because you're not interested in sex but because your arterial (and hormonal) traffic flow isn't quite right. These tips will help keep it moving a little more smoothly.

YOU Tip: Put Your Heart into It. We're not talking about trying harder in terms of needing more foreplay, or more stimulation, or making sure that every lovemaking session has the passion factor of a wedding night (though there's nothing wrong with any of those things). The best thing you can do for your penis is to be good to your heart. That is, follow our guidelines in the previous chapter and throughout the rest of the book about eating heart-healthy and artery-clearing foods and getting at least one hour a week of cardiovascular exercise. While arterial issues aren't the root of every erectile problem, they are the major cause, and the only way to keep the short-lived nitric oxide ready for battle is to keep the troops well exercised. The better your blood pumps, the better other parts of your body will too.

YOU Tip: Go Grape. The polyphenols in Concord grape juice stimulate endothelial cells (the cells that line blood vessels) to release NO, which not only helps protect against cardiovascular disease but helps maintain healthy blood vessels and adequate blood pressure. Only juices with high levels of polyphenols have the beneficial effect, and that depends on the type of grape used and how it's processed.

YOU Tip: Ask for a Quicker Picker Upper. The rise of Viagra-like drugs has basically made most other erection treatments obsolete (see box on page 239). The reason why Viagra's so effective: It stimulates the chain reaction that allows blood to flow into the penis by prolonging nitric oxide's effect. NO stimulates a chain of events that dilates those arteries so much that the return of blood from the penis through the veins is blocked. Rather than answer any of the several dozen junk e-mails selling Viagra that you will receive today, talk to your doc about a prescription that helps stimulate that blood flow. Big caveat: Viagra doesn't cure ED. If you don't treat the underlying cause—be it onion rings, inactivity, or that you smoke more than a five-alarm fire—then you're ultimately never going to fix the problem. Now, if you have the unfortunate side effect of a cement-hard erection that lasts for more than four hours (yes, we said unfortunate), you do need to see a doctor because it means your penis is probably not getting enough new blood and might be starving to death.

YOU Tip: Check Your Labels. Granted, there's a lot we love about pharmaceuticals. Without them, we'd die a lot sooner, feel a lot worse, and spend more time in hospitals than in our homes. But drugs aren't perfect. And many classes of drugs—especially beta-blockers and the SSRI class of antidepressants—list erectile dysfunction as one of the major side effects. (How's that for a trade-off? Take a drug to improve your mood, but risk cutting off your sexual interest and capabilities at the same time.) If you or your partner experience ED while taking a drug, tell your doc so she can switch you to another class that may not have as powerful an effect. For example, switching from an SSRI to Wellbutrin (bupropion) seems to help alleviate arousal and interest issues that are common in people who take SSRIs. So does switching from a beta-blocker for high blood pressure to an angiotensin receptor blocker such as losartan or valsartan.

YOU Tip: Drink This. Research shows that *Rhodiola rosea,* when consumed as a tea or with a light alcohol like vodka, can aid with erectile dysfunction and improve prostate function.

To make tea: Cut fine 5 grams of *Rhodiola rosea* roots. Pour the roots into a cup of boiling water and leave for (brew) at least four hours. Then filter. Drink one-fifth cup three to five times per day. You can also dilute *Rhodiola rosea* tea with juice, tonic, or other herbal teas.

To make vodka mix: Mill 30 grams of *Rhodiola rosea* roots in a coffee grinder, add 150 milliliters of vodka without aromatic additives, agitate, and steep three to five days at room temperature. Separate and filter the extract. Have a teaspoon and a half a day for about three weeks (preferably at night, especially if you're operating heavy machinery).

YOU Tip: Prepare Yourself. Used to be that anything involving the penis caused embarrassment—buying condoms, talking about erection problems, open zippers. But penises should be like any other part of your body: If you've got a problem that can't be fixed with an aspirin, a Band-Aid, or an ice pack, then you ought to seek some attention. At your visit, you can expect a thorough exam, which is the only way to get to the bottom of erectile issues. Here's what you'll do:

❖ *Describe the problem.* The more details, the better. Describe if you have any hardness and for how long, and exactly how long you've been experiencing issues. The more the doc knows, the better he can help.

❖ *Talk about your mind-set.* A doc will want to explore some psychological issues, so speak up about any stresses or changes in your personal life. They may be subconscious contributors.

❖ *Give your full medical history.* As you've seen, a penis problem isn't just a penis problem. A doc needs to know everything so he can see what risk factors may be playing a role. You tell the story; let him connect the dots.

❖ *Go through a physical exam.* A doc will do a visual once-over to see if you have any medical abnormalities that can cause ED, like small testicles or a curved penis, as well as check blood-vessel pulses as an indication of vascular disease.

❖ *Have a lab test.* He'll check important numbers like LDL and HDL cholesterol, triglycerides, glucose, TSH, DHEA, and testosterone to get a better picture of the underlying cause.

Major Ager

UV Radiation

How the Sun Can Nourish or Destroy Your Body

Vampires, inmates in solitary confinement, and third-shift workers may not get all that much exposure to the sun. But you'd *really* have to be living in the dark not to know the value of the largest object in our solar system. It helps us see. It helps plants grow. It makes a mighty fine name for newspapers, yoga positions, and basketball teams from Phoenix. And it can also help you prevent cancer and osteoporosis.

Yet we also know that that bright little bugger can be a real sun of a gun.

Stare into it, and you'll be blinded by the light (just try to get that song out of your head now). Or bathe in it, and you'll be lobstered in no time at all. The ultimate symbol of life can also be a major generator of death (or at least a heck of a lot of wrinkles).

But it would be a mistake simply to say that, yeah, sure, sun is good for your cactus garden but not for your skin (see Figure K.1). The role of the sun and its ultraviolet rays is a little more complex than that—and also gives us great insight into how we age.

The sun acts sort of like one of those machines that shoots out tennis balls.

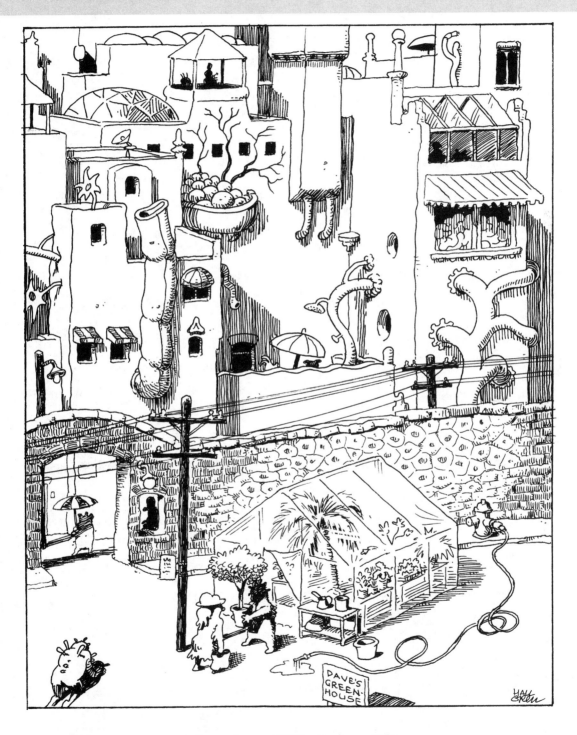

But the sun's tennis balls come in the form of ultraviolet rays that are torpedoed down to earth (see Figure K.2). Now, one type of UV rays—UVC rays—is blocked by the atmosphere (like tennis balls being hit into the net before they reach you), so it has little effect on you. The rays that are constantly being played into your court are the UVA rays and the UVB rays. Now, you have a choice: get pummeled by the rays, or take a swing and block them so that they bounce off of you.

On the surface, it may seem that you're supposed to block every ray that's being served at you. And for good reason. Even though UVB rays are stopped at the level of the skin, they can still cause burning and cancer of the skin, although they cause tanning as well (see more on skin cancer in the cancer chapter). Meanwhile, UVA rays deeply penetrate the skin to cause burns, wrinkles, and skin cancer. To top it off, sunlight also destroys your reserves of folic acid, also known as folate or vitamin B_9. Folate is needed so your body can replicate DNA properly (that's why it helps protect against birth defects). And the rays can damage your eyes—the subject of our next chapter.

How do UV rays cause damage? One way is through connective-tissue breakdown. UV radiation causes the structural protein of our skin, collagen, to break down and disables our ability to repair damage. Another way sun ages our skin is through the formation of free radicals—those aggressive charged compounds that damage cells and break down collagen as well. Free radicals can cause cancer by changing our DNA and preventing our body from repairing it. How? UV destroys the rungs of the DNA ladder so that the DNA ladder posts bind with one another. This makes a bulge so that the DNA doesn't form—or function—correctly. Still another way UV rays cause damage is by thinning the walls of surface blood vessels, leading to bruising, bleeding, and the appearance of blood vessels through the skin.

But the flip side is that we also really need UV rays. Natural sunlight creates active vitamin D, which we need for bone health, since it helps regulate calcium. It also helps ensure the proper function of the heart, nervous system, clotting

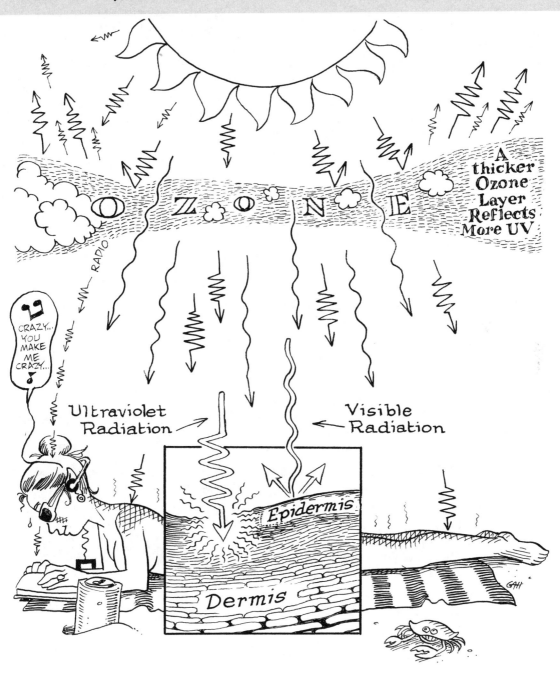

Figure K.2 Burnt Roast Radiation from the sun that passes through the ozone stimulates our eyes (visible rays) and our skin (UV rays). The UV wavelengths either bounce off the dermis or penetrate deeply into our tissues, leading to chemical changes like the creation of active vitamin D or the depletion of folate.

process, and immune system. That's significant because thousands of cancer deaths a year are linked to insufficient UVB exposure and subsequent deficiency of active vitamin D. How does UVB activate vitamin D? From cholesterol. That's why your blood cholesterol levels rise in the winter. Because of the lack of sunlight, you don't have enough active vitamin D, so your body pumps up your cholesterol in the hope of converting as much as possible to active vitamin D. This serves as another example of an evolutionary trade-off between procreation and longevity. To protect us from deficiencies of vitamin D, we've evolved to have higher levels of cholesterol. So now we survive to mate and to be able to stand up strong and look good, only to be felled by high LDL cholesterol and consequent heart disease and stroke.

Here's another interesting way to look at these biological trade-offs: If you have low levels of UVB penetration, then you need higher cholesterol, which can be more readily converted to vitamin D. In this setting of low sun exposure, a substance called Apo E4 rises to help create more cholesterol and subsequent vitamin D. Apo E4 elevations of cholesterol lead to atherosclerosis and Alzheimer's later in life. And in another mutation, those of us whose ancestors lived in areas where the UVB rays were not so plentiful evolved to have less melanin in our skin to allow all those UVB rays to get through. But if the skin color is too light or too much sunlight enters the cells, then folate levels plummet. Without protection from those nutrients, other neurological symptoms increase in people and their offspring are prone to neural tube defects (spina bifida).

This good-and-bad argument is really another example of being balanced. You don't want too much, but you also can't have too little. As is the case with many things we've covered, finding the perfect equilibrium is one of the real secrets to slowing the aging process.

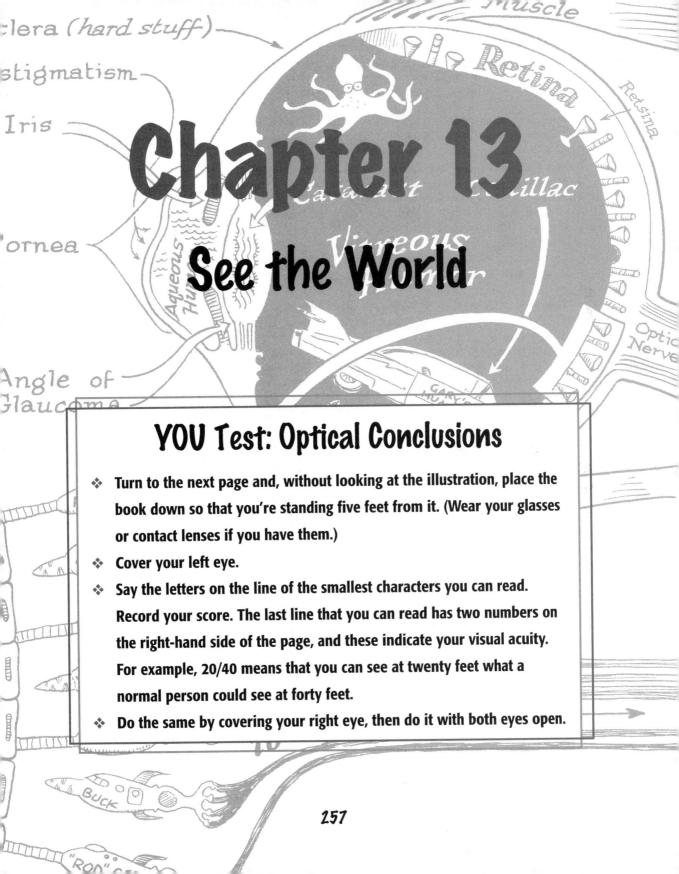

Sclera (hard stuff)

stigmatism

Iris

ornea

Angle of Glaucoma

Muscle

Retina

Retsina

Cataract Cadillac

Vitreous
Humor

Optic
Nerve

Chapter 13
See the World

YOU Test: Optical Conclusions

❖ Turn to the next page and, without looking at the illustration, place the
book down so that you're standing five feet from it. (Wear your glasses
or contact lenses if you have them.)

❖ Cover your left eye.

❖ Say the letters on the line of the smallest characters you can read.
Record your score. The last line that you can read has two numbers on
the right-hand side of the page, and these indicate your visual acuity.
For example, 20/40 means that you can see at twenty feet what a
normal person could see at forty feet.

❖ Do the same by covering your right eye, then do it with both eyes open.

BUCK

"ROD"

Figure 13.1 Eye Chart Hold the page five feet away and read the letters. A score of 20/40 means that you can see at twenty feet what a person with normal vision can see at forty feet.

K	20/200
E E	20/100
P Y O U	20/80
R E Y E	20/70
S O P E	20/60
N F O R	20/50
B O G U S	20/40
E Y E C H	20/30
A R T S	20/20
B O G U S L I N E	20/10

Whether you consider your eyes to be the window to your soul or target practice for stooges' fingers, we can all agree on at least one thing. Those squishy little orbs are just about as precious as a three-week-old puppy. Now, we don't have to sit here and run down all the things you'd miss if you lost your eyesight, because we're certain that you appreciate the landscapes, the family photos, the family faces, the sunsets, the artwork, the hilarity of YouTube, that funny little joke in the illustration on page 238 (go ahead, flip back; we'll wait).

While losing your vision in part or in its entirety isn't a do-or-die issue (though it can certainly make you more prone to accidents, which is), not being able to drive or work your regular job or hit your lips with lipstick can really ruin your day. Still, it seems that we accept age-related decline in vision as much as we accept age-related decline in income—that it's just part of life. While

> **FACTOID**
>
> People with cataracts tend to see illusions, not hallucinations. The difference? An illusion is simply a misinterpretation of data that the brain is receiving—perhaps caused by light being refracted in an odd way. A hallucination, on the other hand, isn't based on any kind of reality.

it's true that some people are predisposed to lose some of their vision, you don't have to resign yourself to a blurry, dark, or colorless world as you get older. By taking steps to protect your eyes—especially from the Major Ager of UV radiation—and feed them with the right nutrients, you'll arm yourself with the optimal optical arsenal (say that three times fast). That's because what we really want you to do is make sure you don't lose sight of losing sight.

A Vision of Loveliness: Your Eyes

When we were young, we all described eyes the same way: There's the white part, the colored part, and the hole in the middle. But now that we're older, wiser, and—thanks to a wealth of TV hospital dramas—able to decipher technical medical lingo, there's a lot more to say about our eyes than how beautiful they are. It

Aging Eyes

Vision loss can be hard to define. Between the extremes of total blindness and binocular vision, there's a whole stream of different ways that our sight may be compromised. As we age, we tend to have trouble with visual-processing speed, light sensitivity, and decreasing field of vision. But vision isn't just about sight; it's about neurological functioning as well. We may be able to see objects, but we have a harder time pulling everything together.

Big example: driving. You can see everything in isolation (pedestrians crossing, light changing, hey, Starbucks on the corner!), but you have a harder time actually focusing on what's important. Add that to the fact that older people have a harder time seeing through dim lights and recovering from bright lights (like oncoming traffic), and you've got the perfect storm of visual problems. You're having trouble making out what you're seeing, but even if you make it out, you can't process it fast enough to realize that the pedestrian, not the venti mocha latte, is what you need to pay attention to. Because it's harder to judge an oncoming moving object as you age, and because left-hand turns account for the biggest incidence of car accidents, we often tell older patients that three right turns really do make a left.

would be a mistake to think that all of our eyes are the same except for the color of the iris (see Figure 13.2). Eyes, which are derived from brain tissue, are different genetically (some populations, like the African Bantu, have lenses that shed particles like dandruff), which means that some of us are more or less predisposed to developing vision problems. Nevertheless, there are some similarities in anatomy to consider. Plus, we all see in the same way. Here's how:

Information (light) from the outside world is transmitted through the cornea, the clear outer covering of the eye. The cornea and the lens behind it bend the light that's coming through to focus on the retina. The retina acts like the film in a camera. Two kinds of retinal cells in the back of your eye connect to neurons in your brain that let you interpret what you think you saw. These two types of brain cells in the retina are rods (which respond to black and white) and cones (which respond to color). Information from the retina travels along the optic nerve so it can be processed by your brain.

Sounds simple enough, right? Well, this momentously amazing process is kind of simple in theory, but—as anyone who's squinted through sun, or blinked from dust, or been blinded by oncoming headlights knows—it's not all that easy. The reason? Subtle changes in our ocular anatomy can shift the way we see and be the reasons why we don't.

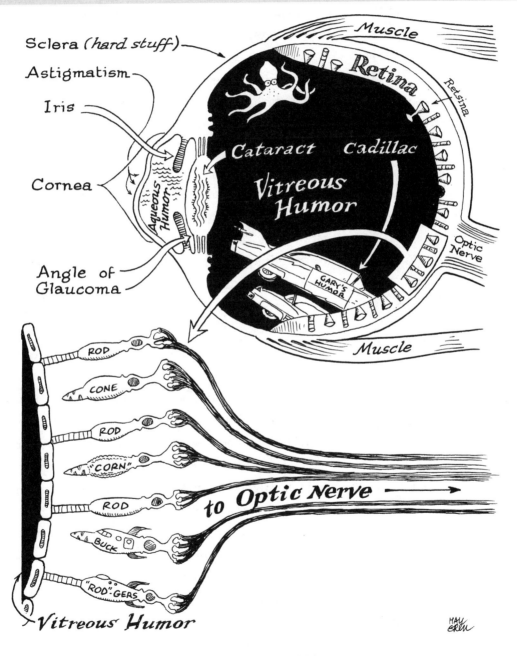

The Cornea: Think of this outer coating as the clear, protective outer covering of a watch. Tears help keep the cornea moist and contain chemicals that fight off bacteria and other vermin. As you age, you produce fewer tears, as well as the antibacterial chemicals contained in them, putting you at risk of dry eyes and infections. You also lose the ability to rapidly develop new corneal cells.

The Lens: Sitting behind the cornea, the lens bends or focuses light into the center. Like a fluid-filled bag, like a water balloon or breast implant, the lens begins to separate—meaning that it scatters the light rays that are coming in, potentially blurring vision. It's responsible for about one-third of the focusing of light that comes to the eye. (The cornea bends, or refracts, the remaining.) UV radiation can cause oxidative stress, which damages vision by clouding our lens and burning through the delicate film and cells of our retina. Prime example: Portland, Oregon, gets a little more than half as much sunlight as Atlanta, and Atlanta eyes have more damage.

> **FACTOID**
>
> Many researchers believe that the reason why so many people are nearsighted (meaning they can't see far away) is because we don't need distance vision anymore. Several generations ago, nearsightedness was nearly unheard of among Alaskans, because they were continually looking out to the horizon for information about the weather. Two generations later, and with the incarnation of TV and computers, 30 percent of Inuit kids are nearsighted. Similarly, the Nepalese people believe that those with problems seeing distance should stare at the moon to help exercise and train their eyes to see far away.

The mass of the lens actually triples from the age of twenty to the age of seventy, which you'd think would be a good thing. But it's not. That thicker lens causes us to become more nearsighted (not being able to see far). The thicker lens becomes unable to change its shape or to focus near, leading to presbyopia (not being able to see up close as well; hence the need for longer arms). And it also makes it more difficult to discriminate colors. Blues get darker, yellows get duller, and you can't make out violet for anything. The other thing that occurs lenswise is the formation of cataracts—a cloudiness of the lens. Often caused by smoking and medication such as steroids in any form, cataracts essentially steam up your optical windows, causing an overall blurriness. They're also caused by our Major Ager of sunlight. The good news is that lenses can be removed and replaced surgically in as little as twenty minutes. Your appointment to determine whether this procedure is right for you should take longer than the surgery.

The Iris: It contains the muscles that control the amount of light that hits the retina through the contraction and dilation of the pupil. As you age, the dilator muscle atrophies, and the pupil ends up smaller, delivering about one-third of the light that it did at age twenty. Interesting note about the iris: Some believe that the health of your brain can be determined by your pupil reflex and response to light.

The Aqueous Humor: Sounds like a description out of a comic book, but this fluid is important because it's what keeps your eyeball inflated to its spherical shape. The production of fluid—turned over every ninety minutes—decreases with age. Glaucoma occurs when the aqueous humor can't drain out of your eye through the meshlike covering where it normally drains, thus building up pressure in the eyeball and cutting off some blood supply to the optic nerve. This clogging of the drain for aqueous fluid can be caused by increased blood pressure in surrounding veins (caused by various diseases and chronic ailments). Glaucoma causes loss of peripheral vision and, if untreated, can lead to blindness. Picture the optic nerve as a tree branch, with the smaller nerve branches reaching to the outer areas; glaucoma affects those outer nerves first, which is why you lose peripheral vision first.

> **FACTOID**
>
> After age sixty-five, you can expect to lose about 5 percent of the vitreous fluid in your eyeball each year. When you lose that fluid, little particles that would be normally pinned in place because of the pressure begin to float. That's what causes those usually harmless black-dot floaters that you may see dancing in your vision. Any change or sudden increase in floaters may also be a sign of a serious retinal problem. Call your eye doctor right away.

The Retina and Macula: This is the part of the eye that houses your rod cells (black and white vision that is associated with your ability to discriminate at night) and cone cells (color vision that is associated with your ability to discriminate during the day)—neurons that carry messages to your brain. A thin film of yellowish pigment lies like Saran Wrap over the retina to absorb dangerous UV rays before

YOU Test: Dot the Eye

To test yourself for macular degeneration, look at the black dot in the middle of the graph. Cover one eye and focus intently only on the dot. Do you see wavy lines, or are parts of the graph missing? If so, that's a sign of macular degeneration.

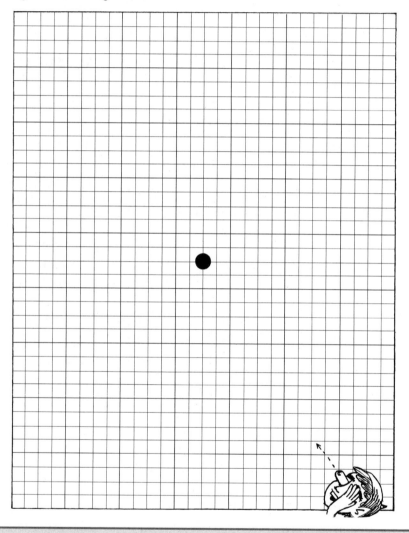

they can damage our rods and cones. The central part of the retina where our vision is focused most is called the fovea. Damage to this area is the major cause of blindness among Americans over age fifty-five. Smoking or high blood pressure cuts off blood vessels that feed the retina (the nerve tissue that converts signals to the brain) and carry vitamins and antioxidants to the back of the eye to repair damage caused by the Major Ager of UV radia-

tion. While genetics do play a role—those with light-colored irises and high blood pressure and low HDL cholesterol are most at risk—lifestyle choices that keep your arteries young will reduce your chances of developing macular degeneration. Similarly, in the case of cataracts and glaucoma, you can help control how fast they develop and whether they'll cause you to lose your eyesight.

As you can see, the Major Ager of UV radiation has a big impact on your eyes by oxidizing the pigments in the retina and decreasing the antioxidants in the thin, yellowish film that protects it, meaning that these delicate cells are always at risk of being damaged through another Major Ager, free radicals. That's why nutrition is so important in rebuilding these antioxidant stores over time, especially when you consider that sunlight damage to the eye is cumulative—particularly in conditions like macular degeneration, where the cells die from oxidative damage.

The above conditions aren't the only reasons to see an eye doctor regularly. By looking in your eyes, your doc gets a small but representative picture of your brain (via your optic nerve), as well as a close-up view of your blood vessels. She'll be able to see kinks in your vessels if your pressure is too high, as well as signs of diabetes where abnormal blood vessels can form under the retina. Now, that's a reason to make regular eye appointments—talk about getting some serious insight.

YOU TIPS!

We all know the most important thing to do to protect our eyes: Cover them when we see an oncoming bug, ball, spear, fist, or any other torpedoing projectile. But we can't rely on eyelids, windshields, and safety goggles for everything. Here are a few ways to protect those baby blues.

YOU Tip: Block Those Rays. Sunglasses do more than hide you from paparazzi and make you look cooler than an Alaskan iceberg. They'll protect your eyes from those nasty UVA and UVB rays. For best protection, follow these strategies:

❖ Find glasses that filter out both kinds of rays (they don't have to be expensive). Look for a label that specifically states 99 percent or 100 percent UV protection. An eye care pro can test them if you're unsure.

❖ They should be dark enough to reduce glare but not dark enough to distort colors, which could affect your recognition of traffic signals. Tint is a matter of personal preference.

❖ People with contact lenses made with UV protection should still wear sunglasses.

❖ Since UV rays can still enter from the sides and top of sunglasses, it's smart to wear a hat with a three-inch brim to help block light.

❖ Make sure you goggle up with UV-protective eyewear, especially when you're on the slopes or in the water. Skiing (water and snow) may be dangerous not only to your knees but to your eyes as well, because they're being pummeled by both refractive and reflective light beams that bounce off the water or snow. So you have higher UV exposure on snow, water, and concrete because these surfaces reflect UV rays. (You also get higher radiation at high altitudes and low latitudes, like near Everest or the Caribbean.) Follow the same rule for your eyes as you do your skin: If you're going to be exposed to the sun, do what you can to block as much as you can.

YOU Tip: See an Eye Doc. That's once every two years after age forty—even if you don't experience any changes in your vision. Besides being able to detect some asymptomatic problems like glaucoma, your doc gets to sneak a peek at the blood vessels in your brain and at your brain itself. As we said earlier, ophthalmologists often are the first docs to detect conditions such as diabetes and high blood pressure.

YOU Tip: Feed Your Eyes. Of course, there aren't too many things you actually want to put directly into your eyes, but that doesn't mean you can't pull the ol' end around: through the digestive system. By getting the right nutrients, you can make sure that enough of them are diverted to your orbs. Our recommendations:

❖ *Lutein:* Found in spinach, leafy green vegetables, and corn, lutein seems to improve the health of your eyes by preventing oxidative damage to your retina. You can also take it in supplement form at 6 to 30 milligrams daily.

❖ *Vitamin C:* Research shows that people who eat more fruits and vegetables (which contain vitamin C and other bioflavonoids) are less likely to develop eye conditions than those who eat fewer.

❖ *Glutathione:* Eggs, garlic, avocados, asparagus, and onions have the free-radical scavenger glutathione, which has been shown to be effective for preventing cataracts (at 500 mg dose). The supplement n-acetylcysteine also helps (also 500 mg daily dose).

❖ *The eye cocktail:* A large study sponsored by the National Institutes of Health found that certain vitamins, when taken together, can help prevent vision loss for those who have age-related macular degeneration. (It wasn't studied to show preventive powers for those who don't have the disease.) The study found that those people who already had wet macular degeneration had a more than 25 percent reduction in their risk of vision loss if they took 500 milligrams of vitamin C, 400 IU of vitamin E, 15 milligrams of beta-carotene (yes, carrots *are* good for your eyes), 80 milligrams of zinc, and 2 milligrams of copper every day in divided doses. P.S.: We think that a lower dose of 30 milligrams of zinc is safer for longer periods of time.

YOU Tip: Sit Back. There's no evidence to suggest that prolonged TV exposure is bad for your eyes (maybe your brain cells, depending on what you're watching, but that's a whole different story). But that's only if you make sure that you're sitting the proper distance away so your eyes can accommodate to the picture. Take the diagonal screen length of your TV and make sure you sit at least that far away from it.

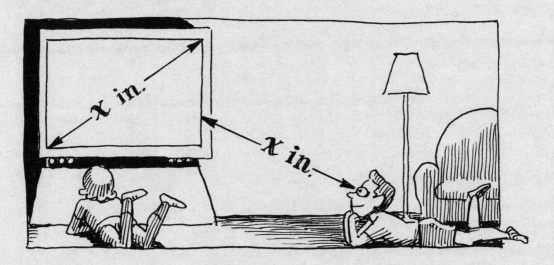

Disuse Atrophy

Prime the Pump to Keep the Body Working Well

We've all heard the "use it or lose it" mantra before. Most often, we hear it in the context of our brains: If you don't give your neurons regular mental workouts with such brain stimulators as crosswords, Sudoku, or work, then your gray matter will age into a skullful of mush. But we also hear it when it comes to everything from our muscles to our sexual studliness. The principle: If you let your body parts shrivel up and die, they'll be happy to take you up on your offer.

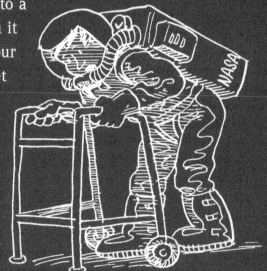

Perhaps the most extreme example of those who don't use it losing it is astronauts who return after space flight. After time without gravity, they lose significant muscle and bone mass—so much so that they have to be helped just to walk on solid ground. They often also lose their mental grounding and perception of where they are. Or another example: Spend any amount of time with your leg in a cast, and the immobility will cause its muscles to wilt like a waterless rose.

The reason? Your body is too efficient to waste energy feeding limbs and organs that aren't being used. So if you ain't using it, then your body says you're losing it. And the nerves that help control those limbs and organs will wilt away too. This mechanism of aging—disuse atrophy—is a classic example of resource allocation. If your body knows that you're using crutches instead of quadriceps, then it figures, forget this, I'll put energy elsewhere—and so your leg muscles atrophy when you don't use them for long periods.

We need to put our bodies to work in our lives: We need to work our muscles, our brains, and virtually every other organ and system in our bodies to make them stronger for longer (see Figure L.1).

When it comes to using your body parts, you've got two extremes: Use them too much, and you suffer from wear and tear; but don't use them enough, and you suffer from disuse atrophy. The ideal, of course, is to find the middle ground, where you do just the right amount to make your body parts grow and thrive—and not age. Here we'll deal with one of the systems most often associated with disuse atrophy in aging: your bones.

> **FACTOID:**
>
> Ballroom dancing and square dancing are two of the few activities shown to involve both physical activity and mental stimulation significant enough to reduce the risk of dementia—a true two-for-one example of using it or losing it.

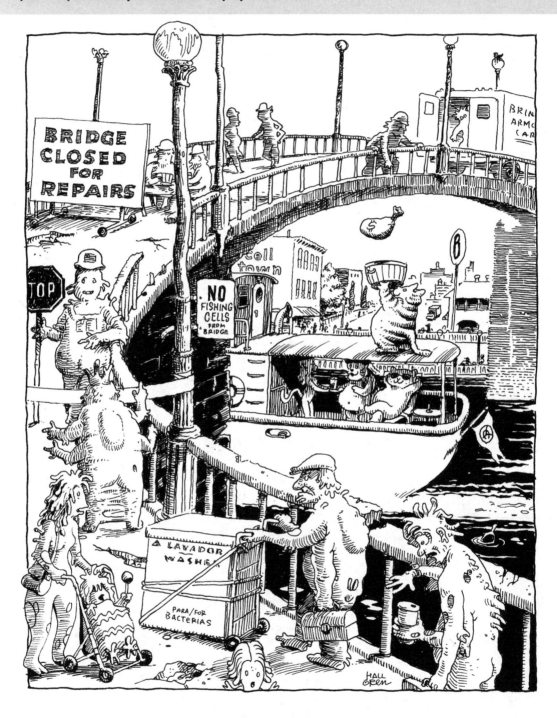

Move Your Body

Bones aren't the only things that grow under stress or activity. Most of your body parts, in fact, become stronger when you use them. A glimpse at what you can and should do to make sure you're doing enough to prime your pumps:

Your Body	Use it	Or Lose It
Heart	Aerobic exercise increases blood flow and trains your heart under stress.	Those who don't do regular aerobic exercise are more prone to suffer from heart disease and heart attacks, and have less ability to fight stress.
Brain	Do crosswords, learn a new skill (or language), read (as opposed to mindlessly waiting for the next great Bud Light commercial). Or *create* the next great Bud Light commercial.	Without mental calisthenics, your brain loses power and memory as you age.
Sex organs, male	Healthy sexual function can be measured in frequent ejaculations (a good goal is about one hundred times a year).	Those who don't have frequent enjoyment of sex have been shown to have increased sexual dysfunction, so don't pass up the chance to have sex, even if you're by yourself. Those who pass it up in middle age may have a harder time trying to have sex in older age.
Sex organs, female	Healthy sexual function can be measured in regular and enjoyable sexual activity.	Postmenopausal women who don't have sex will experience accelerated thinning of vaginal walls and inability to enjoy intercourse later on.

Hormones	Various hormones naturally produce chemicals you need for daily function.	If you replace your normal steroid hormonal function with pills or injectable or inhaled steroids (such as those to fight disease), you could be teaching your glands not to produce the hormones your body craves. For those who need and use steroidal medication, it's wise to take a hormonal holiday and/or take the medication every other day, under medical supervision.
Muscles	Resistance training helps maintain lean muscle mass, which decreases as you age.	Without building muscle, you're more likely to gain weight (because muscle helps speed metabolism), as well as be at increased risk for osteoporosis.
Joints	Walking and any other types of movement stimulate the formation of synovial fluid, which keeps your joints lubed.	A decrease or absence of movement decreases production of synovial fluid, which increases the chances of developing arthritis and other joint conditions.
Gut	In people with mild forms of lactose intolerance, having a little lactose can work to your advantage.	If you avoid lactose altogether, then lactose intolerance worsens because you'll lose production of the digestive enzymes needed to process those foods.

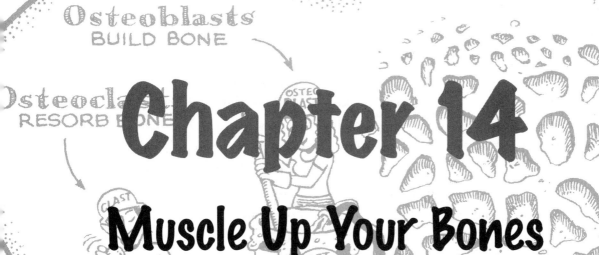

Osteoblasts
BUILD BONE

Osteoclasts
RESORB BONE

Chapter 14
Muscle Up Your Bones

YOU Test: Balancing Act

Stand on one foot, extend your arms out to the sides, and keep yourself balanced. Now close your eyes. Stand as long you can before you have to grab something to get your balance. (Best to do this with a spotter or next to a wall.)

The threshold for success is fifteen seconds at age forty and thirty seconds at age thirty. If you can't make those times, it means that you're about as shaky as a belly dancer—meaning that your lack of balance makes you more susceptible to falling, putting you at a higher risk of breaking your bones.

In the grand scheme of aging, our bones typically don't get much thought. That is, until your life gets flipped upside on its head because your skeleton has more cracks than a city sidewalk.

While women are certainly more in tune to bone loss and bone issues than men, many of us still tend to relegate bone issues to the second tier of medical attention (with heart attacks, cancer, and anything that involves the suffix *-ectomy* typically standing firmly on the first tier). In fact, your bones need care during your youth, as they reach their maximum mass in your twenties. That said, most of us do know that as we age, our bones lose some of their mass, primarily through the Major Ager of disuse atrophy. Loss of estrogen also adds to loss of bone mass in women and loss of testosterone in men, and there's certainly a genetic predisposition to bone loss. Just as important, bone loss is also related to another kind of disuse atrophy: muscle loss, because muscles also play a part in keeping your bones strong. Adding and maintaining lean muscle throughout your life puts the kind of stress on your bones that will strengthen them.

All of us remake our bones every decade. If we don't nurture and challenge them, then the body doesn't bother wasting the energy to keep them and the muscles that pull on them strong as we get older. And that makes us more prone to get shelved like a canned good if we do slip, fall, and break a hip or vertebra. And that's all the more reason to do everything you can to make sure you're not, as George Thorogood would sing, b-b-b-b-bad to your bones.

Forming the Foundation: Your Bones

Our bones serve as more than just a hanger for the rest of our body parts. They form the very foundation of our existence. If you were to slice open a bone and take a look inside (don't try this at home), here's what you'd see: a compact layer (cor-

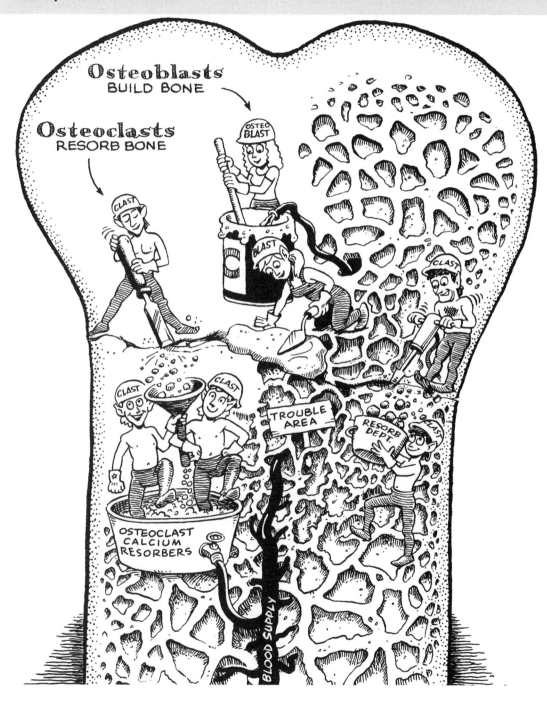

tical bone) forming the exterior of bone with an interior latticework of fine bone structure (trabecular, or spongy bone), as you see in Figure 14.1. It's not the perfectly solid structure that most of us imagine our bones to be. The cortical bone provides rigidity and structural integrity, while the spongy bone on the inside imparts flexibility and compressive strength to the skeleton—similar to the design of the Eiffel Tower. Bone material has both a collagen matrix and a calcium matrix, and bone is dynamic; it's able to remodel itself according to what you need, as in the case of fusing a bone back together after it's been fractured. Bone is so dynamic that you often can't even see in an X-ray where a bone was broken after it's healed.

But even if you never break a bone, your skeleton is perennially remodeling itself. To do this, bone needs a steady supply of protein, vitamins, hormones, and, of course, calcium. You know that you need calcium to mineralize (provide more rigid structure to) the collagen proteins that help build your bone. Now, the flip side is that you stabilize plaque in your blood vessels with calcium reinforcement, which causes stiffening and raises your blood pressure, which forces the heart to work harder. So you want to help move calcium from blood to the bone, and you can do that with your natural vitamin K_2. (You don't have to worry that calcium you take in supplements makes the calcification in arteries worse; research shows that it doesn't.) See the YOU Tip on page 285 for more on vitamin K_2.

Osteoporosis is not just a calcium deficiency disease; it's also a disease of excessive calcium loss. In other words, you can take all the calcium supplements you want, but if your diet and lifestyle choices are unhealthy (like too many caffeine- or phosphate-laden carbonated beverages, or too much protein, and no weight-bearing exercises and no vitamin D), or you're taking prescription drugs such as steroids that cause you to lose calcium, you will end up with a negative calcium balance in your bone account. Nevertheless, you need to take calcium. Inadequate calcium intake sets off a chain of events to ensure normal calcium levels in blood, since normal calcium levels in blood are essential for proper muscle and nerve functioning. To ensure normal levels, you decrease excretion in your urine, increase absorption from your gut, and increase resorption of bone.

Active vitamin D, manufactured when skin is exposed to sunlight, is the key that unlocks the gate and allows calcium to leave the intestine and enter the bloodstream. Vitamin D also works in the kidneys to help prevent the loss of calcium that would otherwise be excreted. You need an abundant supply to remodel bone. Why is it important? As you age, your ability to make vitamin D through the skin decreases. Plus, as you age, you hang out inside more or become housebound and experience less sunlight exposure.

Bone remodeling consists of two stages: resorption, when cells called osteoclasts dissolve old bone, creating small cavities; and bone formation, or remodeling, when cells called osteoblasts build new bone by filling those cavities with calcium. Usually, bone resorption and bone formation occur around the same time and are balanced. When they're not balanced, you lose bone mass. In addition, bone remodeling happens through electricity in the form of low-energy waves that put stress on the bone. To form bone, you need that charge—and that comes from weight-bearing exercise and building muscle that stresses the bone.

That's the reason why any kind of resistance training is so important: to stimulate that charge and put more force on the bone to cause the remodeling (and, importantly, to build muscle and increase your sense of balance, so that you're less likely to fall). This serves as our classic case of the Major Ager, disuse atrophy: If you don't stimulate the charge to recycle bone by putting stress on your bones in the form of weights or other forms of resistance, you will lose bone, muscle, and your sense of balance. Weight lifting turns on a gene that makes a protein that eventually turns on osteoblasts to do the work of building bone (recent evidence in two species of animals indicates that those cells would develop into fat cells otherwise), and that makes your RealAge younger. Like most of us trying to juggle work, home, and catching up on 24, your body is simply too busy to waste its

> **FACTOID**
>
> A supplement of the trace element boron (taken at 3 milligrams) has been shown to reduce the amount of calcium and magnesium that's secreted in urine. Vitamin B_{12} has been shown to help osteoblast function—and those deficient in B_{12} have been shown to have increased rates of osteoporosis.

time and energy remodeling bone, strengthening muscle, and building coordination to avoid falls if you're not going to use it.

Now, this process of remodeling bone isn't important only because you might find yourself in a skateboard accident but because your bone mass naturally declines as you age. As stated, you reach your peak bone mass at age thirty and up until then can increase your banked calcium. After that, men and women lose a half percent of bone per year. For the first five years of menopause (if you're not taking hormone replacement therapy), women's bone loss increases to 2 percent to 4 percent of trabecular bone (the spongy part of bone on the inside) and 1 percent to 2 percent of cortical bone (the hard surface area of bone) per year. After that (or for men of all ages), the decline levels out to a half percent a year again. Still bad, but not so severe, and you can prevent it.

Osteoporosis is caused by a reduction in bone mass or bone density. (The precursor of osteoporosis is called osteopenia; you technically have osteoporosis when your bone density falls low enough that only 5 percent of twenty-year-old women have less than you.) The cause? Risk factors that may be influenced by genes include low vitamin D metabolism and delayed puberty, meaning that you have fewer of years of hormonally stimulated bone growth before you reach your peak. Of course, you influence your vitamin D intake and many other factors. For postmenopausal women, the most common cause of osteoporosis is loss of estrogen. Other risk factors include untreated thyroid disease (especially increased thyroid hormone production, or hyperthyroidism) or overuse of thyroid supplements, kidney disease, inflammation, smoking, certain medications, and especially rheumatoid and other inflammatory forms of arthritis. And, of course, lack of weight-bearing stress, which stimulates bones to remodel.

Besides back pain and a loss of height, the main effect of osteoporosis is that the bones of your spine split faster than a celebrity couple, meaning you're less able to tolerate everyday falls and accidents—and thus severely reducing your chances of being able to live independently. Research shows that the physical energy caused by a fall from a standing position is only about one-twentieth of the amount needed to break a normal hip bone. So if you have kept your bone mass normal, you can easily tolerate usual falls. If you suffer from osteoporosis (or osteopenia), however, your moth-eaten thinned bone is more likely to break. Because of that, you have three jobs: remodeling bone, building muscle, and learning how to fall, which we'll discuss in a moment.

Part of the issue of being more vulnerable to breaks is that you're also more vulnerable to falls; namely, because we lose balance as we age. How? The semicircular canals in our ears are filled with thick viscous fluid with tiny stones floating about. When you turn, these stones slowly move, and nerves in your ears sense this action. However, if the stones have become osteoporotic or the nerve impulses are erratic, the brain cannot rapidly process these clues to movement, and you feel dizzy (see Figure 14.2).

In addition to slowing you down, osteoporotic fractures that happen as a result of falls can have serious—even lethal—consequences. The chance of dying in the six months after a hip fracture is 20 percent to 25 percent, and it's twice as high in men than in women. While men fall less frequently (15 percent of total falls), 40 percent of those men who do fall and break a hip die within the first year. Why? Being prone to falling and fracturing (or fracturing and then falling, which happens much less commonly) signals some other underlying pathology such as inflammation in your body, which makes you more susceptible to other acute types of problems like pneumonia. Ultimately, osteoporosis gives you a sense of frailty that limits your activity and sets off a chain reaction that makes you feel and become old.

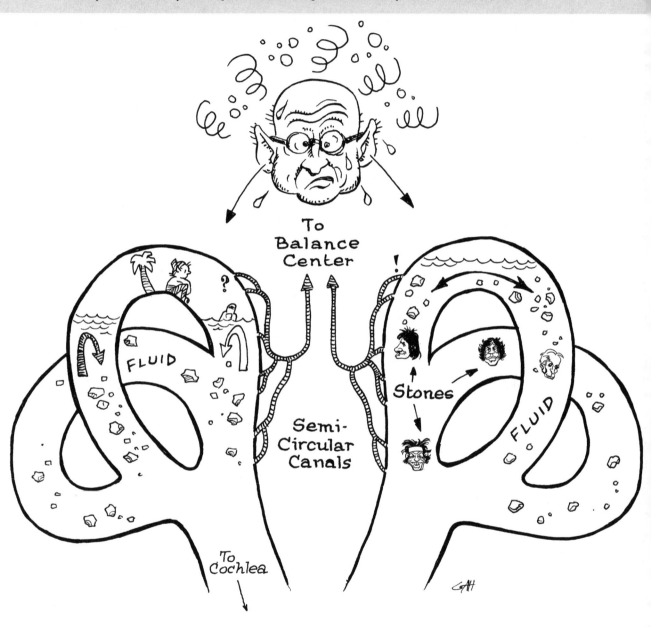

Figure 14.2 **Stay Centered** Tiny stones in the semicircular canals move through Jell-O-like fluid as we bounce around so we can tell up from down. With age, the stones develop osteoporosis and stop moving with us, causing us to feel dizzy, lose our balance, and fall.

To Balance Center

FLUID

Semi-Circular Canals

Stones

FLUID

To Cochlea

YOU TIPS!

Oh, it'd be nice if you could trade in bad bones for good ones. Just go to the store, pick out a nice femur, a jaw-dropping scapula, or a breathtaking phalange, and be on your merry osteoporosis-free way. Building bone isn't *that* easy (yet), but it doesn't have to be all that hard, either. By adding a few things to your workout, chewing a few tablets every day, and knowing that bone *wants* to protect you, you'll feed your skeleton the ingredients it needs to stay strong for a good long time.

YOU Tip: Add Weight. The number one way you can stimulate bone remodeling is with weight-bearing exercise—that is, by doing some kind of resistance training that puts stress on your bones. Now, resistance can come in lots of forms: barbells, dumbbells, resistance bands, exercise machines, other people's bodies. The simplest way (and the way that eliminates excuses) is to use your own body weight as resistance, as in the case of push-ups or the invisible chair form of a squat (see www.realage.com for the YOU Workout). For a full weight-bearing, bone-saving program, see page 366. The step-by-step guide will not only help you build muscle, which will help you burn fat, but it will add meat to your bones. For those with osteoporosis, you may want to try chi-gong, a less bone-stressful form of exercise.

YOU Tip: Stretch It Out. It may seem as if the only reason you need to stretch is because you're about to run a race or because you need to get up from your desk after spending the last thirteen hours following the boss's orders. But flexibility—that is, lengthening your muscles and giving them the ability to adapt to all kinds of situations—is important in the big bone picture. Stretching won't do anything to the physiology of your bones per se, but it will give you the ability to maneuver yourself during a fall or get yourself up after a fall. Oftentimes, people have the strength to get up after falling, but they don't have the flexibility to twist, turn, and wiggle their bodies when they're under chairs or behind toilets. Also, see our chi-gong workout in chapter 18 to prevent that hunched-over look you associate with assisted-living facilities. (Only one-third of people with back fractures know they have them; stretch and strengthen your muscles for this reason as well.) Our suggestions for three good yoga stretches should be incorporated regularly into your life:

Triangle Pose: Stand with your feet spread apart and legs straight; extend your arms straight out to the sides, parallel to the floor. With your right foot pointed to the right and your left foot pointed straight ahead, bend your waist to the right so that your right hand drops to your ankle and your left arm extends toward the ceiling. Hold for ten seconds, return to center, then switch sides. Repeat on the other side. If you have to bend your leg, it's important to keep your knee from going past the heel to prevent injury.

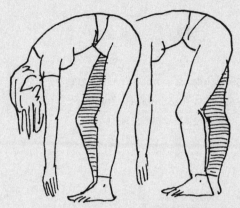

Hippie Stretch: With your feet together and flat on the ground, slowly bend forward at your waist. Alternate bending one knee and keeping the other leg straight (while still keeping your feet flat). Let your relaxed head hang down, releasing all your tension. Stretch each side for fifteen seconds. To maximize stretch, really drop the hip on the side of the bent knee.

Butterfly: Sit on the ground with your back straight and your legs bent so that the bottoms of your feet touch each other in front of you. Let your knees drop toward the floor to stretch the inner parts of your thighs. Take your hands and open the soles of your feet as if you're opening a book, then relax your knees toward the ground on each exhalation. Take thirty seconds to really loosen your hips.

YOU Tip: Find Balance. Granted, all of us are going to take an occasional spill, especially when dealing with rain on the porch or the fist of an enemy. But in many cases, it's not the initial slip that's the problem, it's your inability to right yourself before you land face down on concrete. If you can't prevent the slip, then work to prevent the fall. Train your body to adapt to unstable circumstances. Some ways to do it:

❖ When doing strength training, choose dumbbells over weight machines. The dumbbells will force you to balance the weights as well as lift them. Also, any step-type moves, like lunges or step-ups, require balance.

❖ Try doing any standing exercises (like overhead presses) on one leg at a time. Really. That will help you work your proprioception—your awareness of yourself in space—which will help you develop better balance.

❖ If you like, add in equipment like stability balls to your workout routine. Performing crunches on an unstable surface will force your body to balance. You can also buy balance boards (like mini surfboards) on which to stand and perform exercises.

❖ Perform the YOU Test in this chapter not only as a self-test but as a way to work on your balance.

YOU Tip: Have a Good Setup. Part of being prepared to cope with falls is avoiding them in the first place. That means setting up your home to be the perfect fall-free environment. Make sure that rooms are well lit, don't use slippery rugs, use shower mats, and avoid having shiny floors (glares can be especially problematic for people with cataracts). It's also smart to place enough furniture around your room to help you navigate.

YOU Tip: Learn to Fall. It may seem that a stumble on the sidewalk, a slip on the ice, or a trip over a doggie toy isn't so consequential. But realize that 30 percent of older people fall every year (5 percent or more of those resulting in fracture), falling is the leading cause of accidental death for people over sixty-five, and a woman is more likely to die of complications from a hip fracture than of breast, uterine, and ovarian cancer combined. Nope, falling isn't the minuscule health issue that some people may believe it to be.

In the split second it takes for you to go from slip to sidewalk, it's likely that your world slows way down. Maybe you replay your life, maybe you blurt out seventeen expletives in a row, maybe you recite your grandmother's pineapple cake recipe. Whatever the case, you should be taking that seems-like-an-eternity second to prepare yourself to fall with the least impact possible. There is a right way to fall and a wrong way. (Hint: The wrong way is leading with your nose.) Ideally, you want to minimize the force by falling on as much surface area as possible, and once you are going to fall, don't resist; just try to fall safely. Learn to fall like a martial-arts expert, so the fall won't break your spine or hip.

You can actually practice falling (with an instructor, preferably) on a padded floor. Start by falling from a low position, as in a deep squat. When you fall, don't think, *react.* If these tips exist somewhere in your subconscious and your muscles (muscles have memory), then you might fall correctly and minimize injury (see following page).

YOU Tip: Make a Good Choice. Some brands of calcium supplements have been known to contain lead. It's wise to choose a name brand—such as Caltrate or calcium citrate chewables—over ones in bins from coral, or whatever, in natural-food stores, where you may be unsure about whether or not the companies test for levels of lead. We prefer calcium citrate, since your stomach doesn't need to be acidic for this to be absorbed. Plus, the citrate, combined with the magnesium, reduces the chance of constipation and can even loosen your poop.

How about taking Tums, Rolaids, or another antacid with calcium? Not so fast. As we age, we tend to produce less stomach acid. To be absorbed, calcium requires vitamin D *and* stomach acid. For this reason, it's important to avoid chronic use of antacids, H2-blockers, or proton pump inhibitors, which block or suppress the secretion of stomach acid.

FACTOID

If someone falls and breaks her wrist instead of her hip, it can be a good thing, because it can alert her and her doctor to osteoporosis. But it can also be a sign of something else: that her neurological system is working well. People who fall like a log and break their hips don't put their hands out, indicating that there's some kind of problem getting the message to the brain to stop the fall. (Of course, with a break, you should get a DEXA scan, because it could also be a sign of osteoporosis.)

Figure 14.3 **Free-Falling** Follow these steps no matter what direction you fall.

❖ Tuck your head so that your chin is pointed to your chest.

❖ When you're going down, lean into the direction where you're falling (don't fight it), and bend your knees to lower the center of gravity. Don't stick out your arm or wrist to break the fall.

❖ Aim your landing so that your shoulder and upper back are the first to hit the ground.

❖ Roll over (as in a somersault or forward roll) so that the impact is absorbed over a larger area of your body, rather than just an acute break point at the location of impact.

How To Fall

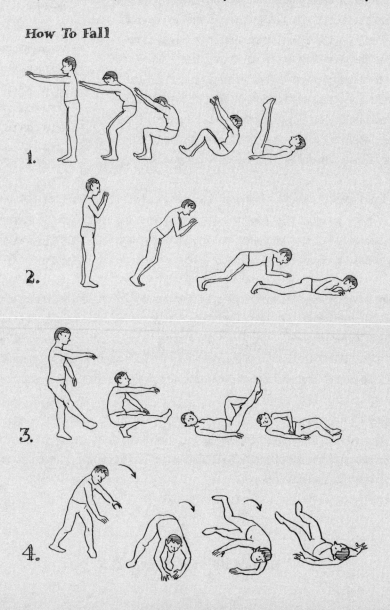

YOU Tip: Chew While You Drive. As if we were going to neglect the obligatory yet necessary tip for adding more calcium into your life. The fact is that most people still don't get enough calcium for optimum bone density. Aim for 1,500 milligrams a day in foods and supplements (though that's on the high side if you're at risk for developing kidney stones).

Tip: Get chewable calcium citrate tablets, put them in the car, and take one every time you put the key in the ignition. Since you can absorb only about 600 milligrams in a two-hour period, this helps make sure the doses are spread out throughout the day. Also, choose calcium citrate or calcium carbonate (if you have GI issues when taking calcium carbonate, switch to calcium citrate). Take calcium carbonate only after a meal. For vitamin D, take 1,000 IU daily (or 1,200 for women older than sixty-five). Plus, it's smart to add 400 milligrams of magnesium a day to prevent the constipation that calcium causes. That's also important because magnesium deficiency may be more common than calcium deficiency in women with osteoporosis. Eat whole grains, leafy green vegetables, and nuts (almonds are rich in both magnesium and calcium). For the most bang for your buck, have something acidic (like OJ) with your calcium. The acidity increases absorption.

YOU Tip: Make Sure the Whole Family Plays. Because peak bone mass is reached in your twenties, your calcium bank needs to be filled in your youth to ensure maximum bone strength and mass (and prevent fractures, especially if you plan on extending your warranty past menopause and andropause). Since genetics drives a lot of osteoporosis, the entire family can play the bone-building game. It's never too early to start. The ideal high-calcium diet sources are fortified low-fat yogurt or milk, soy milk, pink wild salmon (215 milligrams per 4 ounces), kale, spinach (180 milligrams per cup), and tofu (155 milligrams per cube). And remember to pass the supplements with magnesium and vitamin D around the dinner table, so all your relatives get the needed amounts.

YOU Tip: Get a Special K. That is, vitamin K_2, the metabolic product your body makes from vitamin K. It helps move calcium from your blood to your bone if you're calcium deficient. Those who are deficient in vitamin K have been shown to have a 30 percent higher risk of hip fractures than those with higher intakes. A relative of coenzyme Q10, K_2 can be found in something called *natto*—a Japanese fermented soybean dish. (Samurai warriors would eat natto to increase their strength and quicken their reflexes.) K_2 can also be found in low-fat cottage

> **FACTOID**
>
> If you have osteoporosis, you should continue to do resistance exercises, but you should build up before you start lifting very heavy weights. While you may have the muscle to support the weights, you may not have the bone strength. We know of some cases where men with osteoporosis crushed their own bones because they were doing squats with heavy weights.

cheese, chicken, and certain cheeses. It doesn't come from milk and isn't found in yogurt, as it's a waste product of bacteria that ferment milk into cheese.

YOU Tip: Beware of the Supermodel Diet. What's that? Protein and diet soda. Acids from both sources can leach calcium out of bone, accelerating bone loss. Carbonated beverages aren't as bad for bone health as the acid in many other foods, but we do know that children who drink sodas in general have reduced bone mass as adults and fracture more often. The same is true for adults who drink sodas. The reason appears to be that if you drink those kinds of drinks, you're less likely to drink healthy drinks that contain calcium and vitamin D. Evidence shows that if you can get the calcium in other ways, the soda should be OK. Vegetarian protein, interestingly, negatively affects bone strength. All high-protein meals tend to increase the removal of calcium from bones, underscoring the importance of supplementing with calcium whether you get your protein from turkey or tofu. Another big calcium buster: salt. Sodium influences calcium balance by increasing its excretion.

YOU Tip: Know What's Bad to the Bone. Sledgehammers aren't your only skeletal enemies. The others: excessive alcohol, cigarettes, and vitamin A. Having more than 2,500 milligrams of vitamin A in supplements a day could hurt bone formation. You need some vitamin A, but there is such a thing as having too much. (Disregard this advice if you're pregnant or you will be pregnant; your fetus needs even more vitamin A than she gets from you in order to develop her brain.) You can't OD on food sources (carrots, red peppers, sweet potatoes), but make sure your vitamins and supplements don't put you over the limit.

YOU Tip: See the Whole Picture. Around the time of menopause, your doc will suggest that you have a DEXA scan—the preferred standard for screening for osteoporosis and determining bone density. We believe in it too. DEXA commonly measures bone density only at the hip and lumbar spine but can measure it in your wrist too. Ultrasounds, which are safe and cheap, measure only at the heel bones. CT scans use too much radiation for screening but are good for determining the consequences of osteoporosis, like compression factors. Ultrasound and CT scans aren't well correlated with your risk of fracture, while DEXA results are. We suggest one for all women and many men if they're losing height.

YOU Tip: Learn Your Treatment Options. The best treatment for osteoporosis is to build peak bone mass (your bone bank) in your twenties and do weight training, but also to prevent bone loss in the first

FACTOID

Even the thought of the carbonation in colas and soft drinks makes your bones fear their calcium will disappear into your urine. But it's really the sixteen phosphates that are found in caffeinated drinks that may be responsible. So add 20 milligrams more calcium to your intake for every 12-ounce caffeinated soft drink and every 4-ounce cup of coffee. Better: Eat more fruits and vegetables, which may be the best bet for bone health.

place. But if you are prone to it, there are medications available that can help control and slow bone loss, as well as aid in the treatment of symptoms associated with it. In addition to hormone replacement, the bisphosphonates (alendronate, ibandronate, and risedronate), calcitonin, and raloxifene are antiresorptive medications, which slow or stop the bone-resorbing portion of the bone-remodeling cycle without slowing the bone-forming portion of the cycle. So formation is faster than resorption, and bone density may increase as the fracture risk decreases. Teriparatide (Forteo), a form of a parathyroid hormone, is a new osteoporosis medication and the first to increase the rate of bone formation.

Don't think that the consequences of osteoporosis—bone fractures—occur only slowly over time. One in five women who break a vertebra of the spine will have another spinal fracture within the year, possibly leading to a fracture cascade that could leave them with a hump like Grandma. Not only does that make you look old, but vertebral fractures can lead to pneumonia and other causes of warranty shortening. And remember, only one-third of people with vertebral fractures know it. So do the bone-saving strategies as if your independence depends on it—because it does.

Friendly Fat?

While being overweight is death to your joints (not to mention your heart and just about every other organ), it turns out that underweight people tend to get osteoporosis more than others. Fat stores estrogen, which maintains bone density—finally, a benefit! But don't use that to justify the extra portions.

Wear & Tear

How Your Body Handles the Breaking-down Process

Take a look at any city, and you can see signs of wear and tear all around. Paint has faded from houses, sidewalks are cracked, office windows are smudged, and roads can have more potholes than teens have zits. It's the price you pay for actually having people live in, use, and enjoy the city. But you also ask: Where are the repair people?

The more often a city's infrastructure gets used, the more likely it is that it's not going to be able to absorb every bit of shock, trauma, and damage that it was designed to withstand (see Figure M.1). If it's worn down, then likely its use outstripped the ability of the city to maintain it. That probably means that the city hasn't put enough money into repair crews, or maybe the damage has just overrun what extraordinary crews could repair, or maybe the repairs have been made with bad materials. When it comes to many systems in your body, it works the same way. When you grind down your body simply by the act of living—whether it be your joints or your ears—your body is going to experience some kind of damage. It's the slow churning away at the efficiency and productivity of our body's systems that causes many of the ailments we associate with aging.

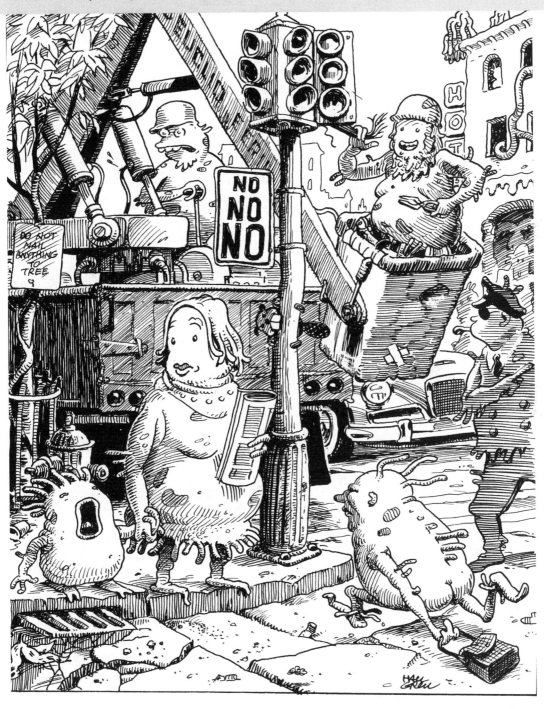

But the problem isn't just the wear and tear of particular body parts. It's the multiplier effect. If a road is shut down because of wear, that puts extra pressure on other roads, or the bus system, or the subway system, to absorb some of the fallout. And then that leads to, yup, more wear and tear on those systems. That multiplier effect is what can lead to a total urban shutdown—and a total bodily one as well. That is, unless you can make the necessary repairs without burdening other systems in the process.

Wear and tear in and of itself won't do you in. What will? Your body's inability to keep up with maintenance as fast as it's needed.

Wear and tear is thought by many to be an obvious reason why we slow down as we get older. Your hearing gets worn down by excessive noise, and wear and tear takes out other systems, from your teeth to your joints. The valves in your heart wear down (and become calcified) after years of letting blood through. They end up working like a door with a rusted hinge. Your liver is subject to wear and tear that can lead to cirrhosis from scarring; in your esophagus, too much wear through reflux problems that haven't been adequately repaired leads to esophageal and throat cancer.

What we have to be careful about is falling into the trap of thinking that deterioration is normal when it comes to aging. Just because it's common to creak like a haunted house as we get older doesn't mean it's inevitable; our bodies ought to be able to make those necessary repairs. It's when we are unable to make those repairs—be it due to chronic disease or damaged DNA—that we slip into what most of us think of as, simply, old age.

Most serious aging happens at the cellular level. The simple act of bending your knee, for example, exposes the cells of your cartilage to physical damage and damaging chemicals. Sometimes those cells are killed directly by the damage (that's called necrosis), while in other instances, damage accumulates over time, and the cells eventually go into retirement. That process is called senescence—when the cells stop dividing permanently, or they undergo apoptosis (the cell death we described earlier in the book), in which they're broken up and reabsorbed.

As cells become senescent, tissues slowly lose their ability to repair and regenerate themselves efficiently and perfectly. Imperfectly repaired cells accelerate damage, which in turn causes more cells to become senescent, which causes even more damage. Imperfectly repaired or replaced or retired cells build up—like those in arthritic joints. And so the vicious cycle of old age keeps spinning, unless you know how to stop it or keep it from starting in the first place.

FACTOID

Continual burning of your esophagus is just like the continual burning of your skin; it causes cellular damage and substantially increases the risk of cancer. As you get heavier, the angle between the esophagus and the stomach (normally, the esophagus enters a side door) straightens out, and acid can easily shoot up into your esophagus. While you're losing weight (which will restore the normal angle), take a course of medications like over-the-counter Prilosec, Zantac, or Pepcid to help heal the injured tissue.

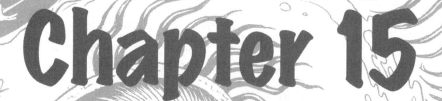

Chapter 15
Hear Ye, Hear Ye

YOU Test: Whisper What

Have someone stand about two feet in front of you. Close your eyes. Ask the person to whisper a sentence of his or her choice at an undisclosed time within a two-minute span, so you don't know when it's coming. Any sentence will do: "Want a turkey sandwich?" "Do you know if your telomeres are frayed?" "Meet me in the bedroom with the canola oil." After two minutes, open your eyes and let your partner know if you heard what was whispered.

If not: You're showing signs of early hearing loss and should be especially aware of taking steps to prevent further damage.

If so: Celebrate and proceed to the bedroom immediately. With canola oil.

This test is easier if a man is the tester, due to the voice tones of most men—see page 297.

We all know (and probably live with) people who have recently added some more words to their verbal repertoire. Namely:

"Huh?"

"Pardon?"

Or, for De Niro fans, "You talking to me?"

At first, we write off such queries as inattentiveness—"You can hear Anderson Cooper just fine, so why do I have to ask you three times to rinse the peanut butter off your spoon?" Or we may just say that our partner is daydreaming or stressed or too wrapped up in his YouTube addiction to actually have what we're saying register in his brain.

While that may be the case sometimes and for some people, it would be a mistake to write off all of these "Whadya say?" statements to simple distraction. Rather, they may be symptoms of the leading ager of all: hearing loss. Hearing loss (or presbycusis if you prefer) affects a whopping one-third of all people over sixty-five and half of people over seventy-five, and the rate of loss accelerates like a hot rod as we age. While hearing loss isn't one of those things that's going to kill you or have you escorted into the back of the ambulance (unless it was a horn you didn't hear), it is one of biggest things that can influence your quality of life and ultimately your health. When you can't hear as well, you limit your social interaction so you don't have to go through the awkwardness of being three conversations behind or missing the punch lines to jokes or constantly asking the barista to repeat herself. The depletion of social networks can cause a tangible decrease in your length and quality of life. In fact, hearing loss can age you at least four years in RealAge terms, mainly due to the social isolation that typically accompanies hearing loss. Bottom line: If you do what you can to save your hearing, you'll feel younger—and be younger.

FACTOID

The reason why doctors wear mechanical watches isn't because they haven't caught up with the digital age (OK, for some, that *is* the real reason). It's because they're a great tool for testing. Just as in the YOU Test at the beginning of this chapter, docs will hold a mechanical watch behind the ears of patients who may be suffering from hearing problems. If they can't hear the ticking, their ears may not be clicking.

Shut the @$#* Up!

If you're going to read this passage aloud to the dude who's sawing wood next to you, your voice will be about 60 decibels (his snoring is about 85). To understand the decibel structure, you have to realize that 70 decibels isn't a small increase from normal conversation. An increase of 6 decibels doubles the noise, and a 20-decibel increase is ten times louder. Forty decibels? That's one hundred times louder. Turning up your iPod headphones to a 70 percent level reaches the 90-decibel range, and that increases by 10 decibels if you use ear buds that go directly into your ear. Think you know your noises? See if you can match up loud sounds to their decibel levels.

A. 80 decibels

B. 100 decibels

C. 110 decibels

D. 140 decibels

E. 160 decibels

1. Front row of rock concert

2. Instant perforation of eardrum

3. Military jet takeoff

4. Vacuum cleaner

5. Large orchestra

Answers: A, 4; B, 5; C, 1; D, 3; E, 2

Your Ears: Turn Up the Volume

Ears can be exposed to some glorious sounds, be it boppy jazz, romantic whispers, waves lapping on your island vacation. But have you ever given thought to how those sounds make their way into your ear and ultimately register in your brain?

Here's how it works (see Figure 15.2): When the sounds from birds chirping or sports fans cursing enter your ear canal, those sound waves hit the skinlike tympanic membrane (that's the eardrum, for those unfamiliar with percussion instruments). That membrane is shiny and reflects lights when it's healthy, but if infected, it appears red with fluid around it. Just as the head of a drum vibrates when hit, so does your eardrum. That oscillation vibrates the smallest bones in your body, which abut the eardrum and are larger than a grain of sand but smaller than a big grain of rice. That then causes the snail-shaped cochlea next to them to quiver as well.

With all due respect to the Beach Boys, these good vibrations—traveling through fluid in the tubes of the cochlea—then stimulate hair cells growing on the insides of these cisterns. Since the hairs are attached to nerves, when they move,

Figure 15.1 **Sound Waves** Sound waves vibrate the eardrum and the adjacent smallest bones in your body, which then cause the snail-shaped cochlea next to them to quiver as well. These good vibrations then stimulate adjacent hair cells to excite the auditory nerves. This is where the message transmission takes place: The nerves send messages to the brain so you can hear. A common cause of hearing loss is fraying of the hairs within the cochlea due to occupational exposure to loud noises that crash into these delicate structures.

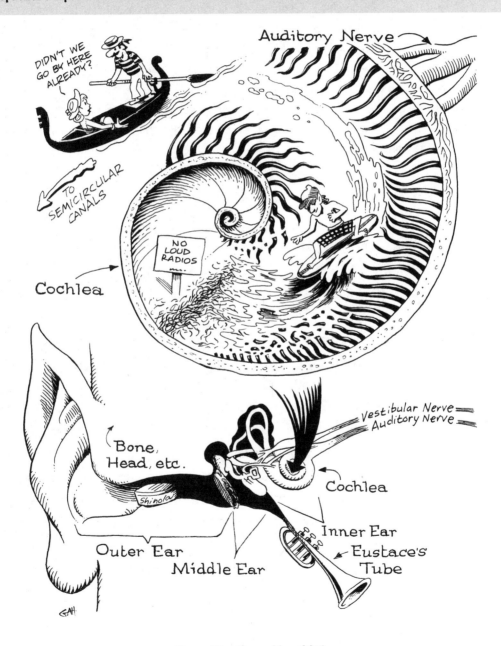

Testing, Testing

In a hearing test, you can expect doctors to use all kinds of diagnostic measures. Some may seem funny, like a tuning fork. They'll test your ability to hear tones versus words and high frequencies versus low frequencies. And they'll also try to get a sense of how your hearing problem developed—what impairment you noticed first and if it was in both ears or just one. So it pays (not just for the doctors) to make some notes about your hearing history.

If you're diagnosed with hearing loss, your doc will talk to you about a number of treatments—everything from cochlear implants, which are implanted in the ear to pick up and process sound, to traditional hearing aids, which amplify sound. The thing you should know about hearing aids: They can be imprecise and expensive, and may not work for all hearing problems. Or they can be less expensive and work perfectly for you. If all the sound you hear is garbled and garbage, a hearing aid will just give you louder garbage. Go to an aid place that lets you return the device within six months if it doesn't work for you. Many say that it takes three months to get used to a hearing aid. So if the first device doesn't work, it's worth trying another brand or solution.

the auditory nerves become excited. These hair cells respond to different frequencies; some to high and some to low. This is where the message transmission takes place: The nerves fire away messages to the brain that allow it to hear the sounds and realize that, yes indeed, that is Ellen DeGeneres doing Dory's voice-over in *Finding Nemo.*

The biggest cause of hearing loss, and the reason why it's such a good example of the Major Ager of wear and tear, is loss that comes from exposure to loud sounds. Loud noises—both sudden and cumulative over a period of exposure—cause the fluid to push through the cochlea too aggressively, thus shearing off the hairs, which, while resilient, don't heal once they're permanently damaged. And the high-frequency hairs are more vulnerable, making the lost ability to hear higher pitches like many female voices one of the signs of age-related hearing loss. Without the hairs, the vibrations can't get transmitted to your nervous system for interpretation. Cochlear damage occurs when we're exposed to more than 85 decibels for eight hours or 100 decibels for one hour (which is why those levels violate the requirements of OSHA, the federal Occupational Safety and Health Administration).

Cochlear hearing loss isn't like turning down the volume on a radio. Rather, it's like listening to a station that fades in and out. When hair cells at the end of the cochlea that transmit high-frequency sounds start to die, the loss of those sounds may go unnoticed at first. Men, who are often affected by hearing loss more than women, since they typically have more workplace exposure to loud noises, may find they can hear low-frequency pulsations but not high pitches and consonants (they have trouble distinguishing between B and P, or T and D). It's not that they don't want to take out the trash or do the dishes (although this is likely the case in some homes); it's that while they can hear the deep male voices shouting out the scores on SportsCenter, they truly can't hear the higher pitches and softer tones of the women they live with. Sounds from women, children, and crowds can be confusing to men—they all tend to blend together like ingredients in a frozen smoothie, so they can't be differentiated.

Another cause of age-related hearing loss is that your ear canal can have more wax than a surf shop. As we age, wax simply gets drier and thicker. Designed to protect your eardrum, wax is supposed to help you by trapping dirt, dust, bugs, and friendly fingers before they reach your eardrum. Wax also helps prevent infections. But too much of a wax buildup works as a roadblock in your ear canal. If the sound waves can't muscle past the wax and onto the drum, they can't start the vibration process that allows your brain to process those sounds, so you experience some hearing loss.

Other things that cause us to lose hearing include wear and tear from viral infections and certain medications that attack hair cells. Sometimes it is actually bad karma. About eighty genes are currently linked to hearing loss as we age; age-related hearing loss is under genetic control, but the details are still unknown.

FACTOID

We tend to think of hearing problems as isolated problems, but more often than not they're accompanied by decreases in vision or balance—all of which work together to chip away at quality of life. Practicing balance and eating the right foods for eye and ear health may not enable you to reenlist, but added together they can dramatically push back the onset of frailty.

YOU TIPS!

We have muffs to protect us from cold and plugs to protect us from snorers. You can stop much of hearing loss by protecting your ears from loud sounds everywhere. That means either wearing plugs or noise cancellation devices, or avoiding excessive noise altogether. The other thing you can do is learn the best ways to manage your ear care so that you can still enjoy the sweet sounds of life—no matter whether your favorite sounds include engines roaring, seagulls chatting, or Yo-Yo Ma playing.

YOU Tip: Trust Your Partner. Here's the thing about hearing loss: How do you know you can't hear something if you don't know what you're missing? So if your partner tells you that your ears seem clogged, resist the temptation to fight back with, "Yeah, and so are your pores." It may feel like nagging at the time, but your partner's frustration with repeating repeatedly is very often the first sign that you should have a medical checkup.

YOU Tip: Get the Wax Out. You probably grew up thinking cotton swabs were the ultimate wax removers. But you've heard it before (assuming you're not suffering from hearing loss): Don't stick any spearlike objects (aka Q-tips) into your ear, as they can perforate your eardrum. Jaw movement naturally forces your ear canal to move and dislodge wax (though we don't suggest a taffy diet to do so). If you experience buildup, you can remove the wax with an over-the-counter softener like glycerine. Or put mineral oil in your ears, let it sit for sixty minutes, then gently flush with saline warmed to body temperature, or just let it fall out on a piece of cotton. You can also see a doctor, who may try to remove it through a vacuumlike device, which is safe if done by an experienced practitioner. The vacuum technique is much safer than a method that used to be commonly used: flushing out the ears with water and high pressure. The water, if not the right temperature, can cause dizziness, and the high-pressure flooding can damage the drum.

YOU Tip: Eat for Your Ears. It appears that two substances—folate and phytochemicals—might have some auditory advantages. Taking 800 micrograms of folate (which is also found in leafy green foods) has been shown to slow the loss of high-frequency sounds. Deficiencies in folate and vitamin B_{12} might affect both the nervous system and the vascular system associated with hearing. Hearing also benefits from phytochemicals, so the stronger the color of the fruit, the better. That means it contains high levels of these protective substances.

YOU Tip: Cover Up. In noisy situations—doing yard work with power tools or maybe dinner with the extended family—it's worth using noise cancellation headphones, which emit energy in a frequency that we can't hear. The sound waves they create have the same amplitude but opposite polarity as the original sound; they combine with the external wave and effectively cancel it out so there's no sound at all. Models available in stores typically cancel lower-frequency noises, while the ear cups themselves protect you from high-frequency noises. (By the way, there's no evidence to suggest that these devices cause any damage of their own.) If you are exposed to loud noises that come and go—sirens, trucks, traffic—cover your ears. And bring earplugs to weddings and bar mitzvahs.

FACTOID

Chronic exposure to noise loud enough to make you raise your voice can increase heart attack rates by 50 percent, especially if this is true at both work and home. And if you work in a noisy place, it's that much more important to make sure you live in a quiet one. So pick an apartment on a higher floor or in a suburban area, or petition for a quieter work environment.

Major Ager

Unforced Errors

Why Our Bodies Can't Withstand the
Crazy Things That Happen in Life

Much of aging certainly is about preventing the decrease in quality of life from chronic disease and long-term wear and tear. But the ultimate form of aging is the kind of aging that bypasses all the details and kills us off immediately: a car crash, a fall from a cliff, or a freak encounter with a rabid antelope.

Most of us like to write off accidents as unfortunate circumstances of fate: The pencil point *had* to be in the exact spot where you stepped. The incoming baseball was perfectly tossed to strike your eye socket. Out of the entire surface area of your driveway, you decided to step in the 3-square-inch spot that still had a patch of ice. An incident like any of these may have you cursing at the gods of fate, wondering why the planets, stars, and moon all had to align at that exact moment in that exact place with you as the exact victim (see Figure N.1). After all, they never align to win the Powerball.

Many accidents, of course, are just that: a small if, and, or but between a close call and a life-or-death situation. Some things you can't always control, but you can take steps to minimize other risks. In fact, many accidents are very pre-

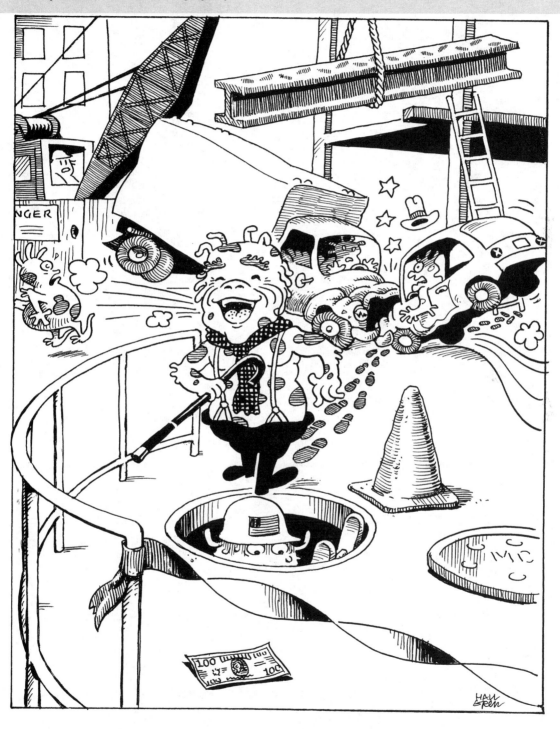

Major Ager: Unforced Errors 301

ventable and not really the end result of some cosmic master plan of evil. While some of us may seem like Mr. Magoo, having accidents follow us wherever we go, the truth is that we're actually responsible through our actions for much of the bad stuff that can happen. Before talking about how you can avoid accidents, however, it's important to know why nature made us so vulnerable to freak accidents, crashes, and ironic incidents of injury.

It's not that our bodies aren't extremely resilient. Just as a city absorbs its share of accidents, be it fires, traffic accidents, or chemical spills, our bodies can also take some hits. But they're not perfect. We die or have a decreased quality of life because we knock our heads, or break our bones, or can't stop bleeding. The reason? Again, it's one of those biological trade-offs. Our bodies certainly could be made to withstand more. If it were necessary to preserve the species, evolution would have made sure that our bones were firm enough to survive a fall from a cliff, or our organs dense enough never to bleed out. But that would be as inefficient as a sleep-deprived college student.

If we had bones heavy enough to withstand falls and crashes, then we wouldn't be able to walk. If our skulls were so thick that we could survive hockey-puck assaults, our heads would be so heavy we'd have to carry them in backpacks. Not all that efficient, right? Evolution had no reason to overbuild us to the point where improvement in one area of biology would sacrifice other areas. For extreme resilience in our bodies, we'd give up our bodies' extreme flexibility and our lifestyles (no more Twister for you).

When it comes to accidents and unforced errors, the big picture is this: It's all about leverage points—tipping life into your favor by doing the things that make your body better equipped to handle the unexpected things that will be hurled your way. And you can do things to tip those scales, as you'll see in Figure N.2. And, at some point, they *will* be hurled your way if they haven't already been. That doesn't mean sitting in your home on a recliner with a frozen dinner and remote control (then you'd subject yourself to that Major Ager of virtually everything: disuse atrophy).

It means making sound decisions in life (nonslip mat in the shower, helmet when you're riding a bike) to stack the odds in your favor. It means knowing where the trouble spots may be, so you can plan to avoid them—and cope with them if you can't.

It's not all about playing life safe. It's about playing to win.

Figure N.2 Accident-proof Your Life Granted, you can't predict when a boulder may drop from a mountainside, roll down the county road, hop a guardrail, and land on your hood on the highway below. Fate is, well, just fate. But that doesn't mean you should accept any accident as karma's way of paying you back for the time you shaved $33 off your taxes in 1994. You can prevent plenty of unintentional problems by intentionally preparing yourself.

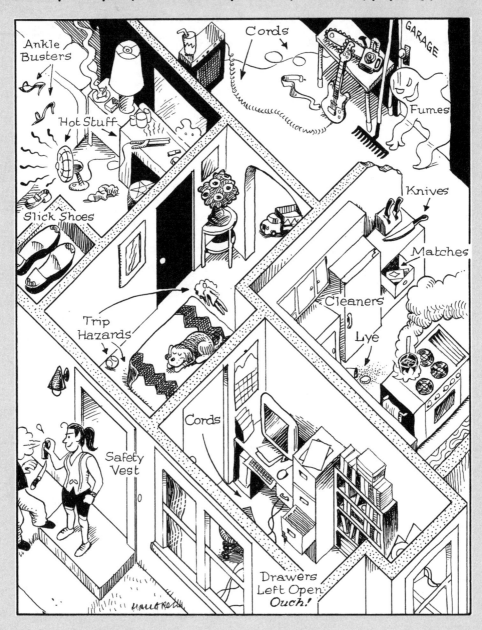

ON SIDEWALK If you're going to run or walk at night, it's worth the twelve bucks to spring for a reflective vest. And depending on where you live, the pepper spray.

IN HOME OFFICE Not counting paper cuts and sadomasochistic stapling, most office accidents happen when people trip over electric cords or drawers left open. Stop looking at the memo you're delivering and keep your eyes up.

IN CLOSET Wearing hard-soled shoes (for men) or high-heeled shoes (for women—and very confident men) can make you more prone to slipping on wet or slick tile, marble, or linoleum floors.

IN BEDROOM The major causes of fire deaths in homes: leaving on a curling iron or heating blanket, dropping a cigarette, or leaving an electric heater too close to flammable material. Make it a habit: Switch it off and pull the plug. (Older homes, by the way, are especially susceptible to faulty electrical wiring, increasing the chance of a fire.)

IN KITCHEN Of course, it's easy to get distracted by kids, cartoons, and doorbells, but an unattended stove or burner being left on accidentally is a leading cause of fire. While you're thinking of it, put all your matches in upper cabinets, not waist-level drawers. Children playing with matches is the leading cause of accidental death for children under two and the third leading cause of death and injury for those under eighteen.

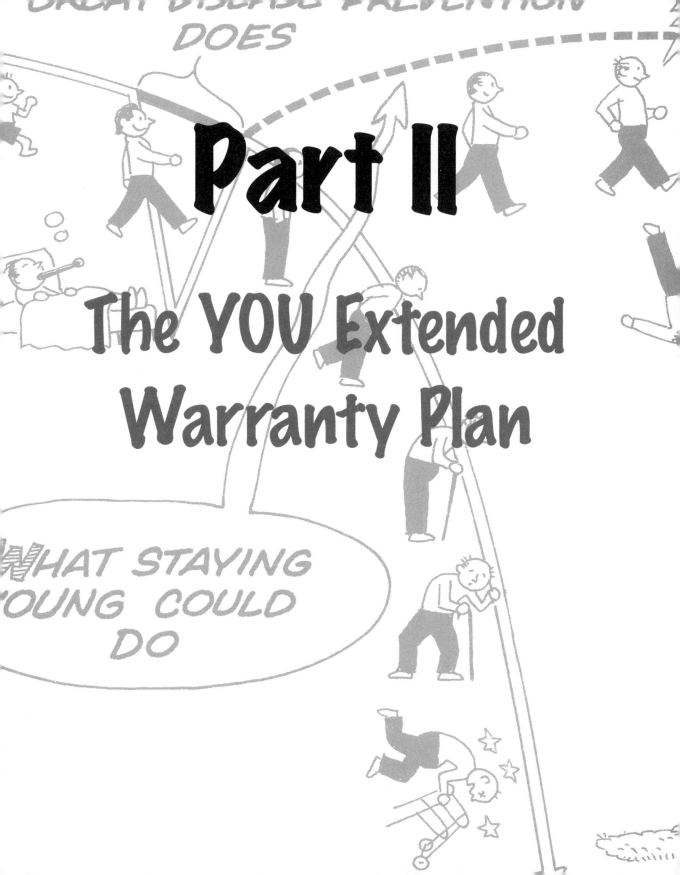

If a city doesn't have a good plan, it goes bankrupt. If a designer doesn't have a good plan, she gets embarrassed. A suitor without a good plan? He ends up with a slap (or a drink) on his face.

Same applies to you. It's not that you have to live your life with a preprogrammed to-the-second schedule that details every time you will eat, sneeze, drink, wipe, work, sleep, and play Bunco. But to live life without a smart plan—especially as you round the corner of your middle years onto the back stretch—you're asking your body to go bankrupt, or be embarrassed, or wind up being slapped upside the head by the effects of aging. And that's why we've constructed this YOU Extended Warranty Plan—to give you a playbook (a YOU-do list, if you will) of the steps you can take to make your life rich, vibrant, and healthy. Follow these guidelines, and you'll be applying the brakes to aging and pressing the gas on living younger.

Our goal here is to help you not only to live to one hundred and beyond but to get there with the fewest health-related roadblocks as possible at a higher quality of life. Before we begin, though, let's recap:

As you now know from your journey through the body and all of the magical cellular processes that happen every day, we age through a variety of Major Agers, which work in a couple of different ways. Some act as outside stressors that wear us down (think UV radiation and toxins). Others age us because they fritz out along the way and are no longer able to defend us (a weakened immune system) or repair us if we're damaged (a slow-

FACTOID

The secret of living to one hundred? Maybe it has nothing to do with fiber, aspirin, or telomere length and everything to do with *American Idol.* Researchers have found that one-third of centenarians watch reality TV shows (gives new meaning to *Survivor,* eh?), a quarter watch MTV or music videos, and some may have even surfed the Web and used an iPod. The researchers also found that this group was into current events, led healthy lifestyles (really, now?), and also considered faith and spirituality a priority. The U.S. Census Bureau says we'll have seven times more centenarians by the year 2040; that's a half million more than we have today. We think the number could be much greater.

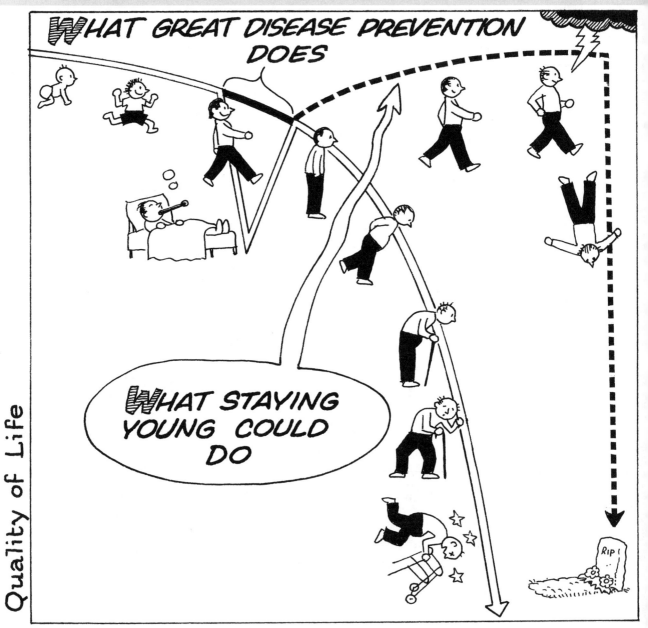

down of stem cells). Our goal in aging is to keep our bodily systems running smoothly. That means not only limiting and defending against outside threats, but, more important, making sure we maintain our reparability. Now, the trick, of course, is that it's not as if we can just flip on some biological switch (right there in the left nostril!) and instantly repair all the damage that we've accumulated over time. Your body's ability to repair takes some energy and can come at the cost of damage itself. These are the trade-offs that we've talked about throughout the book, the perfect example being an autoimmune disease, where your immune system turns on itself. Still, our ultimate goal is to slow that rate of aging—that is, the more we can mitigate or prevent the damage we accumulate over time, the more we can decelerate the rate of aging and the younger we get to stay and feel (see Figure 16.1).

Thankfully, science does have answers that will minimize damage and crank your repair mechanisms to work optimally. We've outlined these answers throughout the book, but we've also brought many of the ideas together here in the YOU Extended Warranty Plan—the plan that will extend the service life of your body so that it continues to work at peak level. What we want you to do is change your mind-set about what kind of "product" your body is. A lot of us treat ourselves as if we were disposable, when we should really start thinking of ourselves as being high-end, with the opportunity to last for a long, long time. After all, no one chucks a disposable camera in the trash and thinks "what a waste." But this YOU Extended Warranty Plan offers the idea that for a specified period of time, if you follow the instructions for good maintenance, your high-quality product will have the reliability and durability and expectations to perform like new.

If you embrace the idea that you can extend your warranty period past what you typically thought was acceptable, then you'll do your part in reversing stereotypes about aging—and your perceptions about aging. After all, aging is about being well enough to do and enjoy the things that you want to do in life. Maybe that means finishing a 5K in at least as good a time as you did five years ago; maybe it's realizing that after decades of dining on takeout, you really want to cook. As you mature, your aspirations should change and develop, because if you're no better today than you were yesterday, then what's the plan for tomorrow? And when you really think about it, what's the point of tomorrow if you're not contributing to the world by improving yourself and your community?

Up next, we're going to give you a Fourteen-day YOU Extended Warranty Plan of tips, quizzes, shopping lists, and action steps that will get your mind and body best prepared to make changes. You'll work on these changes for two weeks—the time it takes for behaviors to become habits. In that time, you'll become accustomed to the foods, activities, and thought processes that will keep you living young for good. Following that, you'll also find more of our YOU Tools and other programs that you will use for the rest of your long and youthful life to enrich your body and your mind.

We're happy that you've made it this far in the book and that you've taken the time to really learn about your body and how it ages from a cellular point of view, a systems point of view, and even an anthropological point of view. But now's the time to apply the information you've digested, so you can go ahead and get the very most—and very best—out of life.

Sound like a plan?

Chapter 16

The Fourteen-Day YOU Extended Warranty Plan

Your Everyday Basics

Your Daily YOU-do List

1 Walk thirty minutes. If you can't walk thirty consecutive minutes at a rate that slightly elevates your heart rate, walk three times for ten minutes. On day one (below), you'll buy a pedometer, so you can also note how many steps you take every day; the total number of steps you take everywhere (including to and from the bathroom), not just those taken during these thirty minutes. A good goal: ten thousand steps. But don't worry as long as you get the thirty minutes (about three thousand steps). You can gradually build up to ten thousand a day. Walk every day. No excuses.

2 Floss and brush the teeth that you wish to keep. Or do it for the heart you wish to nurture, the wrinkles you wish to prevent, or the erection or sexual satisfaction you wish to have.

3 Drink several cups of green tea along with your copious water intake.

4 Take your pills. Specifically, these:

❖ Get into the habit of popping omega-3s in doses of either six walnuts or 1 gram of metabolically distilled omega-3 fatty acids about thirty minutes before lunch and again before dinner. Or have 4 ounces of nonfried nonshell fish three times a week. Or 400 mg of DHA a day.

❖ Take vitamin tablets (see our chart in the YOU Toolbox) by leaving them in a convenient location like your car or by your desk, so you're continuously reminded. Same goes for calcium supplements (more details on day two).

❖ If you are over the age of forty (women) or thirty-five (men), take two baby aspirin at breakfast (162 milligrams) with a half glass of warm water before and after. Get your doctor's approval first.

5 Sleep seven to eight hours a night. Starting with day one, adopt a sleep hygiene program (see page 195) that will help you sleep like a nineteen-year-old cat. About fifteen minutes before bed, finish any must-do tasks still hanging around (even if it's just making a list of what you need to do tomorrow, so you can avoid stress-related sleep problems), do any before-bed hygiene, and spend a few minutes doing breathing and meditation (detailed on page 350). If you have trouble falling asleep, avoid stimulatory acts before bed, like watching TV or working out. But individualize this: Some say a workout helps them go to sleep. Sex, though stimulatory (we hope), is OK. And recommended.

6 Meditate for five minutes at some point during the day; you'll work up to fifteen minutes in future weeks. For some of you, meditation will take the form of prayer (zoning in on ESPN doesn't count). The key is to search for a path that gives you comfort and offers an opening to finding deeper meaning in life. In a world with more noise than a

The Dopamine Jackpot
How to Break Bad Habits

The chemical dopamine has a very important job when it comes to habits: It teaches your brain what you want and then drives you to get it, regardless of whether it's actually good for you or not. That's because dopamine influences memory, desire, and decision making. In other words, it's stimulated by learning. Whenever something unexpected happens, these learning circuits are engaged. So the next time something unexpected happens, we'll know what to do. To break the cycle of bad habits, you need to reset your dopamine cycles. How? By giving yourself robust rewards. We're not suggesting sundaes and sausages here. Instead, reward yourself weekly with shopping (it doesn't matter how little you spend, just that you have an indulgence to look forward to) or a manicure or anything that's not destructive. As you disable the old pathways of bad habits, you'll need to nurture the new ones with new rewards. As you do, your brain will start producing brain-derived neurotrophic factor (Miracle-gro for the brain), which increases brain plasticity to set new pathways for good, long-lasting, and healthy behaviors.

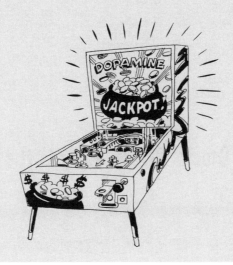

preschool classroom, our brains (and souls) need moments of silence to recharge, refocus, and become rejuvenated. Give yourself a chance to think through your spirituality.

We'll offer you a bunch more habits throughout our fourteen-day starter program so you can adopt them for the rest of your now longer life.

Week One

Day One: Take Stock, Which Way Is the Scale Tipping?

Your YOU-do List

1. Do the everyday basics, uh, every day. See page 313.

2. Get out and go shopping! Buy these items, which should run you less than $125.

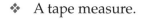

- A tape measure.
- A heart-rate monitor. (We like Polar and Omron products; they have chest straps and monitor watches.)
- A pedometer. (Men typically prefer the type that can be worn on your belt, like Omron; women usually prefer a thin model like the

Accu-Check, which is thin enough to fit on a bra strap. Our patients get much longer life from the belt variety, and it seems more accurate, in our experience.)

❖ A blood-pressure cuff. (Many brands are available that fit on the arm, are easy to use, and have memory and computer download capabilities.)

❖ A good pair of walking or running shoes. (Specialty running-shoe stores can help identify your stride nuances to find a good fit.)

❖ A hand-grip device (from Harbinger, about $15; can find on Amazon.com).

❖ A notebook or access to a computer website to record your results. (See www.mychoicescount.com for such a program. As of now, there is a small yearly charge for this service.) Record and date your answers to all self-tests in your notebook.

3 Determine your RealAge—that is, the actual age of your body (and mind) based on your health and habits, not your calendar age based on when Mama thrust you into the world covered in goop. Take the free test on www.realage.com; it shouldn't take more than about twenty minutes to complete.

4 Measure your blood pressure. If you haven't bought the home device yet, most drug stores have a device that can be placed on your arm.

5 Measure your heart rate in the evening, as well as the highest heart rate you achieve during your most intense exercise.

6 Measure your waist size. Circle the tape measure around your waist at the belly button while you're taking a deep breath and sucking in. (You would anyway, but this is the right way of measuring, as it gets the muscle we do not want to measure out of the way). Also measure your height. The ideal is for your waist to be half your height.

7 Leave a space to record the average number of steps you take this week.

8 Make a doctor's appointment so you can get various blood tests that we're going to tell you about.

9 Answer these questions:

- ❖ Are you living life from (a) fear or (b) passion?
- ❖ Are you playing life (a) to avoid losing or (b) to win?
- ❖ Are your goals based on (a) preserving the status quo or (b) achieving growth?

If you answered (a) to any of them, it's an indication that you're not moving forward in life. Remember, the only times that your vital signs are completely stable are when you're dead. Like sharks, we need to keep moving to live fully.

10 Ask yourself these questions to determine whether you're really enjoying life:

- ❖ Are you happy most of the time?
- ❖ Are you as happy now as you were five years ago?
- ❖ Are you still expecting much from life?
- ❖ Do your days seem to be passing by faster than an express train?
- ❖ Are you sad less than 10 percent of the time?

We obviously want you to have positive answers for these questions. If you're not there, our program, as well as help from a mental health professional, can help you get there.

11 Ask three strangers how old they think you are. (Asking friends and family doesn't count, since they either know or have a vested interest in not hurting your feelings. Think servers, baristas, seatmates on the subway, anyone who won't automatically say "ninety-seven.") That will help give you some kind of baseline as to how others perceive you—based on appearance and demeanor—and it can be a strong indicator of how healthy you actually are. In addition, you can ask a friend you trust to be honest with you about how you are aging compared to others.

12 Ask your friends what your three biggest strengths are. Strengths are invisible to you; because they come so easily, you take them for granted. Identify how you best use these strengths.

13 In your notebook, draw a little box with an amoeba that fills up 70 percent of the box but also goes outside of the box. The box is your job, and the amoeba is you. The empty spots in the box are where we often focus all of our effort, but perhaps you should focus on the part of the amoeba that lies outside the box, as this represents your strengths.

14 Ask yourself this simple question: How have you aged over the last five years? Use a photograph to compare how you looked then as compared to now. Your initial thought:

    A. My oh my, I look like I did in high school, dahling!
    B. I'm steady Eddie—about the same.
    C. I'm about what you'd expect—a little fatter, a little wrinklier, and a little more worn down.
    D. I look like tree bark.

15 Ask yourself this: What activities did you do five years ago that you can't do today? (Keep it clean, slick.)

16 Ask yourself these big-picture stress questions, which can help identify things to work on while using our program:

- Is your perceived level of stress more than you enjoy? Remember that perceived stress is a more predictable driver of aging than our actual stress, so push yourself to be honest with yourself.
- Do you control most of the stress in your life or are you a rat in someone else's experiment?

Day Two: Retool Your Home and Mind

Your YOU-do List

1 Record the results from these YOU Tests:

Push-up test (next page): _____
Sit-up test (next page): _____
Hand-grip test (page 322): _____
Breathing (heart and lung) test (page 322) _____
Hip-flexion test (page 322): _____
Eye test (page 257): _____
Balance test (page 273): _____

2 Trash the nasty food—food that will age you—in your fridge, pantry, and anywhere else you've stashed the Ding Dongs. Toss into a trash can foods containing any of the following as the first five ingredients on the label:

- Saturated fat (any fat that comes from four-legged animals, or palm or coconut oil)
- Hydrogenated fat (trans fat)
- Primary omega-6 fat (corn oil, soybean oil)
- Simple sugars (those ending in -ose, like sucrose, glucose, maltose, and fructose) or sugar alcohols that end in -ol

Optimum results: You can find optimum results for the eye test, balance test, and lung test on the specified pages throughout the book. For the others, these are the norms to shoot for, depending on your age:

Push-up Test: Optimum Number

Calendar Age	Typical Man (Advanced, see page 370)	Typical Woman (Modified Push-ups, on Knees; see page 370)
20–29	More than 35	More than 18
30–39	25–29	13–19
40–49	20–24	11–14
50–59	15–19	7–10
60–69	10–14	5–10
70–79	6–9	4–10
80–89	3–5	2–6
90–99	1–3	1–4

Sit-up Test: Number of Sit-ups in One Minute

Calendar Age	Typical Man	Typical Woman
20–29	More than 45	More than 35
30–39	30–34	25–29
40–49	25–29	20–24
50–59	20–24	15–19
60–69	15–19	10–14
70–79	10–14	7–9
80–89	6–9	4–6
90–99	2–5	1–3

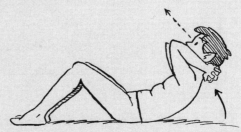

Hand-grip Test: Grab the hand grip and squeeze it, one hand at a time. Do it three times and write down your numbers. If it's too easy, get a stronger exerciser, but you always want your grip strength to be greater than 15 pounds. Higher hand strength correlates with slowing the aging process. Practicing with the gripper (or squeezing a rubber ball) will help you gain hand strength.

Hip-flexion Test: Lie flat on your back with your arms at your sides and your legs straight out on the floor. Without moving your hips or pelvis, lift your right leg up toward the ceiling, keeping your knee straight. Repeat with your left leg.

Results: You should be able to lift your legs until they are almost pointing directly toward the ceiling (about 80 to 90 degrees of hip flexion). If you have less than the desired flexibility, be sure to include hamstring stretches in your workout.

Breathing (Heart and Lung) Test: Take a six-minute walk. You should be able to cover about six hundred yards in that time. Within a few weeks, you should be able to increase your speed to go about fifty yards longer within those six minutes. After the first few weeks, test yourself monthly.

* Syrups (which are simple sugars)
* Any non–whole grain, such as bleached or enriched flour; plus, anything with 4 or more grams of sugars per serving (unless it has a ton of nutritious ingredients to offset it)

3 Shop for healthy foods (see www.realage.com).

4 Shop for vitamins (listed in YOU Tool 5, pages 357–358) and calcium supplements. Specifically, buy calcium tablets that have at least 500 milligrams of calcium, 200 IU of vitamin D, and 150 milligrams of magnesium.

5 Detoxify your home and buy nontoxic products (see YOU Tool 6, page 359).

6 Purchase and install water filters for your kitchen and bathroom.

7 Do the Chi-gong Workout (page 377) to build your coordination and mind-body connection.

8 If you have any addictions, start a cessation program like the smoking cessation program on page 134.

Day Three: Start the Three-Day Body-basic Diet

Your YOU-do List

1 Observe a calorie-restricted diet for three days. The goal of this body-basic diet: Recalibrate your settings to eating better foods—and more sensible amounts.

Here's how it works: Eat about three-quarters the amount of food you usually eat every day (using only healthy foods, now). You can do it by eyeballing, or literally filling your plate as usual, then taking away one-quarter of the meal and storing it for tomorrow. If you find this too difficult, reducing your calorie intake by even 15 percent will work, and if *that* is too challenging, then just eat healthy foods in the usual amount for you. (If you can't even do that, please reread the book.)

Why? We're not trying to deprive you and make you more uncomfortable than wet socks; we're trying to get you to feel what calorie restriction (the only proven senility eraser) feels like. It will be a little uncomfortable, but you'll do it for only three days. Drink as much water with lime or lemon juice or fresh brewed green tea as you want. Those drinks will help clear toxins and prevent dehydration. Please take your vitamin supplements while on the program, since we don't want to starve you if you're already nutritionally depleted from a life of kielbasa with mayonnaise.

You'll find specific foods and nutrients throughout the book and on the website www.realage.com or www.oprah.com. When you add back a little more food on day six, chances are that even in three days you'll have trained yourself and your stomach to need less food than you're accustomed to eating. That's because most of us actually indulge in toxic eating: We eat because we're bored, mad, sad, lonely, depressed, or anything other than actually hungry. We also eat because our bodies are nutritionally starved, even though we're tossing lots of calories into them. This body-basic diet will get you on the right track and remind you what real hunger feels like. This has a centering effect; it's not a coincidence that so many spiritual and meditative practices include a fast. Eat good-for-you foods that we outline below, and avoid foods with the potential for triggering allergies, like gluten (wheat, barley, oats, or rye) and casein (milk products), as well as alcohol, for these three days. And if you feel more lively in the morning, you might have uncovered a subtle (and frequent) allergy.

2 Publicize your goals to your friends and family. You should feel pride in your accomplishments and pressure to stick with the program for two weeks.

3 Do the YOU2 Workout (page 367). Allow your mind to examine new dimensions of your body.

Day Four: Examine Some Habits

Your YOU-do List

1 Continue with the calorie-restricted body-basic diet. To make the experience even more unique (and to challenge your taste buds), you can even try eating vegan for a day. It's all about disrupting old habits by replacing them with viable alternatives plus rewards (remember the dopamine jackpot).

2 Scan your life and home for environmental toxins. For example, check your home for asbestos (around air ducts, pipes, and so forth), lead paint (windowsills are the most common culprits), and radon. See the

YOU Tool beginning on page 359, for more ideas for eliminating toxins. While you're looking, open the windows and vent your home to air out toxins that are locked into modern airtight living spaces.

3 Just for today, turn off the TV and don't read the newspaper. Use the computer only as needed for work or important tasks. No Web surfing. Take the time you saved and practice some stress-reduction techniques (page 353). Take a break from the tube to clear your thought process.

4 List the two things in your life that stress you the most, and for each identify at least two concrete steps you can take to feel better about the issue. (Hint: This means list a total of four behaviors that you can do in the near future, and overthrowing the boss can't be one of them.) Each week, assess how well you've succeeded and make practical adjustments to your plan.

Day Five: Tune Up Your Body and Mind

Your YOU-do List

1 Continue with the last day of your calorie-restricted body-basic diet.

2 Do the YOU2 Workout (page 366).

3 Do something you've never done before, whether it be playing a game, attending some kind of cultural event, or asking your partner to try out position number 119 (use your imagination).

4 Memorize a passage from a poem.

5 In your notebook, write down what you're grateful for. With apologies to David Letterman, list the top ten things that come to mind. While you're at it, it wouldn't hurt to make peace with your biggest enemy at work. You have more important things to do than quibble.

Day Six: Strengthen Your Relationships

Your YOU-do List

1 Carve out at least one hour to do something as a family.

2 Practice a day of nonjudgment, where you live, work, and observe without judging—both inside and outside of yourself.

3 Stop the calorie-restricted body-basic diet. But continue to eat nutrient-rich, calorie-poor healthy foods with ingredients that increase longevity. The key to success is making the process of preparing and eating healthy snacks and meals easy and automatic.

We want you to enjoy your breakfast, lunch, and snacks—but we also want you to get in the habit of automating them, so that you eat healthfully without having to labor over choices. What's automation? It means finding three or so breakfasts, lunches, and snacks (and dinners if you choose) that you like and eating one of them every day. When you can automate your eating behavior with good choices, you'll have mastered one of the crucial steps to fueling your body with ingredients that help you live strong and long.

Day Seven: Detox Your Mind

Your YOU-do List

1 Do something for someone else that you normally wouldn't be doing.

2 Get the tests that we recommend (see page 336), including those that measure intracellular vitamin levels and help us "carbon-date" your body. Also, check the list to see what additional tests you should be having, so you can schedule them with your doctor.

3 Do the Chi-gong Workout (page 377).

4 Stop reading self-help books; start doing what they say.

Week Two

Continue with the Everyday Basics listed on page 313. They're called Your Everyday Basics because, well, uh, they serve as your daily list of fundamentals that provide the basic foundation for healthy living. Of course, you'll also continue to eat healthfully, following our guidelines throughout the book, and not bring bad-for-you foods into your house. Keep at least two of your meals and most of your snacks automated.

Day Eight

1. Measure your blood pressure, heart rate, and waist size.
2. Record the results from these YOU Tests mentioned throughout the book.

Push-up test (page 321): _____

Sit-up test (page 321): _____

Hand-grip test (page 322): _____

Breathing (heart and lung) test (page 322): _____

Hip-flexion test (page 322): _____

Eye test (page 257): _____

Balance test (page 273): _____

3 Restock your kitchen with healthy foods.

Day Nine

1 Do the Chi-gong Workout.

2 Call a high school friend you haven't talked with in years.

Day Ten

1 Do the YOU2 Workout.

2 Write a thank-you note to your significant other or a parent, and tell them how much you appreciate the small things they do.

Day Eleven

1 Take a break day from media and try some of our stress-reduction techniques.

2 Think about and write down why you care about living.

3 Call on someone over the age of eighty whom you might not talk to regularly.

Day Twelve

1 Do the YOU2 Workout.

2 Do something you've never done before.

3 Memorize a passage from a poem (quote it to impress onlookers at a party).

4 Write down three things for which you are grateful.

Day Thirteen

1 Do something as a family.

2 Depending on how many enemies you have, forgive another foe. (Remember Reagan's "trust but verify" line.)

3 Write a thank-you note to someone who helped you—at a hospital or a car service department, for example.

Day Fourteen

1 Do the chi-gong workout.

2 Think about why someone you know over the age of eighty might care about being healthy.

3 Explain to someone else why extending your warranty isn't the same thing as preventing disease.

Today Until Forever

Your YOU-do List

After following our principles for fourteen days—eating well, exercising your mind and body, and taking stock of where you are—you're on your way to continuing the healthy habits you've developed. (Remember, for any behavior to become a habit, it takes at least two weeks.) Don't forget, this plan's goal is to keep you healthy and young, and the steps we've outlined can do just that if you make them a regular part of your life. From here on out, you can follow the steps above for healthy living and the ones below to help guide you along the way.

Once a Week

❖ Go food shopping to make sure your pantry and fridge are stocked with healthy ingredients, to keep you from bringing on pizza deliveries, drive-through heart attacks, and all the spur-of-the-moment foods that can age you.

❖ Measure your blood pressure, waist size, resting heart rate, and maximum heart rate during exercise. Record the results in your notebook.

❖ Record the average number of steps you take in a week.

❖ Repeat these tests and record your results:

Push-up test (page 321):   _____
Sit-up test (page 321):   _____
Hand-grip test (page 322):   _____
Breathing (heart and lung) test (page 322):   _____
Hip-flexion test (page 322):   _____
Eye test (page 257):   _____
Balance test (page 273):   _____

Two to Three Times a Week

❖ Do the YOU2 Workout. This muscle building program, which uses your own body as your gym, will help you build and maintain lean muscle mass, keep your weight under control, and give your muscles strength and flexibility to keep you mobile, limber, and young.

Three Times a Week

❖ Do either the Chi-gong Workout or meditation-relaxation. Both will help balance your body and mind. Depending on your tastes, you can mix and match as you like. We prefer two days or more of chi-gong and at least a day of meditation-relaxation.

Once a Month

❖ Ask yourself the self-evaluative questions from day one on pages 316 to 320—those big-picture questions that measure your stress and your happiness.

If You Get Stuck

❖ Start on day one of The YOU Extended Warranty Plan and go through the pieces of the plan that will help you regain your focus. The calorie-restricted body-basic diet and the self-evaluations should be enough to jump-start you if you run out of juice.

Chapter 17

The YOU Toolbox

Your handyman has tools, your mechanic has tools, and your Microsoft programs have tools. No matter whether those tools come in the form of screwdrivers, hydraulic floor jacks, or spell-checkers, they are all designed for the same purpose: to help you reach some final goal. Same goes here. In our YOU Toolbox, you won't find the duct tape or Band-Aids to make the quick fixes; instead, you'll find the information that you can pull out when you need it to achieve your goal of a rich, vibrant one hundred years of life.

These tools, plus the various ones you'll find throughout the book, are key components of your overall Extended Warranty. You'll use them, you'll love them—and you'll live longer because of them. Bet nobody's been able to say that about a reciprocating saw.

YOU Tool 1
Medical Screening

As you know by now, our mission is to give you the information and education you need to make decisions about how to take care of yourself. Generally, we avoid "See your doc" advice the way supermodels avoid frosting. But the reality is that you need doctors, you need science, and you need lab techs to help you make crucial decisions about your life and health.

Tool 1 consists of an outline of vaccines, lab tests, and medical exams you should have to help guide you; periodic checkups to determine changes in your body and your cells. Remember, you can't test yourself to good health; you can only live to good health. Think of your lab results as the stars that guided old-time sailors to their destination. They're there for navigation—to help steer you in the right direction.

Note: These recommendations are based on people with average risk of disease; if you have increased risk due to genetics or lifestyle, here's one time we're going to say it: See your doc.

Medical Work and Tests by Age

Vaccines

1. Tetanus shot every ten years. While there are fewer than one hundred cases per year in the United States (usually in sick, older people), you should get it so that you don't have to worry about tetanus, especially when you travel.
2. Whooping cough revaccination for all adults: one time only. Get it with your tetanus (Adacel). In adults, whooping cough isn't fatal, but it can cause coughing for months and may result in broken ribs. Yowza.
3. Shingles vaccine: everyone over sixty years old. Though expensive (about $300), it decreases the incidence of the über-painful condition of shingles. Some insurance companies may reimburse for this shot. Check with your insurance provider, and if it's covered, ask for the insurance code and provide it to your doctor—you may find this number makes it easier for all.
4. Pneumovax: for people over fifty. Repeat at sixty-five years old (if five years since first one). Used to prevent the most common cause of bacterial pneumonia in adults.
5. Influenza: yearly. The federal Centers for Disease Control and Prevention (CDC) recommends it for kids, the elderly, pregnant women, and chronically ill persons and those exposed to the above groups, but everyone is exposed, so we recommend it for everyone.

6. Human papillomavirus (HPV) vaccine: Young women up to twenty-six years old should get the series.

General

1. Weight, waist, height, and BMI (Body Mass Index): yearly (we know we asked for waist dimensions weekly, but this is also for your doc's records).
2. Blood pressure: yearly.
3. Cholesterol (HDL, LDL, triglycerides): at least every five years but increasing frequency with age and male gender.
4. Thyroid-stimulating hormone: every other year starting at age thirty-five.
5. Echocardiogram and stress test: once at age fifty as a baseline.
6. Physical exam: yearly.
7. Bone mineral density: around menopause, and every five years after if normal.
8. Eye exam: every two years by an ophthalmologist.
9. Hearing exam: at age sixty-five and yearly in physical.
10. Oral exam: at least yearly by dentist.

Cancer Screening

1. Breast: breast self-exams monthly and by a doctor once or twice a year—once by general doc and once by your gynecologist. You should get a baseline mammogram between ages thirty-five and forty and then yearly ones starting at age forty (higher-risk women use MRI screening). We do not recommend cutting back to every other year in older women. If you have dense breasts, your gynecologist may recommend a sonogram as well as a mammogram, alternating every six months.

2. Prostate: yearly digital rectal exam starting at age forty (yes, really). Yearly PSA to measure change (the change in PSA over time is a better predictor than the absolute number).

3. Colon: colonoscopy starting at age fifty, then every ten years, with additional screening (such as a hemoccult test, which measures blood in the stool) every five years.

4. Cervical: yearly Pap test starting at age twenty-one, or three years after sexual activity starts. Women without uteruses should still have pelvic exams because of vaginal cancers and ovarian issues.

5. Skin cancer: yearly check at every age by someone who is comfortable examining your whole body. For efficiency, tie exam into other activity. Any new or changing moles should be seen by a dermatologist.

See www.realage.com or www.oprah.com if you want to track the tests by age.

YOU Tool 2

The Ultimate Workup

The beautiful thing about most of the self-tests in the book is that, like a few other things we can think of, they're best done in the privacy and comfort of your own home. But to judge how you're aging, it's also important to check what's going on in your blood—and that we don't recommend doing in your own home, no matter how sterile your steak knives.

Your doctor could order all of the following blood tests individually, but the cost would be about $3,500 and likely not be covered by insurance, so to make the process easier and less expensive, we've asked Biophysical Corporation—a company that does innovative biomarker testing (biomarkers are simply chemicals in your blood)—to put all of the key tests for aging into one blood draw, called the BiophysicalYou. (Yes, we use needles, but they're small. Really.)

Biophysical is offering the BiophysicalYou for $1,495. However, the first 250 people who mention that they read this book can order the test for $995. You can sign up on its website (www.biophysicalyou.com) or call them at 866-968-0250, or go to www.realage.com (there is no pop quiz, so honor system here).

We're not really carbon-dating you, but rather are offering a concise test that will provide a robust foundation for figuring out how your body is doing.

The results of your test will come back to you in a private, comprehensive report analyzing 65 biomarkers that indicate how healthfully you are aging, along with lab results you can share with your physician. Remember, if you check sixty-five tests, one or more is probably going to be out of the normal range, so don't call the mortician until you check the out-of-range results with your doctor.

Following the premise of the book, the BiophysicalYou report will highlight your endocrine function, metabolism, cardiovascular status, vitamin and mineral levels, inflammatory condition, and telomere length—along with a brief explanation of what they may indicate, as well as any potential areas that require follow-up with your physician.

More details are available at www.biophysicalyou.com if you are interested.

The Test

Here's the complete panel for what will be measured through the Biophysical YOU test.

Endocrine System and Metabolism

Adiponectin

Bioavailable testosterone

Cortisol

DHEA

Estradiol

Follicle-stimulating hormone

Growth hormone

Insulin-like growth factor-1

Luteinizing hormone

Parathyroid hormone

Progesterone

Sex hormone binding globulin

Testosterone, Total

Thyroid-stimulating hormone

Cardiovascular System

Cholesterol, total

High-density lipoprotein (HDL)

Low-density lipoprotein (LDL)

Triglycerides

Liver, Kidney, and Muscle Function

Alanine transaminase (ALT)

Albumin

Alkaline phosphatase (ALP)

Aspartate aminotransferase (AST)

Bilirubin, total

Blood urea nitrogen (BUN)

Creatine kinase, total

Creatinine

Gamma glutamyl transferase

Globulin

Lactate dehydrogenase

Total protein

Uric acid

Nutrients, Vitamins, and Minerals

Calcium

Carbon dioxide

Chloride

Ferritin

Folic acid

Glucose

Homocysteine

Magnesium

Phosphorus

Potassium

Selenium

Vitamin B_{12}

Vitamin D

Zinc

Inflammation

C-reactive protein

Interleukin-6

Interleukin-8

Tumor necrosis factor-alpha

Complete Blood Count

Basophilis

Eosinophils

Hematocrit

Hemoglobin

Lymphocytes

Mean corpuscular hemoglobin

Mean corpuscular hemoglobin concentration

Mean corpuscular volume

Monocytes

Neutrophils

Platelet count

Red blood cell count

Red cell distribution width

White blood cell count

Telomere Length

Fluorescence hybridization test

What It All Means

Below are the definitions of the tests in this workup; you can find more information about many of these tests throughout the book (see index for references).

Endocrine System and Metabolism

The endocrine system produces hormones, substances secreted by an organ into the blood that travel to other areas in the city to help keep other things young when secreted in the right amounts. Think of hormones as fertilizer. In the right amounts, they keep your hair, skin, and energy system working well. Your hormones can aid repair and help keep you young. As you age, hormone levels may increase, decrease, or remain relatively unchanged. Hormones that are likely to decrease include growth hormone, insulin-like growth factor-1, estradiol, testosterone (total and bioavailable), cortisol, DHEA, progesterone, and possibly leptin. Hormones that typically increase include follicle-stimulating hormone, luteinizing hormone, sex hormone binding globulin, and adiponectin. Hormones that stay about the same or may become slightly decreased include thyroid-stimulating hormones, parathyroid hormone, and adrenocorticotropic hormone.

> **Adiponectin:** Produced by adipose (fat) tissue that influences metabolism. Typically, as the amount of fat tissue increases, the level of adiponectin decreases. Thus, adiponectin levels are lower in overweight people and normal or elevated in lean people. Adiponectin

has anti-inflammatory effects on vascular cells. Researchers have found that centenarians (people over one hundred years of age) have higher adiponectin levels than younger people.

Bioavailable testosterone: This includes all readily available (not tightly bound) testosterone in your blood. Bioavailable testosterone decreases at a rate of about 2 percent to 3 percent per year.

Cortisol: The stress hormone made by the adrenal gland, it kicks in when you're stressed out. Cortisol helps modify numerous body systems, including the response to infection and inflammation, and fat distribution.

Dehydroepiandrosterone sulfate (DHEA-S): A hormone produced by the adrenal glands of both men and women. It's converted into estrogens and androgens (sex hormones). Levels of DHEA-S decline as we age and can be worth supplementing.

Estradiol: An estrogen hormone. Estradiol levels decrease in women after menopause and in men as they age.

Follicle-stimulating hormone (FSH): Produced in the pituitary gland to control reproductive functions in both men and women. In women, FSH stimulates the growth of ovarian follicles and the production of estradiol during the first half of the menstrual cycle. FSH levels increase after menopause. In men, FSH (not dirty pictures) is what stimulates the production of sperm and semen.

Growth hormone (GH): Promotes growth during childhood. In adults, it helps to maintain our tissues and organs. Elevated levels of GH can result in increased bone thickness. Starting around age fifty, levels of growth hormone begin to do exactly the opposite of what the name implies.

Insulin-like growth factor-1 (IGF-1): GH works through this hormone, which stimulates growth of various cells including muscle, bone, and cartilage. Levels of IGF-1—like eyesight and interest in action movies—decline continuously as we age.

Luteinizing hormone (LH): Released by the pituitary gland, LH causes ovulation and stimulates the ovaries to produce estrogen and progesterone (in women) and production of testosterone by the testes (men). Increased levels are seen primarily after menopause.

Parathyroid hormone (PTH): Made by the (duh) parathyroid gland, this functions to regulate calcium levels in the body. PTH levels usually remain stable as you age.

Progesterone: Necessary for proper uterine and breast development and functions, progesterone increases during the reproductive period of a woman's life and becomes lower after menopause.

Sex hormone binding globulin (SHBG): This binds to sex hormones and carries them through the blood. Researchers have found that levels of SHBG start to increase at a rate of about 1.6 percent per year after age forty. And this can reduce the amount of sex hormones free to do their job.

Testosterone, total: This represents all testosterone in your blood—some is bioavailable (free or readily available), and some is bound more tightly to other things. If you couldn't tell by the seventeen-year-old boys prowling the neighborhood, testosterone is the primary male sex hormone. Beginning around the age of thirty, a man's total testosterone level will decline. Testosterone levels in women are typically 5 percent to 10 percent of those in men.

Thyroid-stimulating hormone: Secreted from the pituitary gland, it causes the thyroid gland to produce—who'da guessed—thyroid hormone. If elevated, your thyroid is not responding and needs help.

Cardiovascular System

Cholesterol, total: A fatlike substance that comes from both the body and the diet, cholesterol plays an important role in making some hormones as well as vitamin D and is a part of the cell membrane. Total means it includes healthy cholesterol (HDL), lousy cholesterol (LDL), and some others as well (like VLDL).

High-density lipoprotein (HDL): These are proteins that carry cholesterol from the tissues to the liver, where it is broken down and excreted from the body. High levels of active HDL are considered as protective as a father preparing for his daughter's first date.

Low-density lipoprotein (LDL): These are cholesterol-rich proteins that carry cholesterol into tissues. High LDL levels are a risk factor for cardiovascular disease.

Triglycerides: These are a type of fat made by the liver largely from sugar that can be deposited in the fatty tissues of the body. High triglyceride levels are a risk factor for atherosclerosis and cardiovascular disease.

Liver, Kidney, and Muscle Function

Alanine transaminase (ALT): Reflects liver function in conjunction with other tests.

Albumin: It's a protein made by the liver and monitors the synthetic function of the liver. Decreased levels can be seen in kidney disease, which allows albumin to escape into the urine, or be caused by malnutrition, a low-protein diet, or liver disease.

Alkaline phosphatase (ALP): It's released into blood from many tissues, including liver, bile duct, placenta, and bone. Its level may be elevated in conditions that damage or disrupt the liver, bile ducts, or bone.

Aspartate aminotransferase (AST): An enzyme found in liver, muscle, and heart tissues. Increased levels of AST can be seen after a heart attack and with liver or muscle diseases.

Bilirubin, total: A yellow breakdown product of hemoglobin, which is the oxygen-carrying molecule in red blood cells (RBCs). Bilirubin levels may be elevated in people with liver disease or a blocked bile duct, as seen with gallstones.

Blood urea nitrogen (BUN): This reflects the breakdown of protein (nitrogen containing compounds) and is eliminated by the kidneys. An elevated BUN level may be caused by kidney disease or by poor blood flow to the kidneys, as in congestive heart failure, dehydration, or hemorrhage into the gastrointestinal tract. A decreased level may be seen in liver failure, malnutrition, or anabolic steroid use.

Creatinine: This protein waste product is generated by muscle metabolism and eliminated by the kidneys. Because creatinine is released at a constant rate (depending on muscle mass), its blood level is a good indicator of kidney function. It generally creeps up as you age. Creatinine levels can increase temporarily as a result of muscle injury.

Creatine kinase, total: An enzyme significantly elevated when skeletal or heart muscles are damaged.

Ferritin: Not a small rodent, but a sensitive indicator of the body's iron stores.

Gamma glutamyl transferase (GGT): a liver enzyme elevated in conditions involving liver damage.

Globulin: These proteins are produced in the liver or formed by the immune system. Globulins are the key building blocks of antibody proteins and play an important role in helping to fight infection. High globulin levels may indicate kidney or liver disease, autoimmune disease, infection, cancer, or chronic inflammation. Low globulin levels may indicate immune system dysfunction, malnutrition, liver or kidney disease, or blood disorders.

Lactate dehydrogenase (LDH): These may be abnormally high in heart attack and liver disease, as well as other diseases. LDH plays an important role in energy production in cells.

Total protein: These levels are used in the evaluation of nutritional status, liver synthetic functions, kidney syndromes, malabsorption, and cancers. Protein levels may be elevated due to dehydration, vomiting, and diarrhea. Total protein levels may be decreased in kidney syndromes, salt retention syndromes, severe burns, extensive bleeding, pregnancy, intestinal malabsorption, and severe protein starvation.

Uric acid: Though it sounds as if it belongs more in the toilet than your body, uric acid provides the most antioxidant power in our blood. An overproduction of uric acid occurs when there's excessive breakdown of cells or an inability of the kidneys to excrete uric acid. Uric acid elevations may occur in gout, kidney disease, dehydration, diuretic use, alcoholism, lead poisoning, lymphoma, leukemia, infectious mononucleosis, acute inflammatory state, acidosis, hyperparathyroidism, hypothyroidism, sarcoidosis, chemotherapy, and radiation therapy.

Nutrients, Vitamins, and Minerals

Calcium (Ca): An important component of bone, muscle contraction, heart action, nervous system maintenance, and blood clotting.

Carbon dioxide (CO_2): Measurement of carbon dioxide levels in the blood can help to indicate the blood's acidity and an electrolyte or acid-base imbalance.

Chloride (Cl): A mineral (electrolyte) important in water distribution and general cell function.

Folic acid: Also called folate, folacin, or vitamin B_9, folic acid is a B vitamin involved in producing thymidine for DNA replication. Deficiencies of folic acid may also cause increased homocysteine levels, which in turn are associated with a higher risk for heart disease and stroke.

Glucose: Blood sugar.

Homocysteine: An amino acid that's elevated in cardiovascular disease and stroke. Homocysteine levels can be affected by both diet and genetics. Folic acid and vitamins B_6 and B_{12} have the greatest effect on homocysteine levels.

Magnesium: A mineral key to balancing calcium's effect on constipation and needed to stabilize heart rhythm. It's also critical for almost all metabolic processes because it is involved in the phosphorylation of adenosine triphosphate (ATP), the energy packet that powers the body.

Phosphorus (P): A mineral element found throughout the body, mostly bound to calcium in the bones. Phosphorus is also very important in metabolism.

Potassium (K): An electrolyte with levels that are tightly controlled throughout the body, potassium plays an important role in the electrical conduction in nerve, muscle, and heart tissues and is followed carefully if you are on a water pill. High levels can be caused by adrenal tumors, diabetes, renal insufficiency, congestive heart failure, and gastrointestinal bleeding. Low levels may be caused by vomiting and diarrhea.

Selenium: A trace mineral that is a cofactor for production of active antioxidant enzymes such as glutathione peroxidases and thioredoxin reductase. Research shows a link between low selenium levels and cancer.

Vitamin B_{12}: Important for metabolism, the formation of the red blood cells, and the maintenance of the central nervous system. A deficiency in vitamin B_{12} may occur as a result of an inability to absorb the vitamin from food. It can also occur in strict vegetarians who do not consume any animal foods.

Vitamin D complex: The active component is produced in the skin in response to sunlight. It has important effects on calcium, bone, joints, and prevention of cancer by promoting the immune system's anticancer activities.

Zinc: A trace mineral found in the bones, teeth, hair, skin, testes, liver, and muscles. It is an activator of certain enzymes, and promotes the synthesis of DNA, RNA, and protein.

Inflammation

Without our immune system and the inflammation that it generates, we would die shortly after birth, our bodies consumed by a myriad of infectious agents. Cytokines are the proteins and peptides that participate in the communication that must take place during a clash with an intruding infectious agent. They tell the immune system to produce more of a certain type of cell that will fight off a particular substance or to stop a certain immune response once the problem is resolved. Cytokines are released at the sites of inflammation and facilitate the recruitment cells that participate in the healing process. Circulating levels of cytokines are influenced by age. Some cytokines are pro-inflammatory (such as TNF-alpha, TL-6) and some are anti-inflammatory. Long-term health depends on keeping pro-inflammatory and anti-inflammatory molecules in balance.

C-reactive protein (CRP): A protein produced in the liver whose levels rise dramatically in the presence of inflammation or acute or chronic infection. As a marker of inflammation, CRP has also been established as an important predictor of cardiovascular risk. CRP levels between 3–10 µg/ml are suggestive of the inflammatory process caused by the formation of atherosclerosis. Levels greater than 10 µg/ml suggest other types of inflammation that can occur with such conditions as arthritis or other infection. Common culprits are gingivitis, vaginitis, and prostatitis.

Interleukin-6 (IL-6): It stimulates an immune response to trauma and is strongly associated with cardiovascular disease. Aging is associated with low-grade increases in circulating levels of IL-6.

Interleukin-8 (IL-8): It's involved in a variety of inflammatory processes and may be particularly important in psoriasis (scaly patches of skin) and rheumatoid arthritis, and it increases in old age.

Tumor necrosis factor-alpha (TNF-alpha): Produced by various white blood cells, it's increased in older individuals.

Complete Blood Count

Basophils: A type of white blood cell, basophils make up only zero to 2 percent of the total number of white blood cells. Basophil levels increase response to allergens, myxedema, parasitic infections, and alterations in bone marrow function, such as leukemia or Hodgkin's disease. Corticosteroid drugs, allergic reactions, and acute infections may cause basophils to decrease.

Eosinophils: A type of white blood cell whose levels are most commonly elevated in patients with allergies (for example, hay fever and asthma) and parasitic infections, eosinophils are also active in other disorders, including eczema, leukemia, and autoimmune diseases such as rheumatoid arthritis. Low numbers of eosinophils may be seen in people taking corticosteroid medications, infections that produce pus, or alcohol intoxication. Eosinophils do not respond to bacterial or viral infections.

Hematocrit: This is the percentage of whole blood comprising red blood cells. It's a measure of both the number and the size of these cells and is expressed as a percentage by volume. A low hematocrit may indicate anemia, blood loss, bone marrow failure, destruction of red blood cells, or malnutrition or specific nutritional deficiency. A high hematocrit may indicate dehydration and a few other conditions.

Hemoglobin (Hb): An iron-containing protein that enables red blood cells to carry oxygen from the lungs to body tissues.

Lymphocytes: These are white blood cells that identify foreign substances, bacteria, and viruses in the body—and produce antibodies against them. Lymphocytes are produced in the bone marrow and are divided into T-cell and B-cell lymphocytes. A variety of diseases and drugs and conditions can increase or decrease lymphocyte numbers.

Mean corpuscular hemoglobin (MCH): This is an estimate of the amount of hemoglobin carried by each red blood cell. Hemoglobin is the iron-binding protein that carries oxygen. MCH may be low due to blood loss or anemia.

Mean corpuscular hemoglobin concentration (MCHC): This is an estimate of the level of hemoglobin (the iron-binding protein that carries oxygen) in a given number of red blood cells.

Mean corpuscular volume (MCV): This is the average amount of space occupied by each red blood cell. Causes of a high MCV include liver disease, alcohol abuse, hypothyroidism, reticulocytosis, marrow aplasia, vitamin B_{12} or folic acid deficiency, and myelofibrosis. Causes of a low MCV include lead poisoning, chronic kidney failure, hemoglobinopathy, and certain anemias.

Monocytes: A type of white blood cell involved in the immune response to foreign substances, monocytes are often increased in response to chronic infection, inflammatory bowel disease, leukemia, and certain cancers. They may be decreased in people who have anemia or are taking corticosteroids. Monocytes help to remove necrotic tissues and account for 3 to 11 percent of circulating white blood cells.

Neutrophils: a type of white blood cell whose numbers are elevated in the presence of bacterial and other infections, tissue injury, inflammation, and disorders that cause an overproduction of blood cells in the bone marrow, like cancer.

Platelet count: A measure of the number of platelet cells in a patient's blood.

Red blood cell count (RBC count): This indicates the total number of red blood cells in the blood.

Red cell distribution width (RDW): This measures the variability in size of the red blood cell population.

White blood cell count (WBC count): These are the major infection-fighting cells, but they are also involved in immune system responses to foreign bodies and tissues such as allergens and tumors. The white blood cell count (WBC count) measures the total number of white blood cells present in the blood. A high WBC count is typically seen in response to a sudden onset of infection, trauma, or inflammation. A low WBC count can arise in bone marrow failure (as sometimes occurs with radiation therapy or chemotherapy), overwhelming infections, or the presence of a substance resulting in cell destruction (drugs, heavy metals, and poison). A low WBC count is also seen in diseases of the immune system or autoimmune disease, like systemic lupus erythematosus.

Telomere Length

The long strands of DNA that make up our chromosomes are tipped with repetitive snippets of DNA that act like the hard plastic covering the ends of shoestrings, preventing the strands from unraveling. These snippets progressively shorten each time a cell divides, potentially regulating the life span of an individual cell. These strands become shorter as we age or are stressed by major stressors. Meditation and exercise (and maybe a few other choices) seem to restore this loss by altering the response to stress. (No surprise that cigarette smoking decreases telomere length.)

YOU Tool 3

Deep Breathing and Meditation

Meditation and deep breathing may help modify the messages sent from the gut and the rest of the body to the brain via the vagus nerve. As you learned, controlling the vagus can help you with everything from improving your memory to improving your immune system. We suggest you carve out time each day to breathe deeply and meditate. Before bed is a good time, or else when you're trying to manage stress.

Deep Breathing: Lie flat on the floor, with one hand on your belly and one hand on your chest. Take a deep breath in slowly—it should take about five seconds for you to inhale (imagine your lungs filling up with air; see Figure 17.1). As your diaphragm pulls your chest cavity down, your belly button should move away from

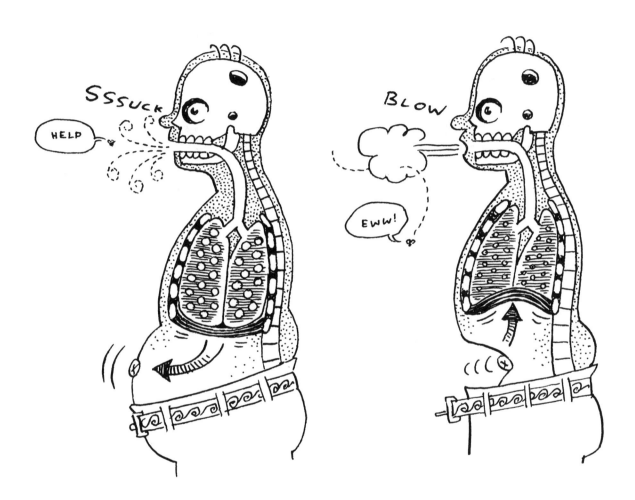

your spine, filling your lungs. Your chest will also widen and perhaps rise. When your lungs feel full, and you even feel a tiny bit of discomfort in the solar plexus, just below the breastbone, exhale slowly (taking about seven seconds). Pull your belly button to your spine to get all the air out.

Meditation: The goal here is to clear your mind of all thoughts. The first step: silence. Even if you use meditation only to sort out headache issues, discipline yourself to squirrel away five minutes of silence a day. To help clear your mind and meditate, pick a simple word (like *ohm* or *Hawaii* or *supercalifrag*—oh, you get the point) and repeat it to yourself over and over. Focusing on the one word helps keep distracting thoughts from seeping into your gray matter.

YOU Tool 4
Stress Management

Many of us have two thoughts about stress: Either you can eliminate it with a bubble bath, or you have to live with your stresses weighing on your mind with the weight of a cement truck. But the truth is that stress management isn't about eliminating it; after all, stress can be *good* for you. It's actually all about regulation—turning the dials of your emotions so you can best handle what life tosses at you. Stress, which is really a complex mix of emotional, physical, and behavioral responses, doesn't have to sideline you from life or send you straight to the ice-cream tub. Here are some tricks to avoid letting your worries burden—or bury—you.

❖ ID the source of your stress. Though some sources are easy to identify, it can be difficult to really determine what's bothering you. Lashing out at your kids may be a reaction not to what your kids did but to an extra assignment piled on at work. The first step to managing your stress is pinpointing the culprit.

❖ Focus on the moment. Though it can be hard, you'll have better stress management by being "mindful"—that is, really paying attention to the present and trying to get out of the gears of the past and the future (both of which are major sources of stress). That means especially noticing the things that you ignore, like your breath, body sensations, and emotions. One way to practice living in the moment: the body scan. How do you do it? Focus on every part of your body, which will help you to relax:

  ❖ Lie down.
  ❖ Close your eyes and notice your posture.
  ❖ Think about the natural flow of your breath, focusing on air filling and leaving the lungs.
  ❖ Notice your toes—any tension, tingling, or temperature change?
  ❖ Move to thinking about your feet, heels, and ankles, all the way up through the knees, thighs, and pelvis.
  ❖ Continue with each body part—going through both the front and back of your body as you work your way up—finishing with the throat, jaw, tongue, face, and brow.

❖ Go through your health checklist. Stress is much more manageable when the other aspects of your life—from your general health, to your sleep patterns, to your eating habits—are in good order. When you don't get enough sleep, for instance, your body produces more stress hormones, making you more vulnerable to the damaging effects of stress. Evaluate what areas in your life need your attention, and work on fixes.

❖ Do the YOU2 Workout (found in the next chapter), walk thirty minutes, stretch, do yoga—just get up and move! Exercise, simply, is one of life's greatest stress relievers.

❖ Do the opposite. Every emotion has an "urge to act" that goes with it. When we feel afraid or anxious, we avoid things; when we are depressed or sad, we withdraw (stay in bed). When we are angry, we want to lash out or yell. Unfortunately, each of these mood-inspired behaviors actually increases an emotion, not decreases it. However, if you can act the opposite way, you can decrease the emotion. Angry at someone? Don't lash out, but, rather, be empathetic. Depressed? Instead of shutting yourself in, go out. Rather than letting your emotions determine what you do, take control and choose how you feel.

❖ Focus on your muscles. By tensing and relaxing your muscles, you can help relieve some of your stored physical stress. While sitting or lying down, tense the muscles of your feet as much as you can and then release the tension. Tense and relax different muscle groups of your body one at a time. Focus on your legs, stomach, back, neck, arms, face, and head. When done, relax for a few minutes.

YOU Tool 5
Your Vital Supplements

If there's one question we are asked more than any other (besides the ones about poop), it's this: What vitamins should I take? Unfortunately, there's no one brand or pill that combines the recommended amount of every vitamin, mineral, and nutrient, but some are close and you can use a liquid or pill form. So you'll have to do a little digging yourself, but we want to make it as easy as possible. So here we've listed our recommendations of pills and supplements that will make your body and mind stronger, healthier, and younger. All of these should be in divided doses. We'd love you to get them from diet, but many have imperfect diets—so consider these recommendations as an insurance policy for an imperfect diet. So you can take half in the morning and half at night to keep a constant vitamin level in your blood during the day.

Vitamins	Optimum
A	More than 2,500 IU is too much (unless you have an eye condition called wet macular degeneration).
B	Get at least the daily value (DV) of all the Bs plus a little more than daily value of these Bs: B_1 (thiamin) 25 mg. B_2 (riboflavin) 25 mg. B_3 (niacin) At least 30 mg, and you can take lots more after speaking with your doctor if you have elevated lousy cholesterol or triglycerides. B_5 (pantothenic acid) 300 mg. B_6 (pyridoxine) 4 mg. B_9 (folic acid or folate) 400 mcg. B_{12} (cyanocobalamin) 800 mcg. Biotin 300 mcg.
C	800 mg or 50 mg twice a day if you're taking a statin drug.
D	800 IU if under age sixty; 1,000 if sixty or over.
E	400 IU in the form of mixed tocopherols. Reduce to 100 IU from supplements if you're taking a statin drug.
K	You should get enough in normal diet (see chapter 14).

Minerals	Get a daily value of all the usual suspects in your multivitamin plus these in higher quantity.
Calcium	This comes from many sources, so total all of them up and get at least 1,600 total mg for women, 1,200 mg for men.
Magnesium	400 mg.
Selenium	200 mcg.

Zinc	15 mg.
Potassium	4 servings of fruit, plus a normal diet should do it.

Additional Vitamin-like Substances You Should Get Daily (Once a Day)

Lycopene	10 tablespoons of tomato sauce a week (400 micrograms).
Lutein	A leafy green vegetable a day (40 micrograms).
Quercetin	Hefty portions of onion, garlic, celery, or lemon juice in addition to the above at least once a day.
Acetyl-L-carnitine	1,500 milligrams (while this comes in dehydrated beef protein, that's not so appetizing, so we recommend the supplement).
Omega-3	Either 1 gram of distilled fish oil or 6 walnuts, preferably twenty-five to thirty minutes before lunch and before dinner, or 2 ounces of fatty fish a day, or 400 mg of DHA.
Cinnamon	½ teaspoon a day.
Red pepper	The more capsaicin, the better for appetite suppression.
Turmeric	As much as you want.

If you're worried about arterial aging and memory, make sure you get the anti-inflammatory/antioxidant vitamins E and C and the homocysteine-lowering vitamins folate, B_6, and B_{12}; vitamin D, magnesium, and calcium; and lutein and lycopene. If you're concerned about osteoporosis, arthritis, or immune aging, pay careful attention to your intake of calcium, magnesium, selenium, lycopene, and vitamins B_6, B_{12}, and D.

Choices you might consider (talk to your doctor about these and all choices):

Coenzyme Q10	200 milligrams day (if on a statin) or for all over age sixty.
Aspirin	162 milligrams a day (check with your doctor) with two glasses of warm water.
Coffee and green tea	2 or more cups of each.
Alpha-lipoic acid	200 milligrams.
Probiotics	2 billion cells of healthy bowel bacteria like bacillus coagulans.

YOU Tool 6
Detoxify Your Life

We tend to think of toxicity as consisting of extreme examples—swallowing poison, smoking exhaust pipes, sticking your head in a microwave. But the truth is that toxicity can happen in less extreme circumstances, and that's why it's important to know the toxicity equation: simply, it's the intersection of the danger of a chemical (don't bathe in dioxin baths) and the duration of your exposure to the stuff.

So be prudent if you're getting a lot of exposure to just about anything in life that *might* be toxic. For many of the dozens of commonly used products on the market, no one honestly knows if they are safe yet, but to be fair, we don't know if they're dangerous either. Here's our advice based on what our families do.

AT FRONT DOOR Leave your shoes here. You can track in toxins such as lawn-care pesticides, which can get trapped in the carpet and contaminate children.

Wash your hands as soon as you enter the house.

IN KITCHEN Don't microwave plastic; you'll get small amounts of it in your food when you heat it. Cover food with ceramic, glass, a paper towel, or waxed paper instead.

Throw away your sponges and replace with ten dishcloths that you clean with bleach weekly.

Don't store foods in open cans for a long period, because the food will be exposed to chemicals such as epoxy resin and aluminum (it will also begin to taste metallic). In fact, reduce the number of canned foods that you consume. Bisphenol A, which mimics estrogen, is leached from the can liners into the foods.

For conga lines of insects, don't resort to toxic cans of bug killer, which is ineffective and unnecessary. Instead, clean the home, remove the clutter, and use boric-acid-based bait stations.

Keep all cleaners up high (oven cleaner can burn the esophagus if children get hold of it).

Filter your drinking water.

Use dishwasher soap without phosphates or chlorine or nonylphenol ethoxylate (NPE), which is called a gender-bender and feminizes fish in the waters where we humans dump our waste. Also make sure they are biodegradeable and nontoxic so kids will survive if they decide to take a swig. Don't have any cleaner anyplace near where anyone could drink it or spill it if it isn't okay to drink.

IN BEDROOM Use products that protect your pillows and mattresses from dust mites. Their excrement, which totals two pounds every two years in pillows, can lead directly to asthma. You can obtain 1-micron pore sheets and pillowcases that filter the air in to keep the microdust from the organisms out.

Commercial brands of carpet and clothing-spot cleaners have largely moved to glycol ethers, which can be inhaled or absorbed through the skin and may cause blood disorders, as well as liver and kidney damage. They can be avoided with a combination of natural oils, alcohol, and oxygen-based cleaners.

IN CLOSETS If you get your clothes dry-cleaned, remove them from the plastic wrap, which traps in the chemicals used to clean them, and air them out on a porch or another covered area that is open to the outside air. Limit dry cleaning to only what absolutely has to be dry cleaned. Use only dry cleaners that have stopped using either trichloroethylene or perchloroethelyene (PERC). These chemicals have been linked to kidney and nervous system damage as well as cancer (in the person wearing the clothes, as well as the person cleaning them).

Moth balls with their naphthalene or p-dichlorobenzene are way too strong for killing insects (they're carcinogens); use cedar chips instead.

GENERAL CLEANING Liquid household chlorine bleaches contain chloride and ammonia, which evaporate into the air and aren't so good for you or the environment (nor are their containers). Reduce use by purchasing concentrated solutions that you dilute as needed (this also cuts the cost of being "green").

Be smart and use nontoxic products to clean your home that are based in alcohol, peroxide, or bicarbonate. Simple baking soda can be great for cleaning sinks and tubs; vinegar in a pump spray bottle cleans windows and mirrors. In the meantime, don't create your own übermixture with bleach and ammonia. Without proper ventilation, that combination creates toxic hydrogen chloride that can kill you. With proper ventilation, it's just a little bit toxic (don't do it).

IN BATHROOM To protect your skin, filter your water with a carbon filter to remove the chlorine and other bad stuff. Do it especially for water that is in contact with your skin for more than a few seconds, like the baby's bathwater, and your bath and hair-rinsing water. Short showers are OK, since there's less exposure to toxins.

Use deodorant instead of antiperspirant, since sweat is normal and blocking the pores is not. Especially avoid aluminum, which is found in high levels in the brain plaques linked to Alzheimer's disease. And with deodorants, avoid phthalates, which are plastics used to help the fragrance stay on our skin and block endocrine function, especially in the male fetus. Parabens, which are used as preservatives in these products, should also be avoided since they could be linked to breast cancer.

Avoid air fresheners, which have gaseous chemicals like those found in moth balls, and the hockey-puck-shaped deodorants in urinals (for those readers lucky enough to frequent the male restroom). They can become toxic when combined with the ozone.

IN BASEMENT Have the level of radon in your home checked (the level needs to be less than 4 picocuries of radon per liter of air, or 4 pci/L). You can measure it with a kit you can get at the National Radon Safety Board website (www.nrsb.org).

In wet environments, use a dehumidifier to reduce mold. Keep humidity under 40 percent.

OUTSIDE HOUSE Hundreds of thousands of kids are exposed to toxic levels of lead paint (you're at risk if your house was last painted before 1978). Big culprit: windowsills, since they tend not to be painted even when the rest of the house is.

Living near the freeway increases respiratory complications in children, and these don't get better when the children grow older. Need evidence? Just look at the state of the trees near the freeway. Recent research that shows people who live near Los Angeles freeways have higher rates of lung complications. And pregnancy near freeways results in smaller babies with a higher rate of asthma.

Wipe your dog's paws and coat. Who knows where he walks?

Lawn and garden pesticides and herbicides often don't stay only where they're applied; many can contaminate groundwater as well as indoor air. Organic, toxin-free products include corn gluten for lawn weed control. (Remember, weeds may cause eyesores, but they won't cause cancer.)

IN DUCTS The best air filter for your home is a high-efficiency particle air filter (HEPA). Replace your air-conditioner filter yearly and clean your air ducts every three years. Partial cleaning of ducts can make your air worse, so do a good job when you attack the clumped-up material. Also, check and clean your humidifiers, because they can harbor toxins.

THE WINDOWS Open your home to the outside world as frequently as you can, since the inside of a home generally has three to four times the pollutants and particles that are most dangerous to us. If you don't air it out, you increase the chance that these pollutants will build up.

Indoor air quality has plummeted because our homes are more airtight and we're using many more products to freshen the air, sanitize the home, and treat fabrics. And remember that your favorite "clean" smell is often caused by chemicals that are present to mask the noxious odor of other chemicals. Plus, 15 percent of us are allergic to the common fragrances. To compound the problem, we're spending more time indoors. So make sure to open your windows as often as possible and bring fresh air in (even once a week in the heat of summer or cold of winter).

IN GARAGE New car smell is more delightful than fresh pie, but it's also ripe with chemicals. Perhaps to the disappointment of your sniffer, it's best to air out new cars.

Don't store any old chemicals, like paint, that contain toluene, a potent reproductive toxin. Buy what you need, then get rid of it when you've finished your project.

ON PORCH Reduce exposure to charred meats, which have PAHs (polycyclic aromatic hydrocarbons). Marinating your meat, chicken, and fish for fifteen minutes beforehand in a vinegar and olive oil mix reduces the danger by over 90 percent.

Citronella is as effective as the neurotoxins often used as insect repellents.

You can find more at www.RealAge.com.

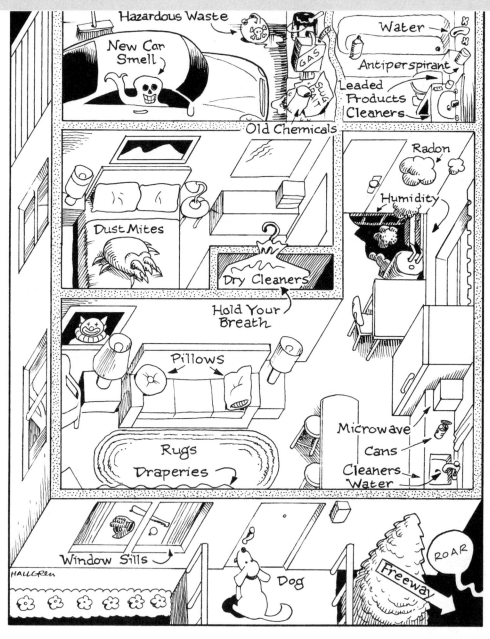

What to Buy

Shop at health-conscious stores, which brag about their "green" products, since at least they'll be embarrassed if their products are toxic. Plus, their employees may be able to help you navigate the toxic terrain of household cleaning products. You can also check for the green seal label (www.greenseal.org).

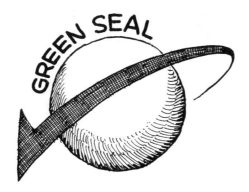

Earth-friendly products include:

Get Clean (available over the Web in concentrated form that might save
   you money)
Seventh Generation
Ecover
Greening the Cleaning
Sun & Earth
Biokleen
Mrs. Meyer's
Orange Plus

Chapter 18

YOU Getting Stronger

Some people exercise because they want to run faster. Some people exercise because they want to be the league MVP. Some people exercise because they want to make oncoming eyeballs pop. But we want you to integrate exercise and activity into your life because you will live longer as a result. The workouts we've detailed below will do just that. The first—the YOU2 Workout—will help you stretch and strengthen your muscles, which will not only help you maintain a healthy weight but will help you do things like build stronger bones. The other workout—chi-gong—not only works your body but will help you de-stress and keep your energy levels high. You can download for free the original YOU Workout featured in *YOU: On a Diet* on www.realage.com; the illustrations should be able to guide you through the moves, but if you prefer to see how they're done with action, you can purchase DVDs of this workout, as well as the following Chi-gong Workout on the website as well. Our frequency recommendations for these workouts are in the Fourteen-Day Extended Warranty Plan. Here we detail the moves you can use.

The YOU2 Workout

The best gym in the world? You're living in it. By using your own body weight to complete a strength-and-stretch workout, not only will you have the ability to transform your body, but you'll have the ability to do so *without excuses.* This eighteen-move workout we made with celebrity trainer Joel Harper is one that you can complete in fewer than twenty minutes—and without equipment (see www.fit packdvd.com for more info). Best of all, though, is the fact that it strengthens your muscles (to make you stronger, leaner, and more equipped to handle the rigors of aging) and stretches them (to make you more flexible and dynamic, for the same reason). In addition to walking thirty minutes a day, which serves as the foundation of any physical activity plan, you should do this workout two to three times a week. Consider it part of your armor against aging. The stronger your body, the longer and better your life. Remember to maintain proper form throughout the exercises and to breathe freely. Keep a strong but relaxed pose as you perform the exercises.

1. **YO-YO** (*Warm-up*)
   Stand with your feet shoulder-width apart and your knees slightly bent. Interweave your fingers and bring your hands and elbows up to shoulder height. Turn your palms out, so now you can see all your knuckles. Keeping your torso upright, slowly twist to the right and left, ten times each side, to where it feels comfortable. Inhale going to one side, exhale back to the other.

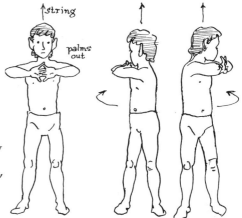

2. **PUNCHING BAG** (*Strengthens Arms and Shoulders*)
Bring your hands and elbows to shoulder
height, and make your hands into fists and
turn your knuckles facing away from you.
Spin your hands around in a circle as far away
from your chest as you can. Keep your shoulders
relaxed, away from your ears. Do it twenty times
clockwise, then twenty counterclockwise. For advanced, do an
additional set double time, balancing on your toes.

3. **PRAYING MANTIS** (*Strengthens Arms, Shoulders, Chest, and Back*)
Bring your forearms flush together in front of you with your
hands in prayer and elbows shoulder height. Your
middle fingers should be in line with your elbows. Pulse
one inch up and one inch down for thirty seconds. For
advanced, clap your hands with your elbows glued
together twenty times while balancing on one leg; then
switch and clap twenty more times.

4. **TITANIC** (*Stretches Chest, Shoulders, and Arms*)
Bring your arms out to your sides, palms facing forward, two
inches below your shoulders. Keeping your torso upright,
stretch your hands out to the sides and back. Hold for twenty
seconds. Breathe into your chest, as if it were one big balloon.
For a deeper stretch, bend your wrists back and reach your
fingers toward one another.

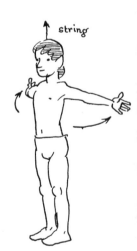

5. **FLAPPER** (*Strengthens Upper and Lower Back*)
With slightly bent knees and feet together,
bend at the waist and lean forward until your
back is flat and as parallel to the floor as possible. (If
you have a bad back, stay up higher.) Keeping your
arms straight and your elbows unlocked, bring your
arms out to the side parallel to the ground, pause,
then lower them down. Do forty times.

6. **HULA HOOP** (*Opens Hips and Balances Back*)
Stand with your feet together and your hands on your
waist. Relax your shoulders and circle your hips
clockwise five times, and counterclockwise five times,
making the biggest circle you can.

7. **DREAM OF JEANNIE** (*Strengthens Quads, Abs, and Shoulders*)
While on your knees, cross your arms and elbows up like a
genie. Keep a straight line from the top of your head to your
knees. Lean back slightly and hold for thirty seconds.
(Advanced can lean back farther.) While pulling your navel in
and squeezing your butt, take deep breaths.

8. **ALL EARS** (*Stretches Neck and Trapezius*)
Sit on your heels and place your palms under your butt (this
prevents you from raising your shoulders during the
stretch). Slightly drop your ear down to one shoulder,
keeping your chin forward. Hold for ten seconds and switch
sides. Do twice, lifting your chest up and taking deep
breaths into the tightest area.

9. **THE FIRE HYDRANT** *(Strengthens Butt and Obliques)*

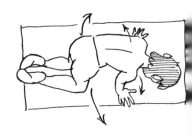

Move onto all fours, with your back flat. Lift your right knee out to the side at hip height and lower it back down to the other knee. Lead with your knee and not your ankle. Do two sets of twenty for each leg. If it feels more comfortable, you can do this exercise with your forearms on the ground and hands clasped. Advanced can kick out to side hip height.

10. **WAG YOUR TAIL** *(Loosens Back, Hips, and Shoulders)*

While on all fours and keeping your back flat and your elbows slightly bent, twist your right shoulder toward your right hip, then switch back and forth for ten times. Look two inches above your fingers the whole time.

11. **SNAIL PUSH-UPS** *(Strengthens Chest)*

Get in the appropriate "up" push-up position for you by either pushing up on your toes or keeping your knees on the ground. Lower yourself until your chest nearly touches the ground and push back up. Lower down on a count of ten, stop one inch off the ground, pause, and come all the way back up on a count of ten. Count out loud to normalize breathing. Build up to ten push-ups in a row. As you straighten your elbows, push your spine toward the ceiling (to help engage your back muscles as well). When doing advanced, pull your heels away from your shoulders, keeping a long, solid body. Don't let your stomach hang down toward the ground, because that will cause unnecessary tension in your lower back. Instead, keep your stomach tight to strengthen your belly muscles. If your lower back starts to hurt, raise your butt slightly.

12. **SUPERMAN TOE TAPS** (*Strengthens Lower Back and Butt*)

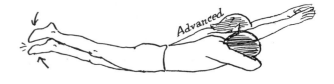

Lie on your stomach with your head turned to the side, resting on your hands. Lift your straight legs off the ground as high as you can and tap your toes together forty times. More advanced can simultaneously scissor your hands and feet. Resist arching your head up and looking down. Breathe normally.

13. **HAMMOCK STRETCH** (*Opens Hips and Hamstrings*)
Sitting on the floor with your hands behind you—palms down, fingers pointing backward, and elbows slightly bent—bring your feet up two feet from your tailbone. Keeping the soles flat on the ground, cross your right leg up on top of your left leg and sit up straight. Focus on pressing your lower back toward your calf. If you want to go deeper, gently press your right knee away from you. Hold for fifteen seconds. Switch sides.

14. **ABDOMINAL BUTTERFLY** (*Stretches Groin and Strengthens Abs*)
Lying on your back, bring your legs into butterfly position, with the soles of your feet touching. Relax your legs. Bring your interwoven hands behind your head, leaving your thumbs on your neck as sensors to keep your neck relaxed. Using your abs only, lift your upper body up two inches and back down twenty-five times. Then hold your upper body up and lift your legs up two inches from the ground, tapping the sides of your feet back on the ground twenty-five times. For more advanced, lift your butterfly legs off the ground and crunch up in sync with your upper body, tapping the sides of your feet on the ground each time.

15. **SCISSOR LEGS** (*Strengthens Abs and Inner Thighs*)

Lying on your back with your head resting on your interwoven palms, lift your legs into the air and point your toes like a ballerina. Pulling your navel in and pressing your lower back into the mat, scissor your legs in the air twenty times, each time bringing your knees two feet apart. For more advanced, straighten your legs and use your arm and ab strength to lift your relaxed head off the ground and separate your knees as far as you can each time.

16. **ELASTIC MAN** (*Elongates Entire Body*)

While lying on your back, interweave your hands and turn your palms so they're facing out. Stretch your arms above your head while taking deep breaths. Try to get the longest distance between your hands and your pointed toes.

17. **BUTT LIFT** (*Strengthens Butt and Hamstrings*)

While lying on your back, and with your crossed arms relaxed on your chest, bring your feet shoulder-width apart underneath your knees. Lift your butt off the ground as high as you can, then drop one inch. This is the highest point you should lift. Tap your butt back on the ground and back up. Curl your tailbone and squeeze your butt twenty times. Then hold your butt up and pulse twenty times. For more advanced, hold one leg straight off the ground, with knees in line with each other, and do one set. Then switch legs for another set. Breathe normally.

18. **CRISS CROSS** (*Stretches Back, Abs, and Hips*)

    Sit with your legs crossed in front of you. Keeping
    your torso upright and the top of your head in line
    with your tailbone, take your right hand to your
    left knee and place your left hand on the
    ground behind you and slowly twist. Take
    two deep breaths and switch sides four
    times. For more advanced, sit in lotus
    position (which is legs crossed with ankles
    on top of your crossed legs).

YOU Getting Stronger Cheat Sheet

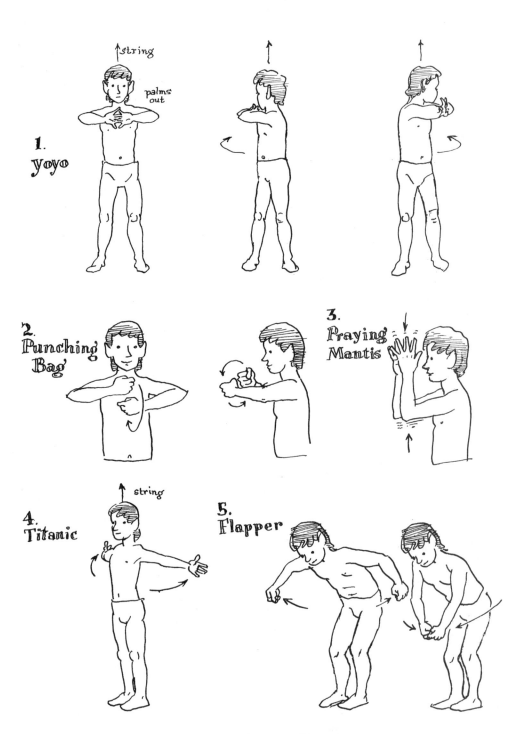

1. Yoyo

2. Punching Bag

3. Praying Mantis

4. Titanic

5. Flapper

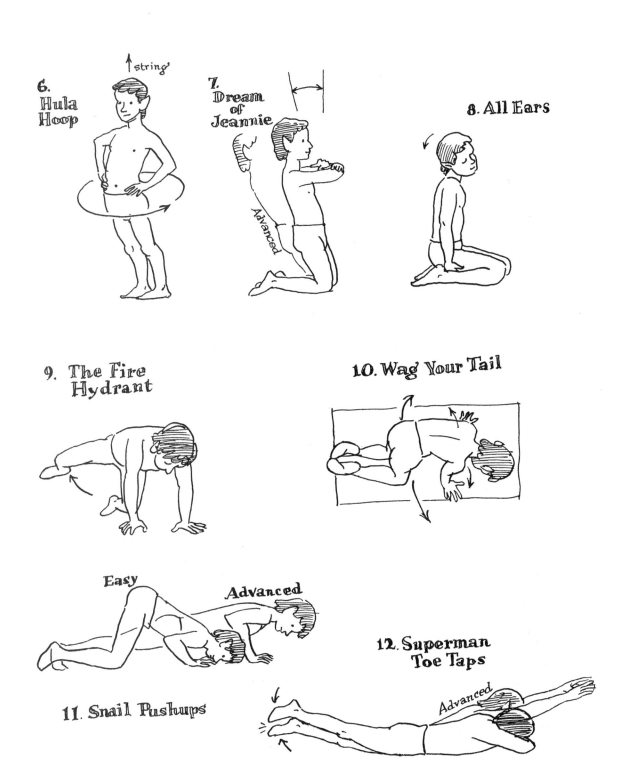

6. Hula Hoop

↑string

7. Dream of Jeannie

Advanced

8. All Ears

9. The Fire Hydrant

10. Wag Your Tail

Easy

Advanced

11. Snail Pushups

12. Superman Toe Taps

Advanced

13.
Hammock
Stretch

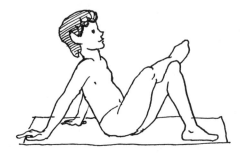

14. Abdominal Butterfly

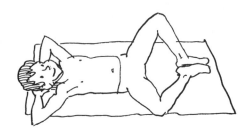

15.
Scissor
Legs

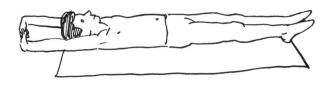

16. Elastic Man

17. Butt
Lifts

Advanced

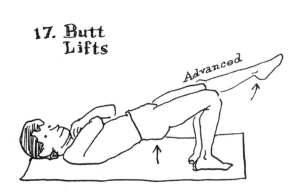

18.
Criss
Cross

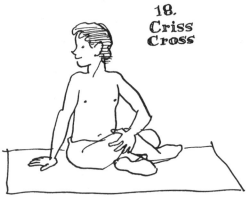

The YOU Chi-gong Workout

Look at any gym brochure or fitness website, and you'll see all kinds of different ways people are concocting to work their bodies. There are all kinds of classes, ranging from spinning to boot camp to cardio striptease. There are all kinds of equipment, ranging from basketballs to stability balls to medicine balls. And there are all kinds of people who want to help you: the zen yogi, the loud-mouthed drill sergeant, and the trainer with accordion abs. While all different types of exercises have their place, as well as their potential benefits, we'd like to suggest that you include a chi-gong routine in your workout. Chi-gong? No, it's not a tea or a percussion instrument but a two-thousand-year-old series of bodily movements and breathing that calms the spirit and the mind. It also has been shown to strengthen the immune system, reduce stress, and improve balance and posture (all important as we get older). Chi-gong works the energy fields we talked about on page 79—by tapping into those intangible life forces that we believe have a profound impact on both our health and the way we feel.

The most important goal of chi-gong is to learn how to breathe correctly—which involves breathing from the *tan tien*—a point two inches below the navel. The deep belly breathing connotes calmness and awareness (as opposed to upper chest breathing, which connotes nervousness and anxiety). By the way, singers and actors use this because they always want their voice to come from a soulful, deep spot.

In each exercise, breathe in slowly. Throughout the following movements, focus on a point on the wall in front of you, with your chin parallel to the ground to help maintain balance. This means that the eyes never drop in any exercise. Ideally, you can do this series of movements, which we crafted with chi-gong master Karl Romain, once daily to help keep your mind and body calm and focused.

Repeat each move three times before moving to the next.

LOOSENING THE NECK

Sink to the ground with your elbows and knees slightly bent, and chin parallel to the ground. Turn your head to the right as you inhale, and exhale as you come back to the middle. Then turn your head to the left and repeat the sequence.

PICKING THE FRUIT

Exhale as you reach for imaginary fruit, and inhale while bringing the fruit down. Reach for the closest fruit first and then progressively move up the imaginary tree. Keep your knees bent and your back straight.

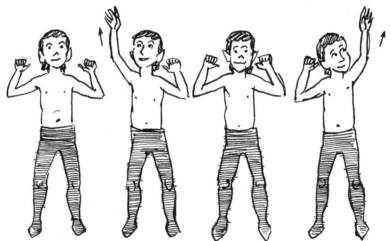

RELAXING THE SHOULDERS

Lift your shoulders first, then elbows, then wrists. Roll your shoulders back; your elbows go out and hands angle toward the middle—as if you're grabbing a pole—with your hands sliding down to the level of your waist. Feel the energy as your hands pass down your body.

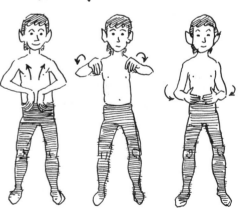

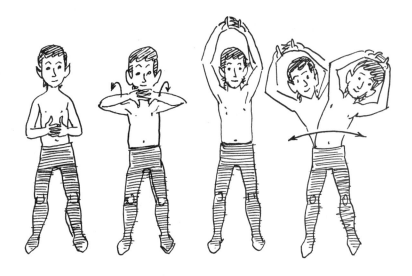

REACHING TO HEAVEN

Inhale and clasp your hands at the level of your navel, and raise your arms as if you're reaching toward heaven. Lean to the right as you exhale, then inhale as you come back to the center. Use the same technique as you lean to the left. Finally, bring your hands down in front of your navel as you exhale.

BOW, BEND, AND STRETCH

As you inhale, bow forward from the waist while your hands slide down your thighs and onto your knees. Bend at your knees and squat with your hands on the insides of your ankles. (You do not exhale until you come back up; this really works the control of the breath.) Then stretch your legs and let your torso hang to the floor, keeping your knees slightly bent. As you slowly rise up, you exhale, allowing your head to be the last part of the body to rise up.

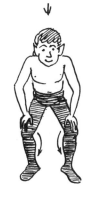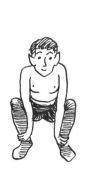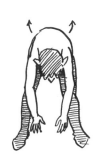

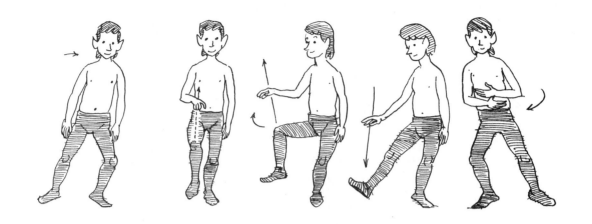

STEPPING OVER THE FENCE

Inhale and deliberately shift your weight to the left until the right leg has no weight on it. Lift your leg only when it is weightless. Pretend that your right hand is attached by a string to the right knee. With your hand over your knee and leg, exhale as you rotate your leg and arm to the right—as if you're stepping over a one-foot fence. Slowly lower your heel, with your foot pointed out, and then rotate your foot frontward as you transfer weight to the right, repeating with your left side.

WHITE STORK KICKS UP

Raise your hands in front of your body, while your elbows remain slightly bent and your hands cross each other in front of your body.

Move them above your head in a circular motion as you inhale. At the same time, lift your right knee, and as you kick out, start to exhale. Your foot should be flexed, kicking out with the heel. You should be kicking at a 45-degree angle, with your

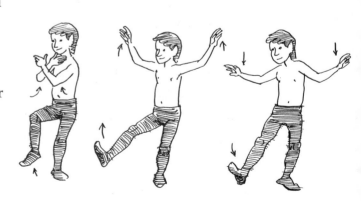

foot moving toward your straight left leg and raised up in the air like a stork. Straighten it as it's rotated to the right. Your arms should move with your leg as you alternate sides.

LIFTING A KNEE

Inhale as you step back, and exhale as you bring your leg back to the center. With your knees bent, lean toward the right as your right leg steps forward with your hands rotating upward. Then lift up your left leg and hold it in the air, as the hands clasp over the knee and pull up. Let go of the leg as you raise your arms back upward and return to your original position.

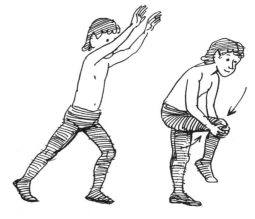

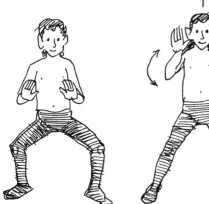

POLISHING THE MIRROR

With your pelvis tucked under and back straight, use your shoulders to circle your arms and squat down as you rotate your arms around in one direction—as though you are cleaning a mirror. After repeating three times (or more), repeat with your arms moving in the opposite direction. Inhale as you squat down, and exhale as you rise.

PICKING UP THE SUITCASE

With your back straight and pelvis tucked, and with your feet shoulder-width apart, squat back with your hands beside your knees and open as if you were reaching for luggage located behind your legs. Go only as low as possible, as if you were grasping luggage handles. (If your knees are strained, your posture is incorrect.) Repeat as if you were putting the luggage back on the floor.

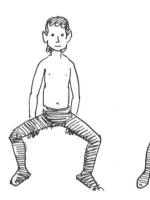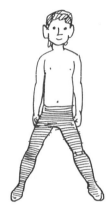

UNIVERSAL POST

With your back straight, step forward with your left leg, and put your arms around an imaginary wide post—elbows bent and shoulders relaxed. Roll the pole to right and then to left. Repeat with the other foot forward.

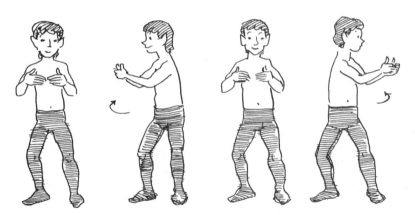

MONKEY HEARS A NOISE

Inhale as you step out, and exhale as you look over your shoulder. With your knees slightly bent, step out to the left and lean forward in a twisted position, with your right arm extended forward and your left hand closed in a fist next to your left hip. Turn your head back over your left shoulder as if you're a monkey running 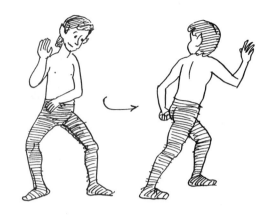 forward while hearing noise behind you. You should feel a stretch in your right calf, lower back, and neck. Then rotate in the opposite direction, with your body facing toward the right.

STANDING MEDITATION

Count your breaths to ten, breathing from the tan tien (that's two inches below the navel). Keep your hands clasped at the tan tien and follow the movement of your belly. Keep your legs bent and spread, and your hips tucked under with a straight back. Do for two minutes, since this is the maximum most can focus.

YOU Chi-gong Cheat Sheet

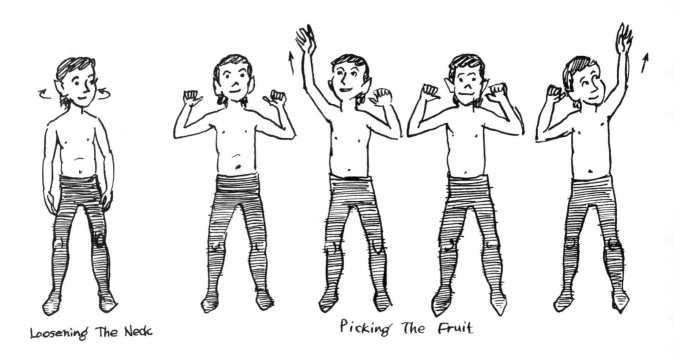

Loosening The Neck

Picking The Fruit

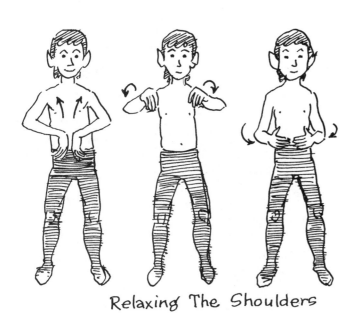

Relaxing The Shoulders

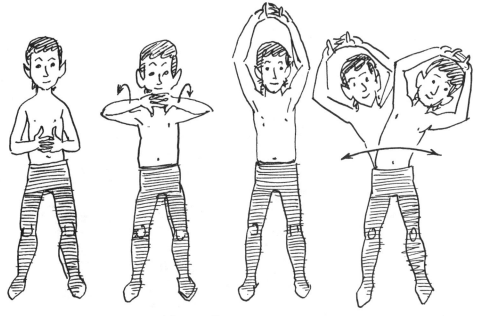

Reaching To Heaven

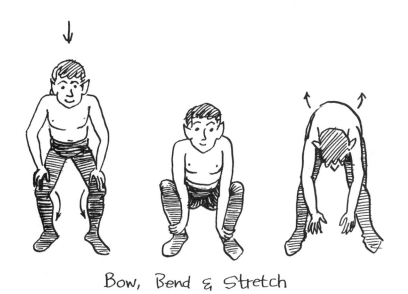

Bow, Bend & Stretch

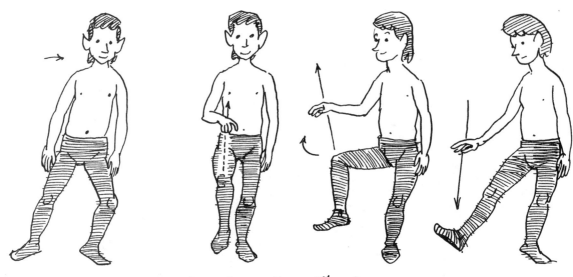

Stepping Over The Fence

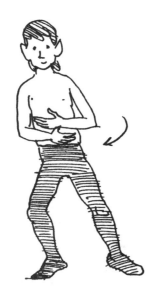

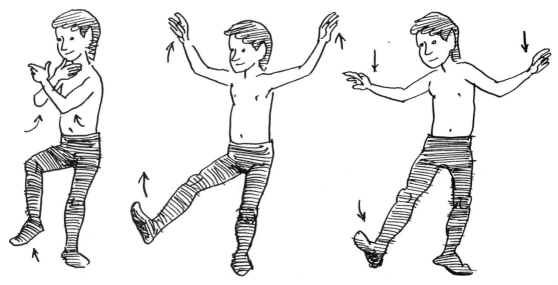

White Stork Kicks Up

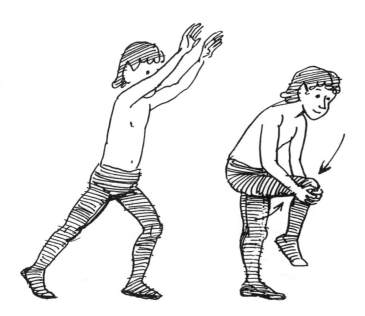

Lifting A Knee

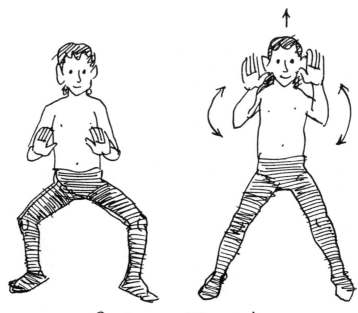

Polishing The Mirror

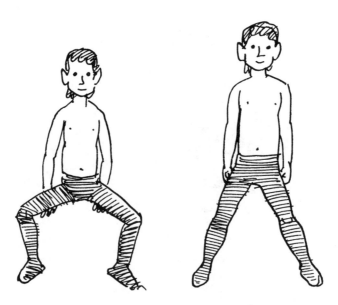

Picking Up The Suitcase

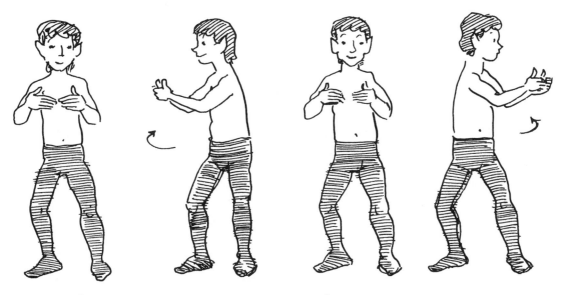

Universal Post

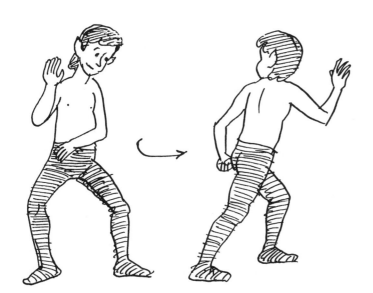

Monkey Hears A Noise

HALLGREN

Acknowledgments

This work has been a true team effort—one that perfectly blended so many people's talents, creativity, thoughts, and wisdom.

Ted Spiker is one of the most unique people with whom we have ever had the honor of working. Ted deserves an honorary doctorate from both our medical schools, but in the meantime, his own University of Florida has wisely awarded him a tenured position in journalism—one of the highest honors in the academic community. As always, he pulled together our random thoughts into an accessible and humorous work that has attitude but is never condescending. Gary Hallgren is a brilliant and witty artist with super medical insights. His cartoons drill *YOU* with riveting insights that bring alive medical breakthroughs. And he always tries to sneak stuff in the small print past us. Craig Wynett's wife is paying the ultimate price for her hubby's bringing us together; she now has to watch him work endlessly with us as a coauthor. Craig transforms us and you with his remarkable insights and pearls of wisdom, now woven through the text. Dr. Mark Rudberg's tireless work and pithy comments brought the perspective of a geriatrician come alive. Jeff Roizen, Alia Menezes, Adam Snavely, and Robin Friedlander answered every esoteric question we could ask as they interpreted the complex studies that we use to teach America about the hard science of vitality and aging. While the hours of conference calls, research, and writing were often exhausting, this powerful group functioned seamlessly to resolve content and style conflicts.

We thank Joel Harper for his remarkable effort to make the YOU2 Workout the perfect tool for us to get procrastinators to exercise. Joel also supervised the great chi-gong video creation by Karl Romain. Erin Olivo crafted a spectacular anger management and relaxation program. Our recipes (see the website www.realage .com/youdocs) were improved by great chefs and artists Jim Perko, Karen Levin, Mindy Hermann, Val Weaver, and Dr. John LaPuma. Finally, our agent Candice Fuhrman's honest commentary and tough advice allowed this book to mature into the manuscript America deserves. Linda Kahn has gained all of our respect once again as she worked tirelessly on multiple revisions of this book. Without Linda, we would have a far inferior product. Lisa Oz lights the path we follow in our quest to educate, and her tough editorial advice keeps us honest. We both love her and one of us got to marry her.

We also want to thank everyone at Free Press (Simon & Schuster) who so enthusiastically supported this material and have dedicated themselves to bringing our ideas to the world. Thanks especially to our insightful editor, Dominick Anfuso, and his assistants, Wylie O'Sullivan and Maria Aupérin. We appreciate the courageous leadership of Martha Levin and the tireless support of Jill Siegel, Carisa Hays, Suzanne Donahue, and Linda Dingler.

We are indebted to our wonderful collaborators at RealAge.com, including Charlie Silver, Val Weaver, Jennifer Perciballi, and its late cofounder, Marty Rom, and at Discovery Health, including Eileen O'Neil, Donald Thoms, Wayne Barbin, and Jonathan Grupper. Billy Campbell: Thanks for always being such an honorable friend.

In a book of this scope based in science, no one human commands all the needed knowledge, so we sought advice from many world experts who selflessly shared their insights in the true academic tradition. We list them all here without details of their contributions to save space for the actual book, but we deeply appreciate your dedication to your specialties and willingness to sacrifice your time in helping craft the most scientifically accurate book on aging possible. We thank Michael Gershon, Tracy Hafen, Evan Johnson, Ivan Kronenfeld, Jon Lapook, Arthur Perry, Paul Rosenberg, Keith Roach, Axel Goetz, Rich Lang, Nancy Roizen, Zeyd Ebraham, Lilian Gonsalves, Paul Katz, Lisa B. Aronson, Marci Anthone, John Petre, Susan Petre, Irwin Davis, Ruth Klein, Roz Wattell, Jane Spinner, Dr. Steve Ross, Jennifer Roizen, Jay Lombard, Judith Reichman, Jennifer Ashton, Freya

Schnabel, Dac Benasillo, Alphonse Gallizia, Aaron Katz, Ferid Murad, Paul Sereno, Ridwan Shapsig, Francis Levin, Robin Golan, Julide Tok, Rob Abel, Rob Kazim, Evan Johnson, Scott Forman, Bill Levine, Ian Storper, Jonathon Levine, Mitch Gaynor, Paul Simonelli, George Roth, Kevin Tracey, Louann Brizendine, Neil Theise, Abby Abelson, Gordon Bell, Linda Bradley, Glen Copeland, Nancy Foldvary, Bryon Hoogwerf, Gordon Hughes, Susan Joy, Cynthia Kubu, Angelo Licata, Izzy Lieberman, Tom Bormes, Jennifer Capezio, Murray Favus, Michael Matheis, David Muzina, Allison Vidimos, Michael Breus, Neil Kavey, Bob Uttl, Bruce N. Ames, Jung Hyuk Suh, Jim Zacny, and Dean Ornish for teaching us about aging and reviewing our work.

From Ted Spiker: My colleagues and students at the University of Florida College of Journalism and Communications, for their talent, enthusiasm, and inspiration. My teachers and friends from the University of Delaware, for sparking and cultivating my career in writing and teaching. Dave Zinczenko and all those I've worked with at *Men's Health* and Rodale, for the opportunities you've given me and for the lessons in health writing. My family, especially my mother, Faith; sisters, Kathy and Kim; and in-laws, Karen and John—for their constant encouragement. My sons, Alex and Thad, who make me smile every time I see them. My wife, Liz, whom I love deeply, not only for her support but for her own gifts and passions that touch so many others. Thank you.

From Craig Wynett: T George Harris, considered by many to be the father of the modern health movement, for his unique insights. Phil E. Pfeifer, the brilliant yet practical professor of quantitative analysis at the Darden School, who made sure we did the math right. My father, Paul Wynett, who taught me to see the world not for what it is but for what it might be. My brothers, David and Ben, and my aunt Sallie Burke. My colleagues Paul Zaffiro, Pete Foley, Faye Blum, Michael Ball, and Jim Bangel. My wife of twenty-four years, Denise, who is forever finding fresh answers to the perpetual question "How do you live with him?" My craziness often overshadows the fact that she is a major force in her own right. She is an artist, musician, and creator of her own beautiful works. To my sons, Ryan and Jim, who are compelling reminders that the purpose of living a long and healthy life is service to others. Thank you all for adding spice and richness to my life.

From Gary Hallgren: Gray's Anatomy, for inspiring the illustration style. Ted Spiker, for breaking me into the land of Oz and Roizen. My wife, Michelle, and daughter, Annabel, for their enthusiastic support of all my endeavors.

From Mark Rudberg: To my many patients, who taught me what is really important for their health and their lives. To my parents, Morrie and Sheila, who encouraged me by being who they are, and to my in-laws, Nancy and Emmett Peck, who showed me the meaning of aging with vitality. To my wife, Ellory Peck, and my son, Leo Rudberg, who have been understanding and encouraging throughout the process, especially for allowing me to run off to our Sunday morning conference calls. Ellory and Leo, you make healthy aging fun and worthwhile.

Acknowledgments of Michael F. Roizen

As you get older, a book on extending your warranty gets personal and up close. So I need to thank—both for their scientific contributions and constructive criticisms, and for allowing me the time and encouraging me to complete this work—the many coworkers, clinicians, scientists, and experts at the Cleveland Clinic both as coworkers in the Division I have chaired, Anesthesia, Critical Care and Pain Management, who are unquestionably the best in the world at what they do (*U.S. News & World Report* probably cannot rank such departments, as there would be a large gap between number one and whoever came next), and in the institute I have just started to chair—the Wellness Institute.

This work started because complications after surgery increase dramatically as you age. Our Division at the clinic wanted to do more than draw your blood and test it before surgery—we wanted to make you ten years younger in the two weeks surrounding your procedure. That is what we try to do daily to many as a result of this work. And the clinic CEO took the position that the Cleveland Clinic cannot continue to just do illness care and thrive as caregivers or consider ourselves a great institution. CEO Toby Cosgrove has said that while the clinic has been and will continue to be known as one of the best, if not the best, in illness care, that wellness (extending your warranty) is part and parcel of what the clinic does and must do for every employee and every person we touch. I am fortunate to work with such a talented and creative group as Dr. Martin Harris, Dr. Brigette Duffy, David Strand, Dr. Mike O'Donnell, Dennis Kenny, Rich Day, Dr. Tanya Edwards, many nutritionists and exercise physiologists, chef Jim Perko, Dr. Rich Lang, Dr. Rene Seballos, Claire and Jim Young, and the Canyon Ranch experts, including Dr. Rich Carmona, Jerry Cohen, Bernard Plishtin, Dr. Mark Liponis (and many more), who span the gamut from inner-city schoolteachers (thank you, Rosalind Strickland, and those who inspire, Reverend Otis Moss) to executive coaches. But most important, I am fortunate to work with many nurses and caregivers who have broken traditional molds and are making the Cleveland Clinic the best place to work and the best place to receive care—especially if you want wellness as a culture and long-term outcome.

Our family was fully engaged—with Jeff as our MD-PhD student research assistant; and Jennifer and Nancy as critical readers, joined at times by the "enlarged family" of the Katzes, Unobskeys, and Campodonicos. I also need to thank Sukie Miller, Linda Defrancisco, Dr. Carl Peck, Rick Cott, Eileen Sheil, Erinne Dyer, Nabil Gabriel, John Maudlin, Zack Wasserman, Rachel Cicurel, and others for encouraging and critiquing the concepts, and especially Anita Shreve, for saying that the early chapters were just what she wanted to read; the many gerontologists and internists who read sections of the book for accuracy; others on the RealAge team who validated and verified the content, and contributed their expertise to the book.

I also want to acknowledge the passion for Staying Young from the staff of the Center for Partnership Medicine at Northwestern Memorial Hospital in Chicago, especially Dr. Lorrie Elliott, Elizabeth Crane, Jeff Klein, Jason Conviser, Dr. Dan

Dermann, Drew Palumbo, and Dean Harrison. And my partners who encouraged the work: Dr. Aaron Gerber, Bob Hurwitz, Jane Spinner, and Mike Kessel.

My administrative associates Candy Lawrence and especially Beth Grubb made this work possible. (Of note, the Cavs almost delayed this work, but thank you also to Dan Gilbert, David Katzman, Steve Cicurel, and LeBron and Booby— you guys almost made the manuscript late, but you taught me that I could tolerate a late two minutes of extreme stress on alternate nights.) It's no accident that *U.S. News & World Report* has ranked the Cleveland Clinic number one in cardiac care thirteen years in a row: Toby Cosgrove, Joe Hahn, Mike O'Boyle, Martin Harris, Paul Matsen, and Jim Blazer are the best at their positions and insist on innovation and simple excellence. They understand the need to do more than prevent illness through promoting wellness every day. And thanks to all the outstanding colleagues at the clinic who answered our many questions. My prior associate, Anne-Marie Prince, deserves special thanks, as does Diane Reverand—she started this process by telling me not to worry about offending medical colleagues. As long as the science was solid, they would understand that we were trying to motivate *you* to understand that you can control your genes.

Having a great partner to ablate stress daily is clearly a magnificent way to make your RealAge younger and extend your warranty. Nancy, just looking at you is a joy and makes my telomeres grow nightly, I'm sure.

I hope and believe this book will help you to live younger and longer—many more people not needing the illness part of our medical system for many years more would be the best reward any physician could want.

Acknowledgments of Mehmet C. Oz

I thank my colleagues in cardiothoracic surgery for supporting the belief that surgeons can heal with our pens as well as with the cold steel of a scalpel edge. They freed me to write and brainstorm, especially Dr. Eric Rose, Dr. Craig Smith, Dr. Yoshifuma Naka, Dr. Mike Argenziano, Dr. Henry Spotnitz, Dr. Allan Stewart, Dr. Mat Williams, Dr. Barry Esrig, and the other superb surgeons on our team. The physician assistants, especially Laura Baer, the nurses in the OR and floor, and our spectacular ICU team cared so meticulously for my patients that in my free time I could turn my mind totally onto this book without the need to "pick up the pieces" from my clinical work. My clinical office manager, Lidia Nieves, has a razor-sharp mind (and memory) that prevented any patient's care from being compromised. My administrative coordinator, Michelle Washburn, not only made sure that all the tasks surrounding the book were done on time, but also read countless drafts of the text and provided incredibly insightful commentary. Thanks to Melanie Fernandi for pitching in whenever we were in need. Finally, as on our other books, our divisional administrator, Diane Amato, was a foil for America as she shared her precious intellect with me without concern for her time and provided broad opinions about the direction of our work.

Thanks to all my colleagues in other specialties who provided quality control by offering thoughtful feedback on our writing. We list them in our joint acknowledgments by name, but your tireless responses to my sometimes tedious questions will always be appreciated. Thanks to the wonderfully talented (and busy) public affairs group at New York-Presbyterian, including Bryan Dotson, Alicia Park, and Myrna Manners, who have taught me to communicate complex messages in an accessible fashion. Thank you, Ivan Kronenfeld, for all your guidance.

My parents, Mustafa and Suna Oz, taught me to work hard for my life goals and keep pushing forward, even when success appears a fading hope. My parents-in-law, Gerald and Emily Jane Lemole, shared their strong value system and passion to look for answers that can change the world. My wife and coauthor, Lisa, who all our friends unanimously agree is the "brains" of the family, kindly shares her remarkable views on health so I can keep my bearings for the authentic family-tested lessons that our readers desire. It is fun to marry and work with one's soul mate. Our siblings Nazlim, Laura, Emily, Michael, Christopher (and especially Samantha, Seval, and Sonya with their workouts) kept us on our toes. Our four children—Daphne, who inherited the bug and has written her first book, Arabella, Zoe, and Oliver—bring joy to our lives with their every breath. We again thank you for sharing your lives with our books.

Index